DATE DUE

APR 2 5 1993			
MAY 2 1 1993			
APR 0 5 1997			
GAYLORD			PRINTED IN U.S.A.

MALARIA

Volume 2

MALARIA

Volume 2
Pathology,
Vector Studies,
and Culture

Edited by

Julius P. Kreier

Department of Microbiology
The Ohio State University
College of Biological Sciences
Columbus, Ohio

ACADEMIC PRESS 1980
A SUBSIDIARY OF HARCOURT BRACE JOVANOVICH, PUBLISHERS
New York   London   Toronto   Sydney   San Francisco

ACADEMIC PRESS, INC.
111 Fifth Avenue, New York, New York 10003

United Kingdom Edition published by
ACADEMIC PRESS, INC. (LONDON) LTD.
24/28 Oval Road, London NW1 7DX

Library of Congress Cataloging in Publication Data
Main entry under title:

Malaria.

    Includes bibliographies and index.
    CONTENTS: [etc.] --v. 2. Pathology, vector
studies and culture.
    1. Malaria. I. Kreier, Julius P. [DNLM: 1.
Malaria--Congresses. WC750 R432 1979]
QR201.M3R47   616.9'362   80-19569
ISBN 0-12-426102-7 (v. 2)

PRINTED IN THE UNITED STATES OF AMERICA

80 81 82 83   9 8 7 6 5 4 3 2 1

Contents

3 Colonization and Maintenance of Mosquitoes in the Laboratory
Woodbridge A. Foster

4 The Transmission by Mosquitoes of Plasmodia in the Laboratory
Jerome P. Vanderberg and Robert W. Gwadz

5 Culture of the Invertebrate Stages of Plasmodia and the Culture of Mosquito Tissues
Imogene Schneider and Jerome P. Vanderberg

6 Cultivation of Erythrocytic and Exoerythrocytic Stages of Plasmodia

William Trager and James B. Jensen

List of Contributors

Numbers in parentheses indicate the pages on which the authors' contributions begin.

Masamichi Aikawa (47), Institute of Pathology, Case Western Reserve University, Cleveland, Ohio 44106

Woodbridge A. Foster (103), Department of Entomology, The Ohio State University, Columbus, Ohio 43210

Yezid Gutierrez (47), Institute of Pathology, Case Western Reserve University and University Hospitals, Cleveland, Ohio 44106

Robert W. Gwadz (153), Laboratory of Parasitic Diseases, National Institutes of Health, Bethesda, Maryland 20014

James B. Jensen* (271), Laboratory of Parasitology, Rockefeller University, New York, New York, 10021

Julius P. Kreier (1), Department of Microbiology, The Ohio State University, College of Biological Sciences, Columbus, Ohio 43210

Imogene Schneider (235), Department of Entomology, Walter Reed Army Institute of Research, Washington, D.C. 20012

Thomas M. Seed (1), Division of Biological and Medical Research, Argonne National Laboratory, Argonne, Illinois 60439

Mamoru Suzuki (47), Department of Parasitology, School of Medicine, Gunma University, Maebashi 371, Gunma, Japan

Jerome P. Vanderberg (153, 235), Department of Microbiology, Division of Parasitology, New York University School of Medicine, New York, New York 10016

William Trager (271), Laboratory of Parasitology, Rockefeller University, New York, New York 10021

*Present Address: Department of Microbiology and Public Health, Michigan State University, East Lansing, Michigan 48824

Preface

The last major effort to review our knowledge of malaria was by Mark F. Boyd whose "Malariology" published by W. B. Saunders of Philadelphia in 1949 is still a valuable resource. The exquisite volume "Malaria Parasites and other Haemosporida" by P. C. C. Garnham published by Blackwell Scientific Publication of Oxford in 1966 is also a valuable review of malariology but in the author's words "is about malaria parasites and not malaria."

This three-volume treatise is appearing in a period of rising activity in malaria research. In the 1950s and 1960s and even into the 1970s funds for this research were scarce and only the hardiest of individuals remained in the field. At present malaria research is again receiving the attention it deserves. The mistaken belief common in the 1950s and 1960s that malaria would soon be eradicated by vector control and chemotherapy and that research was therefore rather pointless has been abandoned in the face of a widespread resurgence of this disease.

A variety of national and international agencies are now funding malaria research. Many individuals attracted by the possibility of funding are turning their efforts to malaria research. Biochemists, immunologists, biophysicists, and molecular biologists among others are entering the field. Many of these individuals, skilled in their specialities, know little or nothing about malaria. It is perhaps to such individuals particularly that this broad review of malariology will be of most value. Even those of us who have worked in some aspects of malaria research for some time may find the reviews of the state of the art in areas other than our own speciality of interest. Those of us actively working in a particular area may find few new facts in the reviews of the areas of our own speciality. I have, however, encouraged the authors to write critical reviews and to relate the facts reported in the literature to each other. Interpretation and speculation are discouraged by the reviewers of most scientific journals in the United States. A book such as this is thus naturally a convenient vehicle for individuals to present their thoughts as well as the facts.

The authors of the reviews of malaria research included in these volumes met in May 1979 in Mexico City with individuals doing research on the closely related disease babesiosis. Babesiosis has an effect on the development of animal husbandry somewhat similar to the effect of malaria on human societies. At this conference current research on malaria and babesiosis was reported and the similarities and differences between malaria and babesiosis were discussed. As an outgrowth of this conference a volume on babesiosis was developed, which will complement these volumes on malaria.

I extend my thanks to the co-organizers of the conference, Dr. Miodrag Ristic of the College of Veterinary Medicine of the University of Illinois with whom I edited the volume on babesiosis, and Dr. Carlos Arellano-Sota of the Instituto Nacional de Investigaciones Pecuarias in Mexico City. I particularly wish to thank the sponsors of the conference for their encouragement and help. Their support made the conference possible and made the preparation of these volumes on research in malaria and babesiosis a more pleasant task.

I particularly wish to thank John Pino, Director of Agricultural Sciences of the Rockefeller Foundation without whose early support the conference and the babesiosis volume would have been impossible. I also wish to thank Kenneth Warren, Director of Medical Sciences of the Rockefeller Foundation, Edgar A. Smith, Health Services Administrator, James Erickson, Malaria Research Officer of the United States Agency for International Development of the Department of State for their support of the conference.

In addition to the Rockefeller Foundation and the United States Agency for International Development several other organizations contributed to the support of the conference and the development of these volumes. These were The Pan American Health Organization, Parke-Davis Corporations, Merck Sharp & Dohme, Anchor Laboratories, Sandoz Ltd., Pfizer Corporation, and the Wellcome Trust.

Last but by no means least I wish to thank all the authors of the reviews that make up these volumes and Academic Press for their unfailing support.

Julius P. Kreier

Contents of Volumes 1 and 3

Contents of Babesiosis

1

Erythrocyte Destruction Mechanisms in Malaria

Thomas M. Seed and Julius P. Kreier

I. INTRODUCTION

The mammalian hemopoietic system is a remarkable piece of biological machinery in terms of its productivity and its intrinsic regulatory processes. In humans, the erythropoietic system produces approximately 2.5×10^6 red cells/second or 2×10^{11} cells/day. This means that about 5×10^{15} cells are produced during an average human life span of 70 years. The erythropoietic system is positively regulated at the level of the committed stem cell by the glycoprotein hormone erythropoietin which is elaborated by the kidney at various rates depending on the oxygen requirements of the individual. Somewhat overlooked, but still equally impressive, is the ability of the reticuloendothelial system (RES) to recognize and eliminate numbers of senescent cells equal to the input in order to maintain a steady level of circulating red cells.

The erythropoietic system can, under stress, increase its productivity approximately seven-fold. When red cell loss exceeds the production rate, anemia occurs. Anemia may be related to either decreased red cell production or enhanced red cell destruction. The length of the anemia bout depends on how efficiently the animal can correct the hemopoietic imbalance. Excessive anemia is a common symptom of ongoing pathology in many types of diseases both of the

Malaria, Vol. 2

infectious and the noninfectious variety. Its causes are many, as are its effects, which are always deleterious. In malaria, as in certain drug-induced diseases, anemia is the result of enhanced erythrocyte destruction, which is in turn a prime contributor to the pathogenesis of the disease. To some degree the enhanced destruction aids the infected animal in ridding itself of the infectious agent. The anemia that ensues is compensated for by the erythropoietic response, the strength of which depends on the degree of anemia and on the condition of the animal.

The course of the infection must be considered when studying the kinetics and consequences of red cell destruction in a process as dynamic as malaria. Various factors need to be considered. These include the changing level of parasitemia, the shift in age composition of the red cell population, and the altered function of specific organ systems of the host, including the RES and the immune and the hematopoietic systems.

Our intent is to review the literature relating to the mechanisms of erythrocyte destruction during malarial infection and to construct a model in which the various destructive and regenerative processes are assigned their proper roles in the pathogenesis of the disease.

II. MECHANISMS OF ERYTHROCYTE DESTRUCTION

A. Hematological and Red Cell Survival Studies

A common denominator in all hemolytic anemias is the shortened life span of circulating erythrocytes. Premature senescence of red cells can be attributed to (1) intrinsic cellular defects, (2) extrinsic defects in the cell environment (Prankerd, 1961, or (3) a combination of these, i.e., intrinsically defective cells circulating within a defective environment. Malaria as a hemolytic disease falls into the latter category. Certainly numerous workers have found that the life span of circulating radiolabeled erythrocytes is shortened during malarial infection (Stohlman *et al.*, 1963; George *et al.*, 1966; Wright and Kreier, 1969; Kreier, 1969; Swann and Kreier, 1973; Rosenberg *et al.*, 1973). To a great extent this is the result of intrinsic cellular defects which enhance sequestration of intact erythrocytes, promote cell fragmentation, and cause hemolysis. Schizogony of intraerythrocytic parasites appears to be a primary cause of hemolysis.

Intravascular hemolysis occurs in varying degrees during plasmodial infections, the extreme being the massive hemolytic crisis of blackwater fever, a not uncommon sequel of quinine-treated *Plasmodium falciparum* infection (Maegraith, 1946). Devakul *et al.* (1969) made a rather detailed study of the relationship of erythrocyte destruction and intravascular hemolysis during experimentally induced *P. falciparum* infections in male Thais. His observations are similar to those made on a variety of laboratory animals infected with plasmodia and include (1) falling total blood hemoglobin levels during periods of rising parasitemia and (2) increased hemoglobin concentrations in plasma during overt infection. The highest plasma hemoglobin concentrations were invariably found during periods of high parasitemia and low hematocrit values. Plasma hemoglobin concentrations reached as high as 147 g% with parasite levels of 16%. The extent of intravascular hemolysis determined by plasma hemoglobulin concentration appeared not only to be related to the absolute level of parasitemia but, like so many other parameters, to be a function of the phase of infection. Intravascular hemolysis is greatest during the crisis and postcrisis periods.

Hemolysis caused by parasites emerging from erythrocytes appears not to be the primary mechanism of red cell destruction, at least during and just after the crisis, but rather it is sequestration which is mainly responsible. The degree of abnormality of parasitized red cells within the circulation appears to be closely associated with the stage of intracellular parasite development. The critical experiments which would confirm this remain to be done, however. These involve the isolation of red cell populations containing parasites in different stages of maturity, radiolabeling them, and subsequently infusing them into compatible drug-treated animals in order to determine the relationship between survival times and the development stage of the intracellular parasites. A variety of indirect experimental studies done by various investigators seem to indicate that erythrocytes containing large parasites are more likely to be sequestered than those containing small parasites. These include (1) morphological ultrastructural studies which indicate that parasitized red cells maintain a normal shape until the intracellular parasites grow and mature beyond the large trophozoite stage (Seed, 1972; Seed and Kreier, 1972; Kreier et al., 1972a,b); (2) histological and ultrastructural studies which indicate that parasitized erythrocytes with larger, more mature parasites are more readily trapped and sequestered by cordal macrophages while, in passage through the splenic cords to the sinuses (Schitzer et al., 1973); and (3) red cell survival studies with radiolabeled infected cell populations. Radioisotope labeling of red cells with either ^{32}P-labeled diisofluorophosphate (DF^{32}P) or ^{51}Cr or both has been done in malarious animals and has provided useful information. A strict proportionality was demonstrated between the percentage of parasitemia and the rates of cell loss when parasitized populations (P. berghei) were radiolabeled with ^{51}Cr and infused into healthy, syngeneic, drug-treated animals (Kreier and Leste, 1967). The biphasic nature of the survival curves strongly suggested preferential removal and destruction of parasitized red cells from the circulation during the first 24 hours (Fig. 1), and the much slower rates of red cell loss thereafter were presumably the result of normal senescence processes acting on the nonparasitized segment of the infused red cell population. Such studies indicate that the intrinsic defects of parasitized red cells are recognizable as such by the normal, uninfected animal. The malarial animal, with its modified hematopoietic and immunological systems, appears to have broader

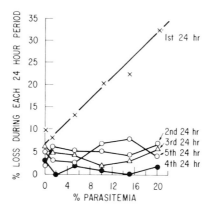

FIG. 1. The degree to which the normal, noninfected animal, in this case the rat, recognizes and removes from its circulation transfused, *P. berghei*-infected red cells. In this experiment red cell samples with various levels of parasitemia were collected, labeled with ^{51}Cr, and infused into healthy, chloroquine-treated, sygeneic rats. Red cell loss was proportional to the parasitemia during the first 24 hours after transfusion, suggesting that the normal animal only recognized as defective the parasitized segment of the infused cell population (data from Kreier and Leste, 1967). It is probable that erythrocyte destruction in malarious animals in crisis is different.

recognition capabilities, making the relationship between red cell destruction and parasitermia more complex.

Red cell survival studies employing radioisotope labeling techniques in humans (Stohlman *et al.,* 1963; Gilles *et al.,* 1969; Voller, 1974) and in a variety of experimental animals (George *et al.,* 1966; Wright and Kreier, 1969; Kreier *et al.,* 1972a,c; Swann and Kreier, 1973) have all indicated enhanced destruction of red cells during active phases of malarial infections. Further, most researchers who have done isotopic labeling studies on erthrocytes now agree that the extent of red cell destruction appears to be in excess of the number of red cells parasitized. These conclusions support similar conclusions based on data gathered by less sensitive hematological methods in which estimates of erythrocyte destruction were made in terms of changes in hematocrit and reticulocyte percentages relative to the percentage of parasitemia of the peripheral blood (e.g., Zuckerman, 1957, 1958, 1960a,b, etc.).

Avivah Zuckerman, for several decades, extensively studied the phenomenon of blood loss and replacement in a number of primate, rodent, and avian host species during plasmodial infections (e.g., Zuckerman, 1957, 1958, 1960b,c, 1964, 1966, 1969, 1977). Her estimates of red cell loss were based on changes in the numbers of mature and immature red cells over the course of infection. Consistent observation of the inordinate loss of mature red cells relative to the level of the parasitemia led her to suggest that a large segment of the erythron was "destroyed by some means other than red cell rupture by emerging parasites"

(Zuckerman, 1960c). The mechanisms responsible for the apparent excessive cell loss have been widely debated and consequently have been the subject of many investigations.

The major hypotheses, including Zuckerman's autoimmune theory (Zuckerman, 1960c, 1964), will be discussed at length in Section II, B. Zuckerman stated many times (e.g., 1957, 1958, 1960,a,b,c) that excessive red cell loss was more apparent in mild, chronic infections than in acute, fulminating ones (Fig. 2). Kretschmar (1969), in several studies, illustrated this point by restricting growth rates of *P. berghei* in NMRI mice by inducing a p-aminobenzoic acid (PABA) deficiency and measuring the net erythrocyte loss. Despite the much lower parasitemias in the mice on the PABA-deficient diet than in the mice of the control group, the erythrocyte loss was approximately the same.

Not all workers, however, have come to similar conclusions concerning the reality of "excessive red cell destruction" during malarial infections. Gilles *et al.* (1969) reported that red cell survival was short in pregnant Nigerian women with untreated malarial infections. Red cell loss, however, was approximately proportional to the degree of parasitemia. Many references in the older literature (Kitchen, 1949) may be found which support the concept that the anemia in malarial individuals is totally attributable to the destruction of red cells brought about by emerging intraerythrocytic parasites.

When "excessive red cell destruction" was detected, the magnitude of the excessive cell loss varied widely. Estimates have ranged from 6% in chickens with experimental avian (*P. gallinaceum*) infections (Swann and Kreier, 1973)

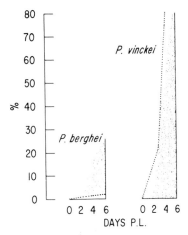

FIG. 2. The relationship of red cell loss to parasitemia in NMRI mice infected with either 5 × 10⁶ *P. vinckei* or *P. berghei* parasites. With the less virulent species the extent of erythrocyte destruction (shaded area) appears incommensurate with the level of parasitemia (dotted line). (Data from Kretschmar, 1969.)

to 300% in rhesus monkeys with *P. cynomologi* infections (Kreier *et al.*, 1972c). Undoubtedly these wide variations are, in part, attributable to differences in species of parasite as well as in the host species. The chickens had high parasitemias of short duration, and the monkeys had low parasitemias and chronic infections.

Kreier and his co-workers studied the kinetics of red cell destruction in rodents (Kreier *et al.*, 1972a), birds (Wright and Kreier, 1969; Swann and Kreier, 1973), and monkeys (Kreier *et al.*, 1972c), using random and cohort radiolabeling procedures with either DF^{32}P or ^{51}Cr radioisotopes. A typical survival curve for randomly DF^{32}P-labeled avian red cells in a healthy chicken is shown in Fig. 3 (right). This curve appears strikingly different from the survival curve of malaria-infected birds (Fig. 3, left). A number of interesting features are immediately evident: (1) Enhanced erythrocyte destruction begins as soon as infection is initiated, despite the apparent lack of detectable parasitemia during the so-called prepatent period; (2) the survival curve might well be a composite of curves representing different survival times. The 32-day survival of the nonparasitized cells is within the range of the normal life expectancy for the red cells of healthy chickens (*Gallus gallus*).

Several attempts have been made to assess directly the survival characteristics of the nonparasitized segment of the erythron during infection. The basic approach has been to estimate the survival time $(T_{1/2})$ of radiolabeled noninfected erythrocytes collected from animals in the postcrisis or recovery phase of infection after they have been infused into normal healthy individuals. Shorter than normal survival times were generally observed. For example, in rats recovering from *P. berghei* infections the erythron, characterized by high basophilia, had an estimated $T_{1/2}$ of only 7.5 days compared to a $T_{1/2}$ of 11.0 days for control red

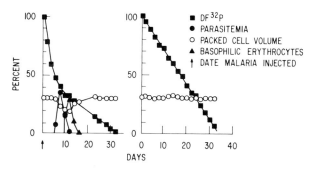

FIG. 3. (Left) A mean survival curve of randomly labeled DF^{32}P-labeled avian erthrocytes from malarial (*P. gallinaceum*) chickens. Note the typical inward bend of the curve and how it is in contrast to the nearly linear survival curve for uninfected chickens (right). Erythrocyte destruction is most rapid early in the course of infection and subsequently slows down later on. This change in the rate of red cell loss as a consequence of malarial infection is evident from the two distinct slopes with the intersection point occurring shortly after peak parasitemia. (Data from Swann and Kreier, 1973.)

cells infused into antimalarial-treated, comparable, healthy rats (Fig. 4) (Kreier *et al.*, 1972c). By comparison erythrocytes from fully recovered rats (20 days after infection with *P. berghei*) had $T_{1/2}$ values comparable to those for the controls, however, the survival curve patterns appeared erratic. This suggests that cohorts of immature red cells, released into the circulation under the severe erythropoietic pressure which occurred as a consequence of massive red cell loss, had mixed survival characteristics. Such experiments indicate the intrinsically defective nature of the noninfected red cell segment of the erythron following the crisis.

In related experiments, the modifying effect of the circulatory environment during infection on noninfected red cells has been demonstrated by radiolabeling and transfusing normal noninfected red cells from healthy individuals into malaria-infected or recovered individuals. A shortened life span for transfused, noninfected red cells has been reported. The various species studied include humans with *P. falciparum* infections (Rosenberg *et al.*, 1973), rats with *P. berghei* infections (Coleman *et al.*, 1976), and chickens with *P. gallinaceum* infections (Schacter, 1968). The work of Rosenberg *et al.* (1973) utilized *P. falciparum*-infected patients who were under treatment with chloroquine, pyrimethamine, and sulfisoxazole. The treatment blocked active infection in the recipient and excluded the possibility that loss of normal transfused red cells would occur as a result of the direct effect of parasitization. A shorter than

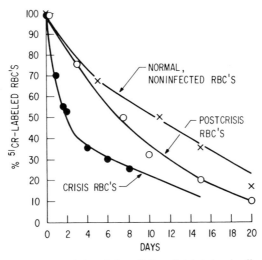

FIG. 4. The survival characteristics of three ^{51}Cr-radiolabeled red cell populations (normal, crisis, and postcrisis) following infusion into healthy, antimalarial-treated, compatible rats. There is a greater than normal red cell loss in the postcrisis phase blood; (in spite of very low parasitemias) but extremely elevated basophilis erythrocyte levels. Characteristically, erythrocytes obtained during postcrisis and recovery exhibit erratic survival characteristics (Kreier *et al.*, 1972a).

normal half-life of the transfused normal red cells was observed in these patients. The extent of reduction in erythrocyte life span was greater in those with severe anemias.

B. Intrinsic Cellular Processes and Effects of Parasitization

1. Events during Penetration

Erythrocyte lesions attributed directly to the parasites can be divided into those associated with (1) merozoite penetration of the host cell and (2) the presence of mature schizonts. The physical processes involved in red cell penetration by merozoites are well described (Ladda, 1969; Ladda *et al.,* 1969; Aikawa *et al.,* 1978) and include specific events which occur in an ordered sequence: (1) merozoite recognition and attachment to susceptible host cells (Miller *et al.,* 1979; Mason *et al.,* 1977; Miller, 1977), (2) junction formation, (3) progressive invagination of the red cell membrane by the invading merozoite, and (4) complete sealing of the formed vacuole over the penetrating parasite. Dvorak and co-workers (1975) demonstrated by interference phase-contrast microscopy that the invasion of susceptible erythrocytes by *P. knowlesi* merozoites consisted initially of apical end attachment followed by surface deformation and subsequent deep invagination of the surface by the merozoites. As the merozoite pushes deep into the red cell, increasing amounts of host cell plasmalemma are consumed as the parasite vacuole is formed. Since the mature erythrocyte has only a finite capacity to expand, this loss of membrane, estimated to be 3% (Holz, 1977), must cause structural strains on the host cell. What effect this has ultimately on red cell survival is unknown, however. A well-defined junction is formed between the invading merozoite and the susceptible host cell (Ladda, 1969; Ladda *et al.,* 1969; Aikawa and Seed, 1973). This junction appears to move around the merozoite, bringing the parasite continually deeper into the invaginated red cell. The final step in penetration is the sealing of the invaginated red cell membrane over the enveloped parasite (Aikawa *et al.,* 1978). Formation and movement of such "tight" junctions appears to be a necessary step in merozoite penetration.

Utilizing an *in vitro* culture system, Miller and co-workers (1979) demon-

---

FIGS. 5 and 6.   These micrographs illustrate red cell surface alterations which appear shortly after merozoite penetration. Figure 5 is a surface view in which a small, circular, shallow depression (arrow) is present precisely in the area where the small, early-stage parasite resides (inset, arrowhead). Figure 6 is a cross-sectional view of the shallow depression and the narrow groove (arrow) that lie directly above the newly penetrated parasite. The penetration channel, although still partially open, appears to be in the final stage of closing over the parasite.

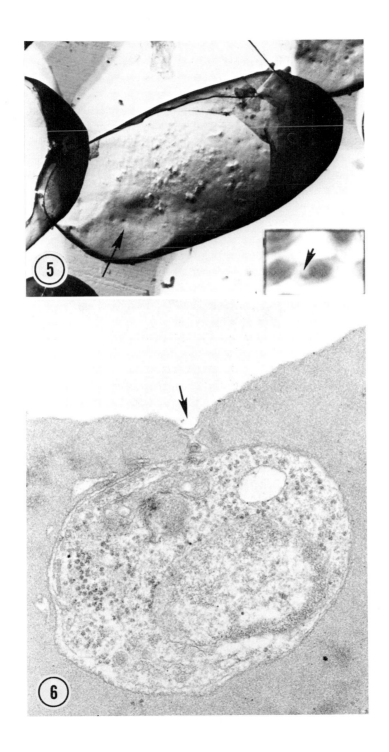

strated that cytochalosin B-treated *P. knowlesi* merozoites were able initially to attach and to deform, but not to penetrate, Duffy-negative human red cells. These nonpenetrating merozoites attached to red cells by way of slender filaments originating from the truncated anterior of the merozoite. The lack of penetrability was attributed to the lack of junction formation.

Small slitlike lesions (Figs. 5 and 6) in shallow surface depressions have been tentatively identified as penetration scars by electron microscopy utilizing various surface-imaging methods (Seed, 1972; Seed and Kreier, 1972; Kreier *et al.*, 1972b). McLaren *et al.* (1977), utilizing the freeze-etching method, observed no apparent modification in distribution of the transmembrane proteins of the red cells' plasmalemma during the initial phases of merozoite penetration. However, by the time the merozoite had completed its invasion, the vacuolar membrane was remarkably depleted of intramembraneous particles. The precise nature and extent of membrane pathology associated with merozoite penetration is not known at this time. However, intuitively it seems that penetration could result in cell surface damage sufficiently great to be recognized by phagocytes of the RES which would then remove the damaged erythrocyte from the circulation. However, this does not seem to be the case since, at least before the crisis, most newly penetrated red cells continue to circulate as intracellular parasites develop.

The extent of damage caused by the penetration of red cells by merozoites during infection is not known. Kreier *et al.* (1972c) calculated that a vast excess of merozoites was produced relative to the number of erythrocytes parasitized during the course of *P. cynomolgi* infection of rhesus monkeys. These workers speculated that the excess red cell destruction seen during the course of these infections might be attributable at least in part to red cell damage due to ineffective merozoite penetration. Hemolytic agents have been isolated from intraerythrocytic parasites and are thought to be derived from the specialized apical organelles of merozoites. These hemolytic agents are believed to function in host cell penetration (Kilejian, 1974, 1976; Kilejian and Jensen, 1977). The action of these agents could damage the erythrocyte membrane sufficiently to cause lysis under some circumstances.

2. *Events during Parasite Growth and Division*

Relationships between red cell morphology and parasitization have been established in *P. berghei* and *P. gallinaceum*-infected mice, rats, and chickens, utilizing a combination of light and electron microscopic techniques (Seed *et al.*, 1971, 1974; Aikawa, 1977; Seed and Manwell, 1977; Kreier *et al.*, 1972a,b; Seed, 1972; Seed and Kreier, 1972).

The general conclusion drawn from these studies was that gross abnormalities in erythrocyte shape occurred only when the parasites developed beyond the trophozoite stage. With the exception of the previously mentioned merozoite "penetration scars," red cells containing parasites in small, early developmental stages had essentially normal shapes and surface structures. As the parasites increased in size, infected erythrocytes became progressively more distorted and their membranes rougher and more irregular (Fig. 7). Red cells containing larger, more mature parasites bear a variety of surface lesions, including pitts, knobs, clefts, large blebs, and deep, broad depressions (Figs. 8–12). The deep surface depressions demonstrated by scanning electron microscopy (SEM) were associated with large underlying parasites (Arnold *et al.*, 1969; Kreier *et al.*, 1972a,b; Seed and Kreier, 1972). Although the integrity of the red cell plasmalemma within these areas was initially questioned (Arnold *et al.*, 1969), the membrane's integrity was later demonstrated by immunocytochemical SEM methods (Reinhart *et al.*, 1971). Many of the alterations in the host cell are characteristic of the parasite, whereas others are not (Aikawa *et al.*, 1975; Aikawa, 1977). Late maturational stages of *P. simium* a vivax-type, nonhuman

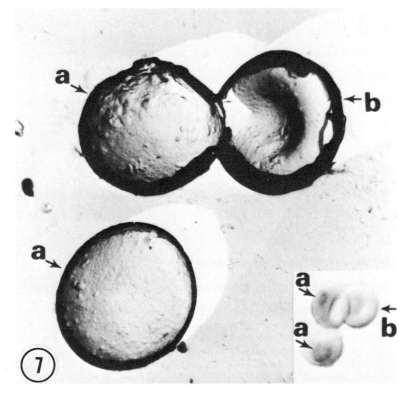

FIG. 7. An electron micrograph of carbon-replicated red cells from a *P. berghei*-infected rat. The inset is a light micrograph of these Giemsa-stained cells prior to replication. Note that the spherocytic cells (a) contain parasites, whereas the noninfected cell (b) maintains its normal biconcave shape.

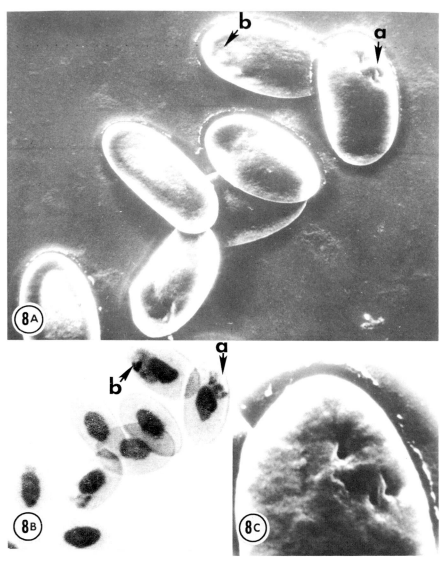

FIG. 8.   The relationship between the location of the intraerythrocytic parasite (*P. gallinaceum*) and the type and degree of surface damage as revealed by scanning electron microscopy. (A) These deep invaginations of the plasmalamma are associated with what appears to be a multiple merozoite invasion (B) Light micrograph revealing the location of the parasites. (C) A higher magnification of the cell shown in (A). The neighboring cell (b) contains a large trophozoite or an early segmenter, and the area overlying the parasite appears as a broad, shallow depression.

FIGS. 9 and 10.   *Plasmodium simium*-infected erythrocytes from a squirrel monkey shown in cross section by transmission electron microscopy (Fig. 9) and topographically by scanning electron microscopy (Fig. 10). This parasite shares many morphological and ultrastructural features with *P. vivax*; it also induces similar types of host cell changes (e.g., microvesicles, cytoplasmic clefts).

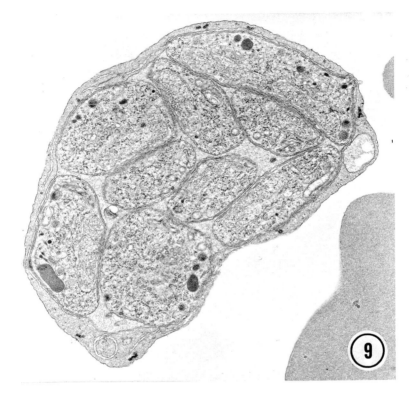

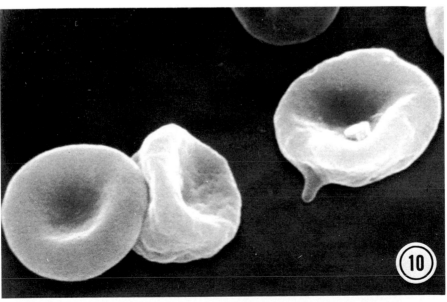

primate species, for example, induce small pinocytotic vesicles (ie., caveola-vesicles) (Figs. 9, 10, and 11c) (Sterling *et al.*, 1975; Seed *et al.*, 1976b), whereas *P. brasilianum,* a falciparum-type plasmodial species in the same host species causes distinct surface knobs called excrescences to be formed (Fig. 12

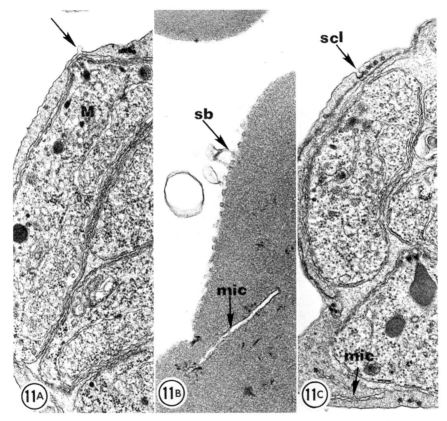

FIG. 11. Some of the typical host cell changes which occur as a consequence of *P. simium* parasitization. (A) Local alterations (blebs, arrow) in the host cell plasmalemma induced by merozoite (M) action. (B) Cytoplasmic clefts (mic) as well as extensive surface blebbing (sb) are illustrated. (C) The distinctive microvesicles (scl) which increase in number during parasite growth and maturation are shown.

FIG. 12. Host cell surface alterations typical of falciparum-type malarias are illustrated in this electron micrograph of *P. brasilianum*-infected erythrocytes from a squirrel monkey. (A) Numerous outpocketings or excrescences (arrow) on the red cell surface are seen; these structures increase in number as the parasite matures. (B) At a higher magnification, the cone-shaped excrescences (arrow) are covered by the intact plasmelemma and contain at times accumulations of dense material. (C) The anionic surface charge of the excrescence-bearing infected red cell is shown. Here a positively charged iron colloid is bound in substantial amounts to the excrescences (arrow). (D) A face-on view of a portion of a carbon-replicated *P. brasilianum*-infected erythrocyte. Multiple, ≈100-nm-wide excrescences (arrow) can be identified.

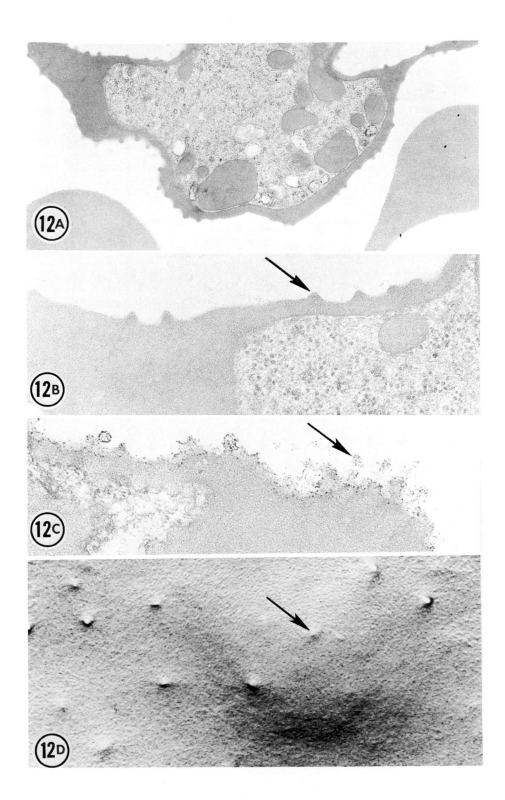

a–d) (Sterling *et al.*, 1972). The plasmodia-induced host cell structures called Schüffner's dots (Figs. 9, 11c), Maurer's clefts (Fig. 11b), and Ziemann's stippling have been recognized by light microscopy in stained blood smears for many decades and are useful diagnostic features for determining the plasmodial species. Many of these structures have been identified and examined by electron microscopy as well (Sterling *et al.*, 1972, 1975; Aikawa *et al.*, 1975; Aikawa, 1977; Seed *et al.*, 1976).

In contrast to the host's apparent inability to detect the minimal damage induced by the penetrating merozoite there is little doubt that the late, more dramatic surface changes induced by the mature parasite are recognized as pathological by the host. For example, a variety of plasmodial species (e.g., *P. falciparum* and *P. coatney*) cause surface excrescences to form on infected red cells. These excrescences contain parasite antigen and bind antibody (Langreth and Reese, 1978), serve as sites of attachment to vascular endothelium, and serve as recognition sites for phagocytic cells within the deep vasculature of various organs (Miller *et al.*, 1971; Aikawa *et al.*, 1972; Sterling *et al.*, 1972;).

3. Alterations in Red Cell Membranes of Biochemical or Biophysical Nature

Various types of erythrocyte dysfunction have been causally incriminated in red cell destruction. These include (1) abnormalities in erythrocyte size, shape and elasticity, (2) metabolic abnormalities, and (3) membrane abnormalities. The changes in red cell shape as a consequence of parasitization are undoubtedly not the result of a single cellular defect but of a cascade of molecular lesions which are responsible for physiological dysfunctions. A list of these disorders and a hypothesis of how these processes interact is given in Fig. 13. It is reasonable to suspect that the parasite initiates these events during its intraerythrocytic development and that the host cell's plasmalemma is the major site of their expression. The actual cellular processes involved, however, are unknown at this time. Recently there have been several reports which might provide an insight into the early events which occur in the erythrocyte membrane during infection. Wallach and Conley (1977), Konigk and Mirtsch (1977), and Weidekamm *et al.* (1973) have reported, respectively, that *P. knowlesi-*, *P. chabaudi-*, and *P. berghei-* infected erythrocytes contain less spectrin than nonparasitized red cells. Although Eisen (1977) failed to confirm the quantitative aspects of the observation, he demonstrated by immunocytochemical methods a redistribution of spectrin within parasitized cells. Spectrin, is a 110,000-molecular-weight protein bound ionically to the cytoplasmic side of the plasma membrane. It is specifically linked to and controls the mobility of the major oligomeric transmembrane complex. The complex is thought to control transport processes and water movement (Nicolson, 1976). Accordingly, it has been termed a permeaphore (Fig. 14) (Pinta da Silva and Nicolson, 1974). Alteration or degradation of spectrin by the

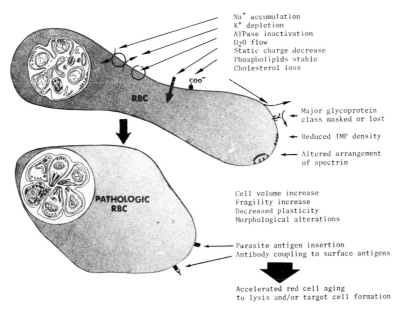

FIG. 13. A partial listing of red cell alterations which occur as a consequence of malarial parasitization. Cumulatively these modifications are responsible for premature aging and sequestration.

intracellular parasite would have a profound effect on red cell membrane function and in turn on red cell survival.

The increased osmotic fragility of the erythrocyte during malaria is a good example of the physiological consequences of molecular dysfunction within the transport complex of the host cell's plasmalemma (Seed and Kreier, 1972; Seed *et al.*, 1976; Fogel *et al.*, 1966; Danon and Gunders, 1962; Bahr, 1969). The extent of increased osmotic fragility is generally proportional to the level of the parasitemia early in the infection and somewhat disproportionate in the postcrisis period (Fogel *et al.*, 1966; Seed and Kreier, 1972). This pattern holds for malaria caused by various species including *P. gallinaceum, P. berghei, P. knowlesi,* and *P. falciparum.*

The transmembrane complex is composed of several major subunits, including a 90,000 to 100,000-molecular-weight glycoprotein (band III), and glycophorin (Segrest *et al.*, 1973). Glycophorin is the major sialoglycoprotein and is of 30,000–50,000 molecular weight. Band III glycoprotein, a trimodal amphipathic molecule, bears the receptors for concanavalin A, whereas glycophorin has receptors for several other lectins also and contains the major isoantigen as well as bearing the major ionogenic sialic acid residues. The complex has been tentatively identified in freeze-cleaved preparations by electron microscopy as a

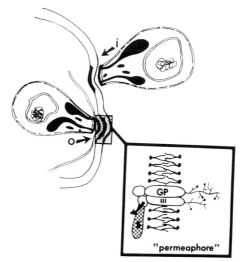

"permeaphore"

FIG. 14. The hypothesis that the processes of red cell entry (i) and release (o) by merozoites are caused by similar mechanisms and involve direct interaction of the merozoite's anterior organelle and the host cell's plasmalemma. The release process would be initiated by the merozoite-induced degradation of spectrin s, which would exert an influence on permeaphore function. As transport systems and osmotic gradients would be affected, a cascade of cellular events would follow, terminating in either cell lysis or formation of a cell easily recognized by macrophages. Therefore the processes of terminal intraerythrocytic development of merozoites, specific host cell plasmalemmal modification resulting in formation of easily phagocytized erythrocytes and merozoite release are temporally related events.

randomly dispersed, 8.5-nm intramembraneous particle (Pinta da Silva and Nicolson, 1974).

The normal density of the intramembraneous particles (IMPs) (Fig. 15) appears to decrease substantially within malaria-infected erythrocytes of certain species during the late stages of parasite development. McLaren *et al.* (1977) examined freeze-fractured schizont-infected (*P. knowlesi*) erythrocytes and observed a 20% reduction in IMPs per square micrometer of internal plasma membrane. Mazen *et al.* (1975) failed, however, to find density differences in IMPs between noninfected and *P. chabaudi*-infected rodent erythrocytes. Seed and co-workers (1971, 1973; and T.M. Seed, unpublished observations) studied *P. gallinaceum*-infected erythrocytes and observed a similar infection-related IMP depletion. An extensive reduction in IMPs was consistently noted in areas where the schizont and the host cell plasmalemma were in close apposition (Fig. 16).

FIGS. 15 and 16. Freeze-cleaved avian erythrocytes. Figure 15 shows the typical uniform array of 8.5-nm intramembranous particles (imp) in an uninfected cell. Figure 16 shows the intramembranous particle depletion (arrows) in membrane areas where the intracellular parasite (p) lies in close apposition.

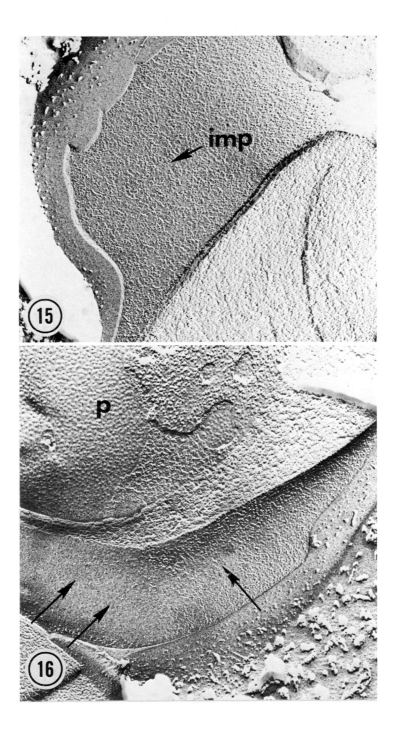

Such IMP depletion is probably the result of both membrane expansion which makes particle density per square unit of membrane less, and lateral movement of the transmembrane components within the plane of the membrane resulting in localized "bare spots."

The ultrastructural rearrangements of IMPs appear to be related to the infection-induced alterations in surface-expressed glycoprotein moieties. Trigg and his colleagues (1977) radiolabeled the surface glycoprotein of noninfected and *P. knowlesi*-infected (schizont stage) erythrocytes. They then fractionated and subsequently isolated plasmalemma glycoproteins. They noted a lack of major galactose- or galactosamine-containing glycoproteins in the infected cells. They suggested that the absence of these various glycoproteins from schizont-infected erythrocytes represented a loss of functionally active surface components. The loss of the high-molecular-weight fractions, for example, might represent the loss of band III-type transmembrane glycoproteins which, as previously noted, carry the concanavalin A lectin-binding receptor (Wallach and Conley, 1977). The presence of fewer concanavalin A-binding sites on *P. knowlesi* schizont-infected red cells than on noninfected red cells supports these findings (P. G. Shakespeare *et al.*, unpublished observations, cited by Trigg *et al.*, 1977).

The pronounced changes from normal of the plasma membrane glycoprotein profiles of infected erythrocytes could have been predicted on the basis of the many ionogenic alterations observed to result from parasitization (Seed and Kreier, 1977). The relationship among surface sialoglycoproteins, ionogenic properties of circulating normal red cells, and survival *in vivo* is well established (Gattegno *et al.*, 1974; Durocher *et al.*, 1975). The removal of charged sialic acid groups by neuraminidase or trypsin dramatically reduces the survival time *in vivo* of treated red cells (Kreier, 1969); such enzyme treatment induces little change in cell shape, cell fragility, or K^+ retention (Gattegno *et al.*, 1974). During both avian and rodent malarial infections, the erythron appears to change its ionogenic character. There is, for example, a precipitous decline in electrophoretic mobility of erythrocytes during the crisis and postcrisis phases (Table I) (Temsuk, 1969; Nirady, 1969). The parasitized segment of the population exhibits a lower mobility than the noninfected segment (Redmond 1948; Heidrich *et al.*, 1979). Surface charge changes also have been demonstrated to occur during the crisis phase of *P. berghei* infection in rats by electron microscopy utilizing a positively charged ion hydrosol as a cytochemical reagent. Postcrisis phase red cells were found to be highly variable with respect to the number of detectable charge sites per unit of membrane. A measure of total red cell sialic acid content revealed an initial drop in the early phases of infection and then an increase at later periods, despite the lower than normal sialic acid content of parasitized red cells (Table II). Basophilic erythrocytes, which comprise a large segment of the erythron during the late stages of the infection, have a high sialic

TABLE I

Electrophoretic Mobility (E_m) of Erythrocytes from *Plasmodium berghei*-Infected and Noninfected Rats

Determination	Number	E_m ($\times 10^{-9}$ cm²/second/V)[a]	MI[b]	PCV[c]	Percentage of IRBC[d]	Percentage of BRBC[e]
Noninfected erythrocytes	48	1.315 ± 0.017	1.00	50	0	0
Infected erythrocytes, low parasitemia	15	1.303 ± 0.015	0.993 ± 0.007	40	12	4
Infected erythrocytes, moderate parasitemia	13	1.311 ± 0.039	0.986 ± 0.006	23	30	4
Infected erythrocytes, high parasitemia	13	1.271 ± 0.044	0.977 ± 0.011	21	51	10
Infected erythrocytes, recovered	7	1.189 ± 0.027	0.916 ± 0.015	ND	1	18
Noninfected erythrocytes, phenylhydrazine-injected rats	2	1.150	1.040	ND	0	37

[a] Average value ± standard mean error.

[b] MI = mobility index = $\dfrac{E_m \text{ (infected)}}{E_m \text{ (normal)}}$.

[c] PCV, Packed cell volume; ND, no data.

[d] IRBC, Erythrocytes infected with plasmodia.

[e] BRBC, Basophilic erythrocytes.

TABLE II

Sialic Acid Content of Malaria-Infected and Noninfected Erythrocytes

Determination	Sialic acid (μg/g tissue)[a]	No. of preparations	Percentage of IRBC[b]	Percentage of BRBC[c]
Noninfected erythrocytes	237 ± 11[c]	26	0	3
Infected erythrocytes, low parasitemia	211 ± 26	5	12	5
Infected erythrocytes, high parasitemia	238 ± 26	7	52	60
Infected erythrocytes, recovered	315	2	3	46
Noninfected erythrocytes, phenylhydrazine-injected)	310 ± 22	5	0	27

[a] Average value ± standard mean error.
[b] IRBC, Erythrocytes infected with plasmodia.
[c] BRBC, Basophilic erythrocytes.

acid content, and consequently their presence provides more than enough sialic acid to compensate for the reduced sialic acid content of the infected red cells. The ionogenic potential of the crisis basophilic erythrocyte present during the recovery phase of malaria appears not to be fully expressed, as the electrophoretic mobility of these reticulocytes is lower than would be expected from their high sialic acid content. It is possible that there is a masking of ionogenic sites by cytophilic macroglobulin, which is produced in high titer during the acute phases of infection (Gautam et al., 1970; Rosenberg et al., 1973) and which has the capacity to reduce dramatically in vitro the electrophoretic mobility of noninfected erythrocytes (Brown, 1933a,b).

Qualitative as well as quantitative abnormalities in the lipid composition of infected red cells have been reported (Lawrence and Cenedella, 1969; Cenedella et al., 1969; Rao et al., 1970; Rock et al., 1971; Seed and Kreier, 1972; DeZeeuw et al., 1972; Seed et al., 1974; Cooper and Miller, 1974; Holz, 1977; Beach et al., 1977), which are thought to contribute to altered red cell form and, in turn, to premature cell senescence. Seed and Kreier (1972) estimated that the phospholipid content of the red cell's plasmalemma changed little during infection, despite the substantial increases in total cellular phospholipid which occurred during the crisis and postcrisis phases of infection. The latter increases were attributed to the increased numbers and growth on intracellular parasites and to the influx into the circulation of immature crisis phase basophils. Plasma membrane cholesterol, in contrast to membrane phospholipid, appears to be depleted as a result of parasitization (Seed and Kreier, 1972). Because cholesterol restricts bilayer fluidity and lateral component mobility and increases the elasticity and strength of membranes (Nicolson, 1976), loss of cholesterol would destabilize the membrane and cause premature cell senescence. The observation of C. R. Sterling (personal communication) of enhanced planar mobility of labeled plasma membrane lipids of schizont-infected erythrocytes by electron spin resonance (ESR) supports the assumption that the membrane of the erythrocyte loses stability during infection.

Further characterization of the phospholipid composition of normal and malaria-infected erythrocytes has been attempted (Beach *et al.*, 1977; Holz, 1977; DeZeeuw *et al.*, 1972). The results obtained indicate a dramatic redistribution of phospholipid within the parasitized red cell. Phosphatidylethanolamine, phosphatidylinositol, and phosphatidylcholine increased about 350, 800, and 175%, respectively (Beach *et al.*, 1977). However, these changes reflect mainly the major contribution by the parasite and do not necessarily reflect an alteration in host cell plasmalemma phospholipids. Two groups of investigators have demonstrated by a more direct ultrastructural approach that there is a redistribution of erythrocyte surface phospholipids during the terminal phase of intraerythrocytic growth. In erythrocytes containing mature parasites the normal uniform mosaic pattern of surface phospolipid appears to be interrupted by enlarged, aggregated phopholipid plaques (Cooper and Miller, 1974; Seed *et al.*, 1974).

A variety of physical and physiological changes accompany the previously described infection-induced alterations in plasma membrane glycoprotein and lipid components. Parasitized red cells become more rigid and less deformable during the terminal phases of intracellular development. Miller and colleagues (1971, 1972) demonstrated that *P. coatneyi*- and *P. knowlesi*-infected red cells were less able to pass through the pores of polycarbonate filter membranes than noninfected cells. The viscosity of infected cells was substantially increased at both low and high shear rates.

We have directly demonstrated a decrease in plasmalemma elasticity with parasitization by employing an assay developed by Marikovsky and Danon (1967) in which elasticity and, in turn, the age of the cell is assessed in terms of its ability to form "stromalytic" surface protrusions when placed under extreme osmotic stress (Fig. 17). When samples of *P. berghei*-infected red cells were tested using this assay, much lower than normal percentages of red cells with highly elastic (stromalytic forms) properties were observed (Table III). This change in red cell deformability and membrane might well play a key role in enhanced splenic and capillary sequestration during malarial infection.

The spleen of both animals and humans has unique anatomical features that make it a highly effective blood filter and monitor of normally senescent or defective erythrocytes (Weiss and Tavassoli, 1970; Chen and Weiss, 1973; Weiss, 1974). It has long been recognized that nonfunctional normacytes with reduced deformability are quickly removed from the circulation by the spleen

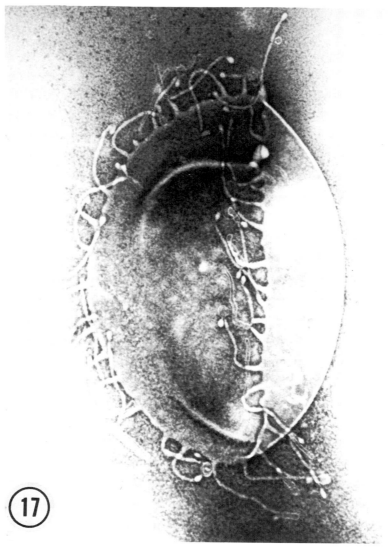

FIG. 17. A "stromalytic" figure is formed by subjecting young red cells with highly elastic plasma membranes to intense hypoosmotic stress. (See Table III for corresponding data.)

(Teitel, 1977); accordingly, highly inelastic red cells are ineffective in performing their primary function of oxygen delivery (Mohandas *et al.*, 1979). During splenic passage red cells are forced to traverse narrow (~0.75 μm) interendothelial slits. Red cells with reduced deformability, because of inelastic membranes or because they contain large, inelastic parasites, are trapped by endothelial

TABLE III

Membranes with Protrusions in Malarious and Nonmalarious Red Cell Populations[a]

Blood sample type	Stromalytic (%)	Intermediate (%)	Smooth (%)	Parasitized (%)	Basophilia (%)
Normal	26.7	47.4	25.8	0	3
Density-fractionated, normal					
Low density (young)	24.5	45.5	30.0	0	
High density (old)	5.5	5.5	89.0	0	
Malarious	7.0	48.9	43.5	57	55

[a] The elastic properties of rat erythrocytes from healthy and *P. berghei*-infected animals were tested by the method of Marikovsky and Danon (1967). Cell samples were osmotically shocked in distilled water, and small droplets were layered on Formvar-coated electron microscope grids and stained with 10% phosphotungstic acid. The prepared grids were examined with an electron microscope, and the percentage of red cells exhibiting many, some, or no stromalytic protrusions determined.

lining cells. "Pitting" of parasites from infected red cells during splenic passage has been reported in spleens of malaria-infected animals (Conrad and Dennis, 1968; Schnitzer *et al.*, 1973). In an analogous fashion, other types of inclusions, e.g., Heinz bodies, can be selectively removed (Weed and Weiss, 1966) as well. In either case, however, the circulating life span of spherocytic pitted red cells is short, as the pitted cell is sequestered in a subsequent splenic passage.

The changes in the physical properties of infected erythrocytes which promote cell entrapment necessarily complement, but do not supplant, specific immunological mechanisms of red cell sequestration.

C. Extrinsic Factors Influencing Erythrocyte Destruction

1. Humoral Factors

Extracorpuscular changes in the circulatory system, occurring as a consequence of malaria infection, are responsible in part for red cell destruction. Because of the intimate relationship existing between intrinsic and extrinsic defects, the magnitude of the extrinsic or environmental effect is often difficult to assess. The following environmental factors seem to contribute to blood pathology.

a. **Chemical and Physical Changes in Plasma Composition.** The changes in total plasma protein, particularly of the strongly acid macroglobulins (Abele *et al.*, 1965), together with the reduction in pH which occurs during the acute phases of infection (Seed and Kreier, 1972) might suppress the ionization of the major charge-bearing sialoglycoproteins on the erythrocytes. The resultant low charge on the erythrocytes, together with the increased plasma viscosity would necessarily promote sludging and capillary blockage. Low plasma pH has been implicated as a cause of red cell rigidity (Murphy, 1967) and reduction of the hemoglobin oxygen-binding capacity (Rigdon and Rostorfer, 1946; Palecek *et al.*, 1967). Both these changes effectively limit the red cell's ability to transport oxygen. A number of the characteristics of red cells from animals with acute malaria, such as increased osmotic fragility, increased agglutinability, and reduced oxygen transport capacity, can be attributed to such pH shifts. *In vitro* adjustment of the pH, or addition of certain metabolites or buffers to the plasma of infected animals, can reverse plasma-induced modifications of red cells (Dunn, 1969a,b; T. M. Seed, unpublished observations).

b. Soluble Toxins Circulating in the Plasma.   A number of plasma factors have been incriminated in hemolysis during the acute phase of the disease; these include lysins, endotoxin-like substances, enzymes, specific parasite products, and autoantibodies.

i. Blood and Tissue Lysins.   Hemolytic octadecanoic fatty acids have been isolated from both normal and infected blood. Laser (1948, 1950) reported increases of 25- to 75-fold in plasma concentrations of octadecanoic acid as a consequence of active *P. knowlesi* infection. Holz (1977) implicated both oleic [18:1 $(n - 7)$] and *cis*-vaccenic [18:1 $(n - 7)$] acids in the prehemolytic and hemolytic episodes associated with *P. lophurae* infections in ducks. *Cis*-vaccenic acid which nearly doubled in cell and plasma concentration during infection, was demonstrated to be twice as active per unit weight in inducing osmotic fragility of red cells as was oleic acid. The mode of action of these hemolytic fatty acids suggested by Holz (1977) is specific modification of plasma membrane fluidity by an alteration in the fatty acid composition of the membrane phospholipids and by the direct influence on adenylcyclase activity. These changes in turn affect membrane protein conformation and ultimately membrane transport.

ii. Endotoxin-Like Substances.   Indirect evidence has been accumulating that endotoxemia is integrally involved in malarial pathology (Cox, 1978; Clark, 1978). This is based on observations that during malaria there is a marked increase in sensitivity to bacterial endotoxin, suggesting prior sensitization. Fife *et al.* (1972) isolated a crude highly pyrogenic lipoidal hemolytic factor from *P. knowlesi*-infected erythrocytes. The factor was of low molecular weight ($\sim$500) and induced osmotic fragility both *in vitro* and *in vivo*.

iii. Enzymes.   Various workers have proposed that during malaria there are increased plasma concentrations of proteolytic and lipolytic enzymes. It has been suggested that these enzymes are elaborated by both parasite and host during infection, the hosts's response being part of a normal physiological response involving degradation and removal of cellular debris (Seed and Kreier, 1969, 1972; Kreier, 1969). Confirmation of this concept by direct assay for enzymes or for antitrypsin factors in the plasma remains to be done. However, the presence of agglutinins to trypsinized normal erythrocytes during infection and the relatedness of red cell surface antigens induced by trypsinization and by natural infection is suggestive of proteolytic modification of circulating red cells (Kreier *et al.*, 1966).

iv. Specific Parasite Products. Endotoxin and enzymes might well be contributed by the malarial parasite, by the host, or by organisms coincidentally present; however, only a histidine-rich protein, a lytic, highly antigenic product associated with the anterior organelles of the merozoite, is known to be contributed by the parasite (Kilejian, 1974, 1976; Kilejian and Jensen, 1977). This rather unusual protein, with $\simeq 70\%$ histidine, no serine, and acid solubility, is thought to promote merozoite invasion of susceptible red cells. It has been isolated in crude form from both *P. lophurae* and *P. falciparum* parasites (Kilejian and Jensen, 1977).

c. Parasite-Directed Antibodies or Autoantibodies. Specific sensitization of either a part or the entire erythron during infection by antibodies with either antiparasitic or autoantigenic specificities has been widely proposed as the cause of red cell destruction (Zuckerman, 1964). However, such antibody-mediated pathological processes have been difficult to substantiate experimentally *in vivo* (George *et al.*, 1966; Kreier and Leste, 1968; Kreier, 1969). The major difficulty has been to demonstrate that the antierythrocytic antibodies present have opsonic activity which enhances cell sequestration *in vivo*. Autoantibodies, primarily of the IgM class (Kreier *et al.*, 1966) but also of the IgG and IgA classes (Kano *et al.*, 1968; Rosenberg *et al.*, 1973; Voller, 1974), with specificity toward uninfected and infected erythrocytes and toward trypsinized erythrocytes have been detected either free in the plasma or cell-bound during the acute anemia phase of malarial infection. This humoral response to malarial infection has been demonstrated in birds (Szilvassey *et al.*, 1969; Seed and Kreier, 1969), in rodents (Cox *et al.*, 1966; Kreier *et al.*, 1966), and in a variety of primates, including humans (Adeniyi-Jones, 1967; Kano *et al.*, 1968; McGregor *et al.*, 1970; Rosenberg *et al.*, 1973). Kano *et al.* (1968) reported in one survey that $\simeq 35\%$ of the Gambian sera collected from individuals with malaria was positive for hemagglutinins against trypsinized human erythrocytes; sera from individuals who did not have malaria were completely negative. The predominance of IgM as the hemagglutinin would explain one of the puzzling and troublesome observations which has plagued proponents of the autoimmune theory, that is, that the Coomb's reaction, which detects cytophilic IgG, is generally negative (Adner et al., 1968; Barrett-Conner, 1967) rather than positive during the phases of the disease during which there is disproportionate red cell loss (Zuckerman, 1977). Rosenberg and co-workers (1973) demonstrated rising titers of IgM (from 100 to 500 mg/100 ml) in P. falciparum-infected U.S. military personnel. The rising titers coincided with falling concentrations of complement (C3), increasing degrees of anemia, and decreasing survival times of noninfected red cells. A study on a battery of other types of infections, malignancies, and autoimmune diseases in which elevated IgM plasma titers also occur failed to exhibit similar correlations. When fluorescent antibody techniques were utilized, the plasma IgM derived from malarious patients was shown to bind to noninfected red cells from healthy individuals. The cells used as antigen in these tests were dried and fixed on microscope slides. Fluorescent antibody tests utilizing fresh, unfixed erythrocytes are considered more appropriate, however.

A similar type of antibody has been observed in chickens with avian malaria and appears to be of the IgM class, as it is sensitive to mercaptoethanol (Kreier, 1969). Using ^{125}I-labeled antiglobulin, Gautam et al. (1970) demonstrated the presence of trypsinized erythrocyte hemagglutinin on P. gallinaceum-parasitized red cells. In contrast to earlier workers (Zuckerman, 1960c; Zuckerman and Spira, 1961, Gautam et al. (1970) took into account the fact that basophilic erythrocytes, which arise in large numbers during the acute stages of infection, normally have surface-bound transferrin, a globulin which interferes with antiglobulin tests by causing false positive Coomb's reactions. With the use of antiglobulin reagents absorbed with basophil-enriched red cells from noninfected, phenylhydrazine-injected chickens, distinct immunological differences were demonstrated between the normal cytophilic globulins coating immature erythrocytes and the infection-induced IgM globulins absorbed to the parasitized erythrocytes.

The cryptic autoantigen, exposed artificially by in vitro trypsinization or by pathological processes during infection, is mainly lipoidal in nature (Seed and Kreier, 1969), in part resembling the VDRL antigen (Kahn, 1949; Kahn and Baribeau, 1949).

Other circulating blood cells including platelets, and cells of tissues such as heart, are probably modified as well during infection and express similar autoantigens (Neva et al., 1970; McGregor et al., 1970). When the pathological sequelae of autoimmune reactions involve blood platelets, they produce a thrombocytopenic condition or perhaps the more rare disseminated intravascular coagulation syndrome known to occur in patients with P. falciparum infections (O'Leary et al., 1972).

Several additional autoantigens have been implicated in the autoimmune disorders occurring during malaria, including modified antigen–antibody complexes (Topley et al., 1973). Opsonic antibodies have been eluted from antigen–

antibody complexes obtained from washed erythrocytes of malarious hosts (Cox, 1973). Surface-adherent antigen–antibody complexes appear to fix complement and induce a prehemolytic or a hemolytic condition. The entire immune complex maybe autoantigenic. Rising titers of immunoconglutinin, which is an antibody, to fixed complement on immune complexes have been identified in patients during the active clinical phases of malaria (Topley *et al.*, 1973).

2. *Organ and Cellular Factors*

a. General Background.   The RES, which has major responsibility for the elimination of aged or damaged tissues, functions during malarial infection as a primary line of host defense by recognizing and phagocytosing not only free parasites but also infected erythrocytes, thus destroying intracellular parasites (Taliaferro and Cannon, 1936; Taliaferro and Mulligan, 1937; Gingrich, 1941; Zuckerman, 1945, 1977; Taliaferro and Taliaffero, 1948; I. N. Brown, 1969; K. N. Brown, 1970, 1971; Brown *et al.*, 1970; Brown and Hills, 1971).

Recent work in our laboratory has demonstrated that macrophages in *in vitro* cultures of *Babesia microti* become hyperactive within 24 hours of the addition of specific antibabesial antibody. These macrophages are spread out on the bottoms of the culture vessels and are filled with parasites, debris, and red cells. In the absence of antiserum the macrophages are much less active and ingest free parasites, some debris, and a few red cells. These results suggest that the activation of macrophages in animals with babesiosis is induced by the ingestion of antigen–antibody complexes. The system may be an *in vitro* model for study of the crisis in babesiosis and malaria (Bautista and Kreier, 1979, 1980).

The RES, through its phagocytic activity, is one of the regulators of the humoral immune response and thus exerts profound influence on the outcome of malarial infection. The function of the RES changes with both the stage and degree of infection. In the early stages of avian (Cox *et al.*, 1964) and rodent infections (Cox *et al.*, 1963; Cantrell and Elko, 1966; Cantrell *et al.*, 1970; Kitchen and DiLuzio, 1971; Loose *et al.*, 1972), there is an increased rate of vascular clearance of various types of injected particles, including colloidal carbon and sheep erythrocytes. Sheagren and co-workers (1970) observed enhanced rates of vascular clearance of ^{125}I-labeled microaggregated serum albumin in 10 patients with active malarial infections, two of which had *P. ovale* infections, one a *P. falciparum* infection, and the rest *P. vivax* infections. Reduced blood flow through the tissues of the RES occurred concomitantly with infection, and blood flow returned to normal upon cure. Loose *et al.* (1972) reported that ^{51}Cr-labeled sheep erythrocytes were cleared from the circulation of *P. berghei*-infected mice at a rate 47% greater than from noninfected control mice. Increased uptake by the spleen and by the liver accounted for most of the increase. However, when the data were adjusted for organ weight differences between infected and noninfected animals, the differences in rate were small and often a negative correlation occurred.

There are reports in the literature which indicate that at very high parasitemias there is a decline in the rate of vascular clearance of foreign substances. Cox *et al.* (1963, 1964) demonstrated this in both *P. gallinaceum* and *P. vinckei*-infected animals when parasitemias rose above ≈ 25 and $\approx 90\%$, respectively. Such reduced phagocytic activity and in turn antigen processing by macrophages, during the acute phases of infection might be temporally related to the now well recognized immunosuppressive condition occurring as a consequence of acute infection. A reduced capacity of the infected animal to produce antibody to specific heterologous particulate antigens such as heterologous erythrocytes (Salaman *et al.*, 1969; Greenwood *et al.*, 1971b; Loose *et al.*, 1972; Barker, 1971; Sengers, 1971), aggregated IgG (Greenwood *et al.*, 1971a), tetanus toxoid (McGregor and Barr, 1962), murine leukemia and sarcoma viruses (Salaman *et al.*, 1969), and *Salmonella typhimurium* (Kaye *et al.*, 1965) has been demonstrated.

A nearly normal antibody response to certain antigens, such as keyhole limpet hemocyanin (Greenwood *et al.*, 1971b), which do not require macrophage processing for immunogenicity, suggests that the lymphocyte–plasma cell compartment which is in the afferent limb of the humoral response, remains functionally intact during malaria. It is probably the antigen-processing step by the macrophage which is impaired as a consequence of infection (Loose *et al.*, 1972). If at the time of the suppression of function the processing of plasmodial antigen has not been adequate to induce antibody production, the host's ability to limit the infection may be compromised.

b. Spleen and Splenic Macrophage Function. The enhanced clearance of inert substances from the blood has been considered indicative of nonspecific hyperactivity of the RES. Phagocytic indexes of primary blood-filtering organs increase in proportion to the severity of the malarial infection (McGregor, 1971, 1974; Brown, 1969). Splenic enlargement occurs during active malarial infection. Epidemiologically there is an association between chronic malarial infection and the tropical splenomegaly syndrome. Big-spleen disease is characterized pathologically by intense lymphoreticular proliferation, greatly elevated plasma IgM levels, associated plasmodial antibodies, and erythrocytic autohemagglutinins (Zuckerman, 1977). Lymphoreticular hyperplasia of the bone marrow and spleen is believed to contribute to anemia by lowering red cell production (Dokow *et al.* 1974). The increased commitment of the pluripotent hemopoietic stem cell compartment to the production of granulocytes and macrophages for host defense purposes might well prevent red cell production. In rodents with experimental infections it is not uncommon for an up to a 20-fold increase in spleen size to occur, with phagocytic indexes elevated 200-fold (Zuckerman, 1977).

Hypersplenism is purported to cause accelerated red cell destruction and anemia in a number of hemolytic diseases in addition to malaria (Motulsky *et al.*, 1958; Jandl *et al.*, 1961). Splenic enlargement during malaria is an undisputed finding. However, whether it causes abnormal red cell loss is unclear. George *et al.* (1966) was unable to demonstrate the presence of circulating autoantibodies or an effect of immune sera on the *in vivo* survival of red cells and suggested that excessive red cell destruction during the acute phases of infection was caused solely by the hypersplenic response. Zuckerman *et al.* (1969) attempted to test this hypothesis by inducing a sterile-type hypersplenic condition within normal, noninfected rats with protracted methylcellulose treatment. The treatment produced mild anemia, however, the degree of anemia as well as the hypersplenic response to methylcellulose was less than that observed during malarial infection. Consequently, Zuckerman *et al.* (1969) suggested that other factors such as autoimmunization (Table IV) probably contributed to excessive red cell loss and the severe anemia commonly associated with malaria.

Although various reports indicate different degrees of phagocytosis of both nonparasitized as well as parasitized erythrocytes during infection with plasmodia, some amount of erythrophagocytosis has been consistently reported in both humans and animals with plasmodial infection (Taliaferro and Cannon, 1936; Taliaferro and Mulligan, 1937; Taliaferro and Taliaferro, 1948; McGhee and Corwin, 1964; Zuckerman, 1966; Giles *et al.*, 1969; Wells, 1970). Splenic phagocytes increase in number, in avidity, and in phagocytic efficiency during infection (Neva *et al.*, 1970; Zuckerman *et al.*, 1973). The specificity recognition during infection is thought to be broadened to include nonparasitized erythrocytes, and this is considered to contribute to excessive red cell destruction and development of a degree of anemia disproportionate to the parasitemia (Zuckerman, 1977). Zuckerman (1974) recounted her observations on the phenomenon of erythrophagocytosis when reporting the results of one of her experiments during a meeting in 1973:

> Erythrophagocytosis in *P. berghei*-infected outbred sabra rats is marked just before, at, and particularly after crisis, remaining slightly above normal during latency. This is precisely

TABLE IV

Factors Contributing to Malaria Anemia

1. Direct damage of red cells by invasion and growth of parasites
2. Indirect damage by circulating toxic substances
3. Hypersplenism
4. Autoimmunity

the temporal pattern of peripheral anemia. The ingestion of parasitized red cells rose and fell exactly with parasitemia. When present, infected red cells were ingested in their normal proportions within the total population. But erythrophagocytosis was not specifically oriented to infected cells and the ingestion of unparasitized red cells always far outstripped that of parasitized cells. Normal controls (i.e., noninfected rats) have negligible erythrophagocytosis, representing the normal removal from the circulation of effete cells.

c. Macrophage Targeting Mechanisms. The precise molecular mechanisms are not known by which macrophages recognize and remove defective erythrocytes from the circulation during infection. Many of the infection-induced red cell changes are internal and as such are probably not directly involved in the macrophage recognition processes. It is more than likely that the macrophage recognizes surface modifications rather than activities or concentrations of internal enzymes or metabolites. It seems logical, therefore, that the mechanisms responsible for red cell sequestration involve the changes in structure and distribution of surface components occurring during the course of the infection. It has been noted that malaria induces red cell alterations which biochemically and biophysically mimic normal red cell aging, but the development of which is accelerated (see Fig. 13) (Seed and Kreier, 1972). The recognition processes by which macrophages discriminate between normal mature self and aged, senescent self are part of the normal physiological homeostatic processes of all animals. As a consequence of plasmodial infection, the finely tuned discriminatory processes by which the RES makes this discrimination appear to be partially lost. If specificity is not lost, at least the sensitivity is greatly increased and the specificity broadened to such an extent that some workers have considered some of the activated processes of the RES pathological phenomena (Zuckerman, 1964, 1977). One might just as well consider autoimmunity an exaggerated but normal physiological response designed to clear the circulation of senescent cells and debris. The latter would necessarily aid the host defense by eliminating cells containing blood parasites.

In the healthy animal the processes by which the RES recognizes senescent cells are under strict control and require a functionally intact macrophage population. Proteolytic modification of the macrophage surface can effectively eliminate the ability of the macrophage to recognize senescent cells by destroying specific membrane receptors which are regenerable under proper environmental conditions. Trypsinization abolishes the macrophages ability to bind plasmodia also, and treatment with serum will restore this ability (Chow and Kreier, 1972).

There is yet some question as to the nature of the surface structures of aged or defective red cells which the macrophage receptors recognize. Anionic charge-bearing major sialoglycoproteins have been implicated in recognition (Danon 1967; Skutelsky and Danon, 1969), as have bound IgGs (Kay, 1975). Selective elimination of defective red cells by the RES is considered a two-stage process involving, first, recognition and attachment which appears to be serum-independent, and second, engulfment and degradation, a serum-dependent (C3b and immunoglobin) process. The age- or infection-modified surface moiety might itself be the recognition site, or immunoglubulin coupling at this site might be necessary to initiate engulfment. The terminal carbohydrate moiety exposed by the removal of sialic acid (Nicolson, 1973) to which immunoglobulin binds avidly has been proposed as the macrophage recognition site (Kay, 1975).

It is not entirely clear how and to what extent these normal recognition systems are operative during malarial infection. One would predict that such mechanisms are not only operative but that their actions are enhanced in infected animals. There is, however, only partial presumptive evidence to support the concept that red cell destruction during plasmodial infection is caused by systems similar to those which remove senescent cells. Electrophoretic mobility studies and cyto- and biochemical analyses (See Tables I and II) (Heidrich et al., 1979) indicate that the sialoglycoprotein surface moieties of erythrocytes, especially those of parasitized erythrocytes, are modified. Erythrocytes whose membranes have undergone alteration have reduced survival times and are easily phagocytized. Other membrane intercalated antigens of either parasite or host origin might also serve as macrophage recognition sites. Opsonizing immunoglobulins of the IgM class have been eluted from parasitized erythrocytes and have been shown to be cross-reactive with surface antigens of trypsinized normocytes (Kreier et al., 1966; Gautam et al., 1970). Trypsinization, in many ways, induces membrane alterations which mimic those induced by the infectious process. Trypsinization reduces electrophoretic mobility of the cell (Seed, 1969), reduces net sialic acid content, and curtails normal cell survival in vivo (Kreier, 1969). It has been suggested, although not documented experimentally, that infection-activated proteolysis may be responsible for sensitization of the erythron (Kreier, 1969).

The question still unanswered is whether or not the surface lesions induced naturally in the aging process, by malarial infection, or by enzyme treatment are chemically and biologically equivalent and whether they are recognized by the same macrophage membrane receptors and serum factors. In vitro, in a totally autologous, serum-free system which allows only for the attachment steps of the phagocytic process to occur, it has been shown that isolated macrophages have difficulty distinguishing parasitized erythrocytes from nonparasitized cells of the population (Table V; Figs. 18 and 19). However, the parasitized (P. berghei) erythrocytes bound by macrophages consistently contained the larger, more fully differentiated parasites. By cytochemical electron microscopic analysis, it was shown that the plasmalemmas of parasitized erythrocytes which attached to macrophages had a less luxuriant glycocalyx, fewer anionogenic surface groups, and fewer concanavalin A-binding receptors than erythrocytes which did not attach to macrophages. The cytochemical changes did not appear to be associated with much obvious gross structural abnormality in the membrane. The erythrocyte plasmalemma within the zone of macrophage attachment was not obviously

TABLE V

Targeting of Erythrocytes by Autologous Macrophages[a]

Cell sample	Treatment	Red blood cells bound per 200 macrophages (±SEM)	n
Light fraction (young)	Gradient	8 ± 5	8
Heavy fraction (old)	Gradient	27 ± 9	8
Control 1 (fresh)	None	7 ± 3	6
Control 2 (top)	Gradient	7 ± 1	4
Control 3 (bottom)	Gradient	3 ± 1	2
Aged, in vitro	5 days, 4°C	24 ± 9	4
Aged, in vitro	12 days, 4°C	40 ± 12	2
Aged, in vitro	15 days, 4°C	103 ± 41	2
Aged, in vitro	49 days, 4°C	256 ± 23	2
Enzyme-digested	Trypsin	128 ± 35	5
	Chymotrypsin	117 ± 56	4
	Neuraminidase	130 ± 51	4
Parasitized	None	8.3 ± 2.1	3
Parasitized	10 mg/ml cloroquine	15.0 ± 7.2	3
Parasitized	100 mg/ml chloroquine	20.5 ± 9.1	3
Parasitized	10 mg/ml primaquine	5.0 ± 1.4	3
Parasitized	100 mg/ml primaquine	22.5 ± 3.5	3

[a] Peritoneal macrophages were collected from exudate washings of adult albino rats 72 hours after intraperitoneal injection with sterile mineral oil. Exudate cells were washed three times and resuspended in medium 199–10% bovine serum albumin–100 U/ml penicillin-streptomycin. Aliquots of these suspensions were plated out in 35-mm petri dishes, placed in a carbon dioxide incubator (7.5% carbon dioxide, 37°C) for five hours, and subsequently removed from the incubator and washed to remove the nonadherent cells. Aliquots of the red cell suspension to be tested were then added to the macrophage cultures (in a final concentration of 100 red cells per macrophage), and the dishes were then returned to the incubator for 30 minutes. The cultures were thoroughly washed to remove the nonadherent erythrocytes and processed for either light or electron microscopic examination. Normal or modified red cells to be assayed for their targetability were treated as follows: (1) Aged cells—suspensions of washed red cells were stored in a refrigerator at 4°C for periods of 0–49 days. (2) Enzyme treatment—cells were trypsinized in 0.25% (w/v) trypsin for 30 minutes at 37°C; cells were digested in chymotrypsin at an enzyme concentration of 8.3 U/ml; a mixture of neuraminidase from *Clostridium perfringens* (0.012 U/ml) and *Vibria cholerae* (3.7 U/ml) was used for 30 minutes at 37°C to digest red cells. (c) Density fractionation—mixtures of phlalate esters with final specific gravities ranging from 1.07376 to 1.10598 were used to fractionate light (young) and heavy (old) erythrocytes from normal blood samples (Marikovsky and Danon, 1967). (d) Parasitization—parasitized red cell samples were collected from *P. berghei*-infected rats with parasitemias averaging ≈20%. Cells were washed and preincubated for 30 minutes at 37°C in either normal growth media alone or media containing 10 or 100 mg/ml of antimalarial. The samples were then washed, resuspended in normal media, and added to the macrophage cultures.

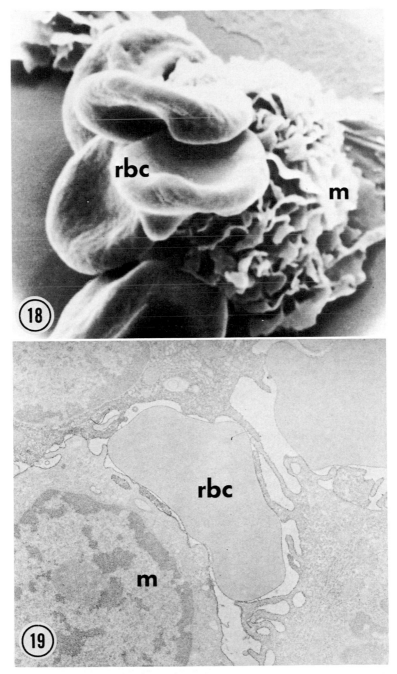

FIG. 18 and 19. A scanning electron micrograph of macrophages (m) and red cells (rbc). The cells are from a parasitized (*P. berghei*) red cell sample. A comparable cross-sectional view by electron microscopy of two nonparasitized erythrocytes. (See Table V for corresponding data on targetting assays.)

different from that in the nonattached areas as no localized surface alterations were detected (T. M. Seed, unpublished observations, 1975). In contrast to the bulk of the parasitized population, normally aged erythrocytes separated by buoyant and density centrifugation, or those artificially aged by storage in the refrigerator, are readily recognized as being inherently defective and are readily bound by macrophages *in vitro*. Similarly, treatment of normal erythrocytes with trypsin, chymotrypsin, or neuraminidase can produce surface defects easily recognized by macrophages (Table V) (Seed and Kreier, 1977).

The discrepancy between the degree of macrophage binding of parasitized erythrocytes *in vitro* and *in vivo* suggests that *in vivo* humoral and cellular factors not duplicated in our *in vitro* systems are operating. Interestingly, parasitized erythrocytes can be made highly susceptible to binding by normal or immune macrophages *in vitro* by pretreatment with small quantities of antimalarial drugs (Table V) (Seed and Kreier, 1977). Perhaps, in an analogous fashion, natural cytotoxic agents such as endotoxin (Cox, 1978) elaborated *in vivo* during certain phases of the infection (e.g., at crisis) alter the host cell in a way which increases macrophage recognition. Our recent observation that macrophages in *in vitro* cultures of *B. microti* become very actively phagocytic within hours of the addition of immune serum suggests that *in vivo* a change which enhances the macrophages' ability to ingest red cells may occur at the time of the onset of the immune response (Bautista and Kreier, 1980).

III. PROPOSED MODEL OF THE RELATIONSHIP BETWEEN ERYTHROCYTE LOSS AND PARASITEMIA

Our working model is based on the premise that the events of red cell alteration which ultimately result in either hemolysis or sequestration are temporally related to the terminal events of the developmental cycle of the intraerythrocytic malarial parasite. It is possible that one of the initiating events involves the degradation or rearrangement of spectrin, a functional stabilizing component of the permeaphore complex, by the fully segmented parasite during the release phase of mature merozoites from the entrapping host cell (see Fig. 14). It is also quite possible that the processes of host cell invasion by merozoites and merozoite release from the host cell are mechanistically related; i.e., both processes mediated by the release of membrane-modifying substances from the merozoite's specialized anterior-end organelles (Fig. 20a and b).

Rearrangement of intramembranous particles within membranes of schizont-containing red cells, depletion of lectin surface receptors, specific galactose- and galactosamine-bearing structures, and reduced surface sialic acid content indicate a modification of the permeaphore complex. The parasite-induced dysfunction of the major transport complex within the host cell's plasmalemma would result in a

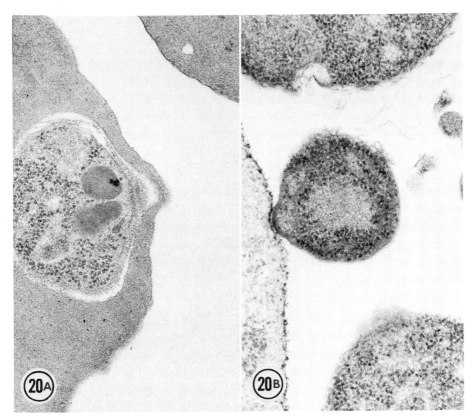

FIG. 20. Intraerythrocytic (A) and extraerythrocytic merozoites (B) inducing localized disturbances in the host cell plasmalemma. Merozoite entry and release may be functionally related processes in the life cycle of the malaria parasite. (See Fig. 14 and text for further discussion.)

cascading sequence of biochemical and biophysical changes, the more important of which affect erythrocyte permeability and osmotic regulation. Inactivation of the cationic transport enzymes of the Na^+-dependent, Mg^{2+}-activated ATPase system probably causes an influx of Na^+ and in turn water. The ensuing changes in cell volume, cell fragility, and cell shape, together with a modified lipid structure would result in a less deformable, more readily targeted and phagocytized red cell. To a large extent the changes resemble those which occur with normal red cell aging, (Danon, 1967) but during malaria they occur prematurely (Seed and Kreier, 1972).

As a consequence of the change in red cell membrane permeability, an increased outflux and surface localization of soluble parasite antigen might be expected. This process alone, or coupled with specifically bound immunoglobulin, would affect the targeting of such modified red cells by immunocompetent cells.

The parasite-initiated production of surface autoantigens and the subsequent loading of the cell surface with autoantibody of the IgM class have been considered to play a role in red cell destruction in malaria (Seed and Kreier, 1969; Kreier, 1969). Similar mechanisms for the recognition and sequestration of normally aged red cells within healthy individuals have been reported (Kay, 1975), however, the class of immunoglobulin implicated in the sequestration of normally aged erythrocytes is IgG.

The changes which contribute to sequestration of parasitized red cells may also occur in the nonparasitized segment of the erythron. Many noninfected red cells are obviously sufficiently modified during infection that during the crisis they are destroyed. The factors responsible for the modification of uninfected erythrocytes may include plasma-soluble toxic and enzymatic substances of parasite and host origin, exposed autoantigens, and parasite materials absorbed onto and inserted into the membranes of the erythrocytes. The abnormalities of the erythrocyte membrane may be recognized directly or through constitutive opsonins, antiparasitic antibodies, autoantibodies, or complement components.

The destruction by the RES of the modified erythrocytes is facilitated by changes in the circulatory system during infection, including increased plasma viscosity, reduced plasma pH, and reduced blood flow through RES organs. Destruction of parasitized and nonparasitized erythrocytes becomes prominent just before and during the crisis. Activation of phagocytes at the crisis is probably induced by the phagocytes ingestion of antigen–antibody complexes. The activated phagocytes develop an increased capacity to ingest modified red cells.

Loss of nonparasitized cells late in the infection can in part be attributed to the loss of noninfected crisis reticulocytes which may have short life spans. These reticulocytes are produced under the extreme stress of intense anemia and aid the host in returning its erythropoietic system to equilibrium. If these reticulocytes did not have a range of survival characteristics, recurrent bouts of anemia would occur at the end of the life span of the replacement cohort.

The massive destruction of erythrocytes which occurs during the malarial crisis aids the host by coincidental destruction of parasites. If the host is then able to replace the destroyed erythrocytes quickly enough, it will recover and the parasites will be controlled by more specific antiparasitic mechanisms.

REFERENCES

Abele, D. C., Tobie, J. E., Contacos, P. G., and Evans, C. B. (1965). Alterations in serum proteins and 19S antibody production during the course of induced malarial infections in man. *Am. J. Trop. Med. Hyg.* **14**, 191–197.

Adeniyi-Jones, C. (1967). Agglutination of tanned sheep erythrocytes by serum from Nigerian adults and children. *Lancet* **1**, 188–190.

Adner, M. M., Altstatt, L. S., and Conrad, M. E. (1968). Coomb's-positive hemolytic disease in malaria. *Ann. Intern. Med.* **68**, 33–38.

Aikawa, M. (1977). Variations in structure and function during the life cycle of malarial parasites. *Bull. W.H.O.* **55**, 139–156.

Aikawa, M., and Seed, T. M. (1973). Cytochemical surface properties of malarial parasites enhancing penetration of host erythrocytes. *In* "Progress in Protozoology," p. 8. Université de Clermont, Clermont-Ferrand.

Aikawa, M., Rabbege, J. R., and Wellde, B. T. (1972). Junctional apparatus in erythrocytes infected with malarial parasites. *Z. Zellforsch. Mikrosk. Anat.* **124**, 72–75.

Aikawa, M., Miller, L. H., and Rabbege, J. R. (1975). Caveola-vesicle complexes: The plasmalemma of erythrocytes infected by *Plasmodium vivax* and *Plasmodium cynomolgi:* Unique structure related to Schüffner's dots. *Am. J. Pathol.* **79**, 285–300.

Aikawa, M., Miller, L. H., Johnson, J., and Rabbege, J. R. (1978). Erythrocyte entry by malaria parasites: A moving junction between erythrocyte and parasite. *J. Cell Biol.* **77**, 72–82.

Arnold, J. D., Balcerzak, S. P., and Martin, C. D. (1969). Studies on the red cell-parasite relationship. *Mil. Med.* **134**, 962–971.

Bahr, G. F. (1969). Quantitative cytochemistry of malaria infected erythrocytes (*Plasmodium lophurae* and *Plasmodium berghei*). *Mil. Med.* **131**, 1013–1025.

Barker, L. R. (1971). Experimental malaria: Effects upon the immune response to different antigens. *J. Infect. Dis.* **123**, 99–101.

Barrett-Conner, E. (1967). *Plasmodium vivax* malaria and Coombs-positive anemia. *Am. J. Trop. Med. Hyg.* **16**, 699–703.

Bautista, C. R., and Kreier, J. P. (1979). Effect of immune serum on the growth of *Babesia microti* in hamster erythrocytes in short term culture. *Infect. Immun.* **25**, 470–472.

Bautista, C. R., and Kreier, J. P. (1980). The action of macrophages and immune serum on growth of *Babesia microti* in short-term cultures. *Tropenmed. Parasitol.* **31** (in press).

Beach, D. H., Sherman, I. W., and Holz, G. G., Jr. (1977). Lipids of *Plasmodium lophurae* and of erythrocytes and plasmas of normal and *P. lophurae*-infected Pekin ducklings. *J. Parasitol.* **63**, 62–75.

Brown, H. C. (1933a). Preliminary observations on electric charge of the erythrocytes in bird malaria. *Trans. R. Soc. Trop. Med. Hyg.* **26**, 515–522.

Brown, H. C. (1933b). Further observations on the electric charge of the erythrocytes in certain protozoal diseases. *Br. J. Exp. Pathol.* **14**, 413–421.

Brown, I. N. (1969). Immunological aspects of malaria infection. *Adv. Immunol.* **11**, 267–349.

Brown, K. N. (1970). Cell-mediated protective immunity in trypanosomiasis and malaria. *J. Parasitol.* **56**, 36–37.

Brown, K. N. (1971). Protective immunity to malaria provides a model for the survival of cells in an immunologically hostile environment. *Nature (London)* **230**, 163–167.

Brown, K. N., and Hills, L. A. (1971). Macrophage activation and action of opsonizing antibodies in malaria. *Trans. R. Soc. Trop. Med. Hyg.* **65**, 6.

Brown, K. N., Brown, I. N., and Hills, L. A. (1970). Immunity to malaria. I. Protection against *Plasmodium knowlesi* shown by monkeys sensitized with drug-suppressed infections or by dead parasites in Fruend's adjuvant. *Exp. Parasitol.* **28**, 304–317.

Cantrell, W., and Elko, E. E. (1966). Effect of splenectomy on phagocytic activation by *Plasmodium berghei*. *J. Infect. Dis.* **116**, 429–438.

Cantrell, W. F., Elko, E. E., and Hopff, B. M. (1970). *Plasmodium berghei:* Phagocytic hyperactivity of infected rats. *Exp. Parasitol.* **28**, 291–297.

Cenedella, R. J., Jarrell, J. J., and Saxe, L. H. (1969). Lipid synthesis *in vivo* from 1-^{14}C-oleic acid and 6-^{3}H-glucose by intraerythrocytic *Plasmodium berghei*. *Mil. Med.* **134**, 1045–1055.

Chen, L. T., and Weiss, L. (1973). The role of the sinus wall in the passage of erythrocytes through the spleen. *Blood* **41**, 529–537.

Chow, J. S., and Kreier, J. P. (1972). *Plasmodium berhei:* Adherence and phagocytosis by rat macrophages *in vitro. Exp. Parasitol.* **31**, 13-18.

Clark, I. A. (1978). Does endotoxin cause both the disease and parasite death in acute malaria and babesiosis? *Lancet* **2**, 75-77.

Coleman, R. M., Rencricca, N. J., Ritterschaus, C. W., and Brissett, W. H. (1976). Malaria: Decreased survival of transfused, normal erythrocytes in infected rats. *J. Parasitol.* **62**, 138-140.

Conrad, M. E., and Dennis, L. H. (1968). Splenic function in experimental malaria. *Am. J. Trop. Med. Hyg.* **17**, 170-172.

Cooper, G. W., and Miller, L. H. (1974). Propanoic acid-ferric oxide hydrosols: Differential cell surface binding and its relation to membrane lipid. *J. Histochem. Cytochem.* **22**, 856-867.

Cox, H. W. (1973). The spleen in babesiosis, malaria and other red cell infections. *In* "Progress in Protozoology," p. 97. Université de Clermont, Clermont-Ferrand.

Cox, F. E. G. (1978). Malaria, piroplasmosis and endotoxin. *Nature (London)* **274**, 312.

Cox, F. E. G., Nicol, T., and Bilbey, D. L. J. (1963). Reticulo-endothelial activity in *Haemamoeba* (=*Plasmodium*) *gallinaceum* infections. *J. Protozool.* **10**, 107-109.

Cox, F. E. G., Bilbey, D. L. J., and Nicol, T. (1964). Reticulo-endothelial activity in mice infected with *Plasmodium vinckei. J. Protozool.* **11**, 229-236.

Cox, H. W., Schroeder, W. F., and Ristic, M. (1966). Hemagglutination and erythrophagocytosis associated with anemia of *Plasmodium berghei* infection of rats. *J. Protozool.* **13**, 327-332.

Danon, D. (1967). Structural changes associated with red cell aging. "John G. Gibson II," Lect. XVII. Columbia University, College of Physicians and Surgeons, New York.

Danon, D., and Gunders, A. (1962). On the relationship between parasitemia and increased osmotic fragility of erythrocytes in rodent malaria. *Bull. Res. Counc. Isr. Sect. E* **10**, 59-64.

Devakul, K., Harinasuta, T., and Kanakakorn, K. (1969). Erythrocyte destruction in *Plasmodium falciparum* malaria: An investigation of intravascular hemolysis. *Ann. Trop. Med. Parasitol.* **63**, 317-325.

DeZeeuw, Wijsbeek, J., Rock, R. C., and McCormick, G. J. (1972). Composition of phospholipids in *Plasmodium knowlesi* membranes and in host rhesus erythrocyte membranes. *Proc. Helminthol. Soc. Wash.* **39**, 412-418.

Dokow, S. J., Golenser, J., Greenblatt, C., and Spira, D. (1974). Changes in rat splenocyte population during infection with *Plasmodium berghei. J. Protozool.* **31**, 463.

Dunn, M. J. (1969a). Alterations of red blood cell sodium transport during malarial infection. *J. Clin. Invest.* **48**, 674-675.

Dunn, M. J. (1969b). Alterations of red blood cell metabolism in simium malaria: Evidence for abnormalities of non-parasitized cells. *Mil. Med.* **134**, 1100-1105.

Durocher, J. R., Payne, R. C., and Conrad, M. E. (1975). Role of sialic acid in erythrocyte survival. *Blood* **45**, 11-20.

Dvorak, J. A., Miller, L. H., Whitehouse, W. L., and Shiroishi, T. (1975). Invasion of erythrocytes by malaria merozoites. *Science* **187**, 748-750.

Eisen, H. (1977). Purification of intracellular forms of *Plasmodium chabaudi* and their interactions with the erythrocyte membrane and with serum albumin. *Bull. W.H.O.* **55**, 333-338.

Fife, E. H., von Doenhoff, A. E. Jr., and D'Antonio, L. E. (1972). *In vitro* and *in vivo* studies on a lytic factor isolated from *Plasmodium knowlesi. Proc. Helminthol. Soc. Wash.* **39**, 373-382.

Fogel, B., Shields, C., and von Doenhoff, A. E., Jr. (1966). The osmotic fragility of erythrocytes in experimental malaria. *Am. J. Trop. Med. Hyg.* **15**, 269-275.

Gattegno, L. Bladier, D., and Cornillot, P. (1974). The role of sialic acid in the determination of survival of rabbit erythrocytes in the circulation. *Carbohydr. Res.* **34**, 361-369.

Gautam, D. P., Kreier, J. P., and Kreier, R. C. (1970). Antibody coating on erythrocytes of chickens infected with *Plasmodium gallinaceum. Indian J. Med. Res.* **58**, 529-543.

George, J. H., Stokes, E. F., Wicker, D. J., and Conrad, M. E. (1966). Studies of the mechanism of hemolysis in experimental malaria. *Mil. Med.* **131**, 1217–1224.

Gilles, H. M., Lawson, J. B., Sibelas, M., Voller, A., and Allan, N. (1969). Malaria, anemia and pregnancy. *Ann. Trop. Med. Parasitol.* **63**, 245–263.

Gingrich, W. D. (1941). The role of phagocytosis in natural and acquired immunity in avian malaria. *J. Infect. Dis.* **68**, 37–45.

Greenwood, B. M., Muller, A. S., and Valkenburg, H. A. (1971a). Rheumatoid factor in Nigerian sera. *Clin. Exp. Immunol.* **9**, 161–173.

Greenwood, B. M., Brown, J. C., De Jesus, D. G., and Holborow, E. (1971b). Immunosuppression in murine malaria. II. The effect on reticuloendothelial and germinal centre function. *Clin. Exp. Immunol.* **9**, 345–354.

Heidrich, H. G., Rüssman, L., Bayer, B., and Jung, A. (1979). Free-flow electrophoresis for the separation of malaria infected and uninfected mouse erythrocytes and for the isolation of free parasites (*Plasmodium vinckei*): A new rapid technique for the liberation of malaria parasites from their host cells. *Z. Parasitenkd.* **58**, 151–159.

Holz, G. G., Jr. (1977). Lipids and the malarial parasite. *Bull. W. H. O.* **55**, 237–248.

Jandl, J. H., Jacob, H. S., and Daland, G. A. (1961). Hypersplenism due to infection: A study of five cases manifesting hemolytic anemia. *N. Engl. J. Med.* **264**, 1063–1071.

Kahn, R. L. (1949). Universal serologic reaction with lipid antigen. V. In malaria. *Am. J. Clin. Pathol.* **19**, 414–418.

Kahn, R. L., and Baribeau, B. J. (1949). Universal serologic reaction with lipid antigen. II. In animals. *Am. J. Clin. Pathol.* **19**, 361–368.

Kano, K., McGregor, I. A., and Milgrom, F. (1968). Hemagglutinins in sera of Africans of Gambia. *Proc. Soc. Exp. Biol. Med.* **129**, 849–853.

Kay, M. M. B. (1975). Mechanisms of removal of senescent cells by human macrophages *in situ. Proc. Natl. Acad. U.S.A.* **72**, 3521–3525.

Kaye, D., Merselis, J. G., and Hook, E. W. (1965). Influence of *Plasmodium berghei* infection on susceptibility to *Salmonella* infection. *Proc. Soc. Exp. Biol. Med.* **120**, 810–813.

Kilejian, A. (1974). A unique histidine-rich polypeptide from the malaria parasite, *Plasmodium lophurae. J. Biol. Chem.* **249**, 4650–4655.

Kilejian, A. (1976). Does a histidine-rich protein from *Plasmodium lophurae* have a function in merozoite penetration? *J. Protozool.* **23**, 272–277.

Kilejian, A., and Jensen, J. B. (1977). A histidine-rich protein from *Plasmodium falciparium* and its interaction with membranes. *Bull. W. H. O.* **55**, 191–197.

Kitchen, A. G., and DiLuzio, N. R. (1971). Influence of *Plasmodium berghei* infections on phagocytic and humoral recognition factor activity, *RES, J. Reticuloendothel. Soc.* **9**, 237–247.

Kitchen, S. F. (1949). Symptomatology of malaria: General considerations. *In* "Malariology" (M. F. Boyd, ed.), Vol. 2, pp. 966–994. Saunders, Philadelphia, Pennsylvania.

Konigk, E., and Mirtsch, S. (1977). *Plasmodium chabaudi*-infection of mice: Species activities of erythrocyte membrane-associated enzymes and patterns of proteins and glycoproteins of erythrocyte membrane preparations. *Tropenmed. Parasitol.* **28**, 17–22.

Kreier, J. P. (1969). Mechanisms of erythrocyte destruction in chickens infected with *Plasmodium gallinaceum. Mil. Med.* **134**, 1203–1219.

Kreier, J. P., and Leste, J. (1967). Relationship of parasitemia to erythrocyte destruction in *Plasmodium berghei* infected rats. *Exp. Parasitol.* **21**, 78–83.

Kreier, J. P., and Leste, J. (1968). Parasitemia and erythrocyte destruction in *Plasmodium berghei*-infected rats. II. Effect of infected host globulin. *Exp. Parasitol.* **23**, 198–204.

Kreier, J. P., Shapiro, H., Dilly, D., Szilvassy, I. P., and Ristic, M. (1966). Autoimmune reactions in rats with *Plasmodium berghei* infection. *Exp. Parasitol.* **19**, 155–162.

Kreier, J. P., Mohan, R., Seed, T. M., and Pfister, R. M. (1972a). Studies of the morphology and survival characteristics of erythrocytes from mice and rats with *Plasmodium berghei* infection. *Z. Tropenmed. Parasitol.* **23,** 245–255.

Kreier, J. P., Seed, T. M., Mohan, R., and Pfister, R. (1972b). *Plasmodium* sp.: The relationship between erythrocyte morphology and parasitization in chickens, rats, and mice. *Exp. Parasitol.* **31,** 19–28.

Kreier, J. P., Taylor, W. M., and Wagner, W. M. (1972c). Destruction of erythrocytes in monkeys (*Macaca mulatta*) infected with *Plasmodium cynomolgi*. *Am. J. Vet. Res.* **33,** 409–414.

Kretschmar, W. (1969). Anemia in experimental malaria. *Ann. Soc. Belge Med. Trop.* **49,** 253–264.

Ladda, R. L. (1969). New insights into the fine structure of rodent malarial parasites. *Mil. Med.* **134,** 825–865.

Ladda, R. L., Aikawa, M., and Sprinz, H. (1969). Penetration of erythrocytes by merozoites of mammalian and avian malaria parasites. *J. Parasitol.* **55,** 633–644.

Langreth, S. G., and Reese, R. T. (1978). Antigenicity of the infected erythrocyte surface in falciparum malaria. *J. Cell. Biol.* **79,** C1406.

Laser, H. (1948). Hemolytic system in the blood of malaria-infected monkeys. *Nature (London)* **161,** 560.

Laser, H. (1950). The isolation of a hemolytic substance from animal tissue and its biological properties. *J. Physiol. (London)* **110,** 338–355.

Lawrence, C. W., and Cenedella, R. J. (1969). Lipid content of *Plasmodium berghei*-infected rat red blood cells. *Exp. Parasitol.* **26,** 181–186.

Loose, L. A., Cook, J. A., and DiLuzio, N. R. (1972). Malarial immunosuppression—A macrophage mediated defect. *Proc. Helminthol. Soc. Wash.* **39,** 484–491.

McGhee, R. B., and Corwin, R. M. (1964). Bone marrow dycrasia in malarious ducklings. *J. Parasitol.* **50,** 12.

McGregor, I. A. (1971). Immunity to plasmodial infections: Considerations of factors relevant to malaria in man. *Int. Rev. Trop. Med.* **4,** 1–52.

McGregor, I. A. (1974). Mechanisms of acquired immunity and epidemiological patterns of antibody responses in malaria in man. *Bull. W.H.O.* **50,** 259–266.

McGregor, I. A., and Barr, M. (1962). Antibody response to tetanus toxoid inoculation in malarious and non-malarious Gambian children. *Trans. R. Soc. Trop. Med. Hyg.* **36,** 364–367.

McGregor, I. A., Rowe, D. S., Wilson, M. E., and Billewicz, W. Z. (1970). Plasma immunoglobulin concentrations in an African (Gambian) community in relation to season, malaria and other infections and pregnancy. *Clin. Exp. Immunol.* **7,** 51–74.

McLaren, D. J., Bannister, L. H., Trigg, P. I., and Butcher, G. A. (1977). A freeze-fracture study on the parasite-erythrocyte interrelationship in *Plasmodium knowlesi* infections. *Bull. W.H.O.* **55,** 100–203.

Maegraith, B. G. (1946). Blackwater fever—Modern theories: A critical review. *Trop. Dis. Bull.* **43,** 801–809.

Marikovsky, Y., and Danon, D. (1967). Structural differences between old and young negatively stained red cell membranes. *J. Ultrastruct. Res.* **20,** 83–90.

Mason, J. J., Miller, L. H., Shiroishi, T., Dvorak, J. A., and McGinniss, M. H. (1977). The Duffy blood group determinants: Their role in the susceptibility of human and animal erythrocytes to *Plasmodium knowlesi* malaria. *Br. J. Haematol.* **36,** 327–335.

Mazen, L., Gull, K., and Gutteridge, W. E. (1975). A freeze-fracture study of the host/parasite interface of the malarial parasite, *Plasmodium chabaudi*. *J. Protozool.* **22,** 54a (abstr. 156).

Miller, L. H. (1977). Hypothesis on the mechanism of erythrocyte invasion by malaria merozoites. *Bull. W.H.O.* **55,** 157–162.

Miller, L. H., Fremount, H. N., and Luse, S. A. (1971). Deep vascular schizogony of *Plasmodium knowlesi* in *Macaca mulatta*. *Am. J. Trop. Med. Hyg.* **20,** 816–824.

Miller, L. H., Chien, S., and Usami, S. (1972). Decreased deformability of *Plasmodium coatneyi*-infected red cells and its possible relation to cerebral malaria. *Am. J. Trop. Med. Hyg.* **21,** 133–137.

Miller, L. H., Aikawa, M., Johnson, J. G., and Shiroishi, T. (1979). Interaction between cytochalasin B-treated malaria parasites and erythrocytes. *J. Exp. Med.* **149,** 172–184.

Mohandas, N., Phillips, W. M., and Bessis, M. (1979). Red blood cell deformability and hemolytic anemias. *Semin. Hematol.* 16, 95–114.

Motulsky, A. G. F., Casserd, E. R., Giblett, G. D., Brown, S. R., and Finch, C. A. (1958). Anemia and the spleen. *N. Engl. J. Med.* **259,** 1164–1169.

Murphy, J. (1967). The influence of pH and temperature on some physical properties of normal erythrocytes and erythrocytes from patients with hereditary spherocytosis. *J. Lab. Clin. Med.* **69,** 758–775.

Neva, F., Sheagren, J. N., Shulman, N. R., and Canfield, C. J. (1970). Malaria: Host-defense mechanism and complications. *Ann. Intern. Med.* **73,** 295–306.

Nicolson, G. L. (1973). Anionic sites of human erythrocyte membranes. I. Effects of trypsin, phosphilipase C and pH on the topography of bound positively charged colloidal particles. *J. Cell Biol.* **57,** 373–387.

Nicolson, G. L. (1976). Transmembrane control of the receptors on normal and tumor cells. I. Cytoplasmic influence over cell surface components. *Biochim. Biophys. Acta* **457,** 57–108.

Nirady, K. (1969). The electrophoretic mobilities of erythrocytes of malaria-infected chickens. M.Sc. Thesis, Ohio State University, Columbus.

O'Leary, D. S., Barr, C. F., Wellde, B. J., and Conrad, M. E. (1972). Experimental infection with *Plasmodium falciparum* in *Aotus* monkeys. III. The development of disseminated intravascular coagulation. *Am. J. Trop. Med. Hyg.* **21,** 282–287.

Palecek, F. M., Palecekova, M., and Aviado, D. M. (1967). Pathologic physiology and chemotherapy of *Plasmodium berghei*. II. Oxyhemoglobin dissociation curve in resistant strains. *Exp. Parasitol.* **21,** 16–30.

Pinta da Silva, P., and Nicolson, G. C. (1974). Freeze-etch localization of concanavalin A receptors to the membrane intercalated particles of human erythrocyte ghost membranes. *Biochim. Biophys. Acta* **363,** 311–319.

Prankerd, J. A. J. (1961). "The Red Cell." Blackwell, Oxford.

Rao, K. N., Subrahmanyam, D., and Prakash, S. (1970). *Plasmodium berghei:* Lipids of rat red blood cells. *Exp. Parasitol.* **27,** 22–27.

Redmond, W. B. (1948). The electric charge of red blood cells in malaria. *Science* **107,** 199–200.

Rigdon, R., and Rostorfer, H. H. (1946). Blood oxygen in ducks with malaria. *J. Natl. Malar. Soc.* **5,** 253–262.

Reinhart, J. J., Balcerzak, S. P., and LoBuglio, A. F. (1971). Study of the malarial parasite-red cell relationship with use of a new immunological marker. *J. Lab. Clin. Med.* **78,** 167–171.

Rock, R. C., Standefer, J., and Little, W. (1971). Incorporation of ^{32}P-orthophosphate into membrane phospholipids of *Plasmodium knowlesi* and host erythrocytes of *Macaca mulatta*. *Comp. Biochem. Physiol. B* **40,** 543–561.

Rosenberg, E. B., Strickland, G. T., Yang, S., and Whelan, G. E. (1973). IgM antibodies to red cells and autoimmune anemia in patients with malaria. *Am. J. Trop. Med. Hyg.* **22,** 146–152.

Salaman, M. H., Wedderburn, N., and Bruce-Chwatt, E. J. (1969). The immune depressive effect of a murine plasmodium and its interaction with murine oncogenic viruses. *J. Gen. Microbiol.* **59,** 383–391.

Schachter, S. W. (1968). Survival of ^{51}Cr-labeled erythrocytes tranfused from *Plasmodium gallinaceum*-infected inbred chickens to drug treated inbred chickens. M.Sc. Thesis, Ohio State University, Columbus.

Schnitzer, B., Sodeman, T. M., Mead, M. L., and Contacos, P. G. (1973). An ultrastructural study of the red pulp of the spleen in malaria. *Blood* **41,** 207–218.

Seed, T. M. (1969). Autoimmune reaction in chickens with *Plasmodium gallinaceum* infection: The isolation and characterization of a lipid from trypsinized erythrocytes which reacts with serum from acutely infected chickens. M.Sc. Thesis, Ohio State University, Columbus.

Seed, T. M. (1972). Erythrocyte membrane alterations and associated plasma changes induced by *Plasmodium gallinaceum* infection. Ph.D. Thesis, Ohio State University, Columbus.

Seed, T. M., and Kreier, J. P. (1969). Autoimmune reaction in chickens with *Plasmodium gallinaceum* infection: The isolation and characterization of a lipid from trypsinized erythrocytes which reacts with serum from acutely infected chickens. *Mil. Med.* **134**, 1220–1227.

Seed, T. M., and Kreier, J. P. (1972). *Plasmodium gallinaceum:* Erythrocyte membrane alterations and associated plasma changes induced by experimental infections. *Proc. Soc. Helminthol. Wash.* **39**, 387–411.

Seed, T. M., and Kreier, J. P. (1977). Macrophage mediated red cell destruction during experimental malaria. *58th Conf. Res. Workers Anim. Dis.* Abstract No. 168.

Seed, T. M., and Manwell, R. D. (1977). Plasmodia of birds. *In* "Parasitic Protozoa" (J. P. Kreier, ed.), pp. 311–357. Academic Press, New York.

Seed, T. M., Pfister, R. M., Kreier, J., and Johnson, A. (1971). *Plasmodium* gallinaceum: Fine structure by freeze-etch technique. *Exp. Parasitol.* **30**, 73–81.

Seed, T. M., Aikawa, M., Prior, R. B., Kreier, J. P., and Pfister, R. M. (1973). *Plasmodium* sp.: Topography of intra- and extracellular parasites. *Z. Tropenmed. Parasitol.* **24**, 525–535.

Seed, T. M., Aikawa, M., Sterling, C. R., and Rabbege, J. R. (1974). Surface properties of extracellular malaria parasites: Morphological and cytochemical study. *Infect. Immun.* **9**, 750–761.

Seed, T. M., Brindley, D., Aikawa, M., and Rabbege, J. R. (1976a). *Plasmodium berghei:* Osmotic fragility of malaria parasites and mouse host erythrocytes. *Exp. Parasitol.* **40**, 380–390.

Seed, T. M., Sterling, C. R., Aikawa, M., and Rabbege, J. R. (1976b). *Plasmodium simium:* Ultrastructure of erythrocytic phase. *Exp. Parasitol.* **39**, 262–276.

Segrest, J. P., Kahne, I., Jackson, R. L., and Marchesi, V. T. (1973). Major glycoprotein of the human erythrocyte membrane: Evidence for an amphipathic molecular structure. *Arch. Biochem. Biophys.* **155**, 167–183.

Sengers, R. C. A. (1971). Immunosuppression in malaria. *Lancet* **1**, 594.

Sheagren, J. M., Tobie, J. E., Fox, L. M., and Wolff, S. M. (1970). Reticuloendothelial system phagocytic function in naturally acquired human malaria. *J. Lab. Clin. Med.* **75**, 481–487.

Skutelsky, E., and Danon, D. (1969). Reduction in surface charge as an explanation of the recognition by macrophages of nuclei expelled from normoblasts. *J. Cell Biol.* **43**, 8–15.

Sterling, C. R., Aikawa, M., and Nussenzweig, R. (1972). Morphological divergence in mammalian malarial parasites: The fine structure of *Plasmodium brasilianum. Proc. Helminthol. Soc. Wash.* **39**, 109–129.

Sterling, C. R., Seed, T. M., Aikawa, M., and Rabbege, J. R. (1975). Erythrocyte membrane alterations induced by *Plasmodium simium* in *Saimiri sciureus:* Relation to Schüffner dots. *J. Parasitol.* **61**, 117–188.

Stohlman, F., Contacos, P. G., and Kavin, S. F. (1963). The abnormal life span of the red blood cell. *J. Am. Med. Assoc.* **184**, 1020–1021.

Swann, A. I., and Kreier, J. P. (1973). *Plasmodium gallinaceum:* Mechanisms of anemia in infected chickens. *Exp. Parasitol.* **33**, 79–88.

Szilvassy, I. P., Kreier, J. P., and Ristic, M. (1969). Autoimmune reactions of chickens infected by *Plasmodium gallinaceum. Avian Dis.* **13**, 528–534.

Taliaferro, W. H., and Cannon, P. R. (1936). The cellular reactions during primary infection and superinfections of *Plasmodium brasilianum* in Panamanian monkeys. *J. Infect. Dis.* **59**, 72–125.

Taliaferro, W. H., and Mulligan, H. W. (1937). The histopathology of malaria with special reference to the function and role of the macrophages in defense. *Indian Med. Res. Mem.* **29**, 1.

Taliaferro, W. H., and Taliaferro, L. G. (1948). Reduction in immunity in chicken malaria following treatment with nitrogen mustard. *J. Infect. Dis.* **82**, 5–30.

Teitel, P. (1977). Basic principles of the filterability test (Ft) and analysis of erythrocytic flow behavior. *Blood Cells* **3**, 55–70.

Temsuk, P. (1969). The electrophoretic mobility of the red blood cells of rats infected with *Plasmodium berghei*. M.Sc. Thesis, Ohio State University, Columbus.

Topley, E., Knight, R., and Woodruff, A. W. (1973). The direct antiglobulin test and immunoconglutinin titers in patients with malaria. *Trans. R. Soc. Trop. Med. Hyg.* **67**, 51–54.

Trigg, R. I., Hirst, S. I., Shakespeare, P. G., and Tappenden, L. (1977). Labelling of membrane and glycoprotein in erythrocytes infected with *Plasmodium knowlesi*. *Bull. W.H.O.* **55**, 205–209.

Voller, A. (1974). Immunopathology of malaria. *Bull. W.H.O.* **50**, 177–186.

Wallach, D. F., and Conley, M. (1977). Altered membrane proteins of monkey erythrocytes infected with simium malaria. *J. Mol. Med.* **2**, 119–136.

Weed, R. I., and Weiss, L. (1966). The relationship between red cell fragmentation occurring within the spleen and cell destruction. *Trans. Assoc. Am. Physicians* **79**, 426–438.

Weidekamm, E., Wallach, D. F., and Lin, P. S. (1973). Erythrocyte membrane alterations due to infection with *Plasmodium berghei*. *Biochim. Biophys. Acta* **323**, 539–546.

Weiss, L. (1974). A scanning electron microscopic study of the spleen. *Blood* **43**, 665–691.

Weiss, L., and Tavassoli, M. (1970). Anatomical hazards to the passage of erythrocytes through the spleen. *Semin. Hematol.* **7**, 372–380.

Wells, J. V. (1970). Immunological studies in tropical splenomegaly syndrome. *Trans. R. Soc. Trop. Med. Hyg.* **64**, 531–546.

Wright, R. H., and Kreier, J. P. (1969). *Plasmodium gallinaceum:* Chicken erythrocyte survival as determined by sodium radiochromate[51] and di-isopropyl-fluorophosphate[32] labeling. *Exp. Parasitol.* **25**, 339–352.

Zuckerman, A. (1946). *In vitro* opsonic tests with *Plasmodium gallinaceum* and *Plasmodium lophurae*. *J. Infect. Dis.* **77**, 28–59.

Zuckerman, A. (1957). Blood loss and replacement in plasmodial infections. I. *Plasmodium berghei* in untreated rats of varying ages and in adult rats with erythropoietic mechanisms manipulated before inoculation. *J. Infect. Dis.* **100**, 172–206.

Zuckerman, A. (1958). Blood loss and replacement in plasmodial infections. II. *Plasmodium vinckei* in untreated weanling and mature rats. *J. Infect. Dis.* **103**, 205–224.

Zuckerman, A. (1960a). Blood loss and replacement in plasmodial infections. III. *Plasmodium cynomolgi, Plasmodium gonderi,* and *Plasmodium knowlesi* in *Macaca mulatta mulatta,* the rhesus monkey. *J. Infect. Dis.* **106**, 123–140.

Zuckerman, A. (1960b). Blood loss and replacement in plasmodial infections. IV. *Plasmodium gallinaceum* and *Plasmodium lophurae* in untreated and prebled mature chickens and in untreated chicks. *J. Infect. Dis.* **107**, 137–148.

Zuckerman, A. (1960c). Autoantibody in rats with *Plasmodium berghei*. *Nature (London)* **185**, 189–190.

Zuckerman, A. (1964). Autoimmunization and other types of indirect damage to host cells as factors in certain protozoan diseases. *Exp. Parasitol.* **15**, 138–183.

Zuckerman, A. (1966). Recent studies on factors involved in malarial anemia. *Mil. Med.* **131**, 1201–1216.

Zuckerman, A. (1969). Current status of the immunology of malaria and of the antigenic analysis of plasmodia: A five-year review. *Bull. W.H.O.* **40**, 55–66.

Zuckerman, A. (1974). Functional aspects of immunity in malaria rats. *In* "Basic Research on Malaria" (J. N. Bateman, eds.), Tech rep. Eur Res. Office-5-74, pp. 87–96, European Research Office and Chelsea College, London.

Zuckerman, A. (1977). Current status of the immunology of blood and tissue protozoa. II. Plasmodium (a review). *Exp. Parasitol.* **42,** 374–446.

Zuckerman, A., and Spira, D. (1961). Blood loss and replacement in plasmodial infections. V. Positive antiglobulin tests in rat anemias due to the rodent malarias *Plasmodium berghei* and *Plasmodium vinckei,* to cardiac bleeding, and to treatment with phenylhydrazine hydrochloride. *J. Infect. Dis.* **108,** 339–448.

Zuckerman, A., Abzug, S., and Burg, R. (1969). Anemia in rats with equivalent splenomegalies induced by methyl cellulose and *Plasmodium berghei. Mil. Med.* **134,** 1084–1099.

Zuckerman, A., Spira, D. T., and Ron, H. (1973). A quantitative study of phagocytosis in the spleen of rats infected with *Plasmodium berghei. In* "Dynamic Aspects of Host-Parasite Relationships" (A. Zuckerman and D. W. Weiss, eds.), Vol. 1, pp. 79–115. Academic Press, New York.

Pathology of Malaria

Masamichi Aikawa, Mamoru Suzuki, and Yezid Gutierrez

I. INTRODUCTION

Even before the discovery of the causative agent, *Plasmodium*, the presence of a characteristic brownish pigment in the spleen, liver, and brain was noted by most pathologists who conducted necropsies on people who had died of malaria. In 1847, Meckel pointed out that the brownish condition of the organs was caused by the accumulation of pigment removed from the blood and, later, Frerichs and Virchow confirmed this observation. This finding was of importance because it was the starting point of Laveran's research leading to the discovery of plasmodial parasites.

There have been many reviews of malaria pathology in the past, such as those by Thayer (1897), Marchiafava and Bignami (1900), Mannaberg (1905), Craig (1909), Marchoux (1926), Taliaferro and Mulligan (1937), and Maegraith (1966). These reviews contain detailed descriptions of the gross and microscopic changes produced by malarial parasites in humans. In recent years, new knowledge has accumulated in many fields of medicine because of the use of modern techniques such as electron microscopy and immunofluorescence microscopy. This new knowledge has increased the understanding of many disease processes including some aspects of malaria. Moreover, the successful infection of nonhuman primates by human malarial parasites has recently been accomplished, allowing studies of the morphological or immunological changes which may occur at any stage of infection.

Pathological changes in malaria result primarily from the infection of erythrocytes by *Plasmodium* and from the host's response. To understand these changes three factors contributing to the development of pathological lesions in various organs must be considered: (1) parasitemia, (2) destruction of damaged erythrocytes, and (3) the defense response of the host against the infection, including phagocytosis and the development of immunity. Malarial parasites invading erythrocytes initiate the pathological process, and the consequences of this infection influence the host's other tissues and organs. Destruction of host red blood cells occurs not only when plasmodia rupture the erythrocytes at the end of schizogony, but also through phagocytosis of infected and noninfected erythrocytes. The destruction of erythrocytes can result in some degree of anemia and contribute to anoxia. However, profound tissue anoxia resulting in shock and death occurs in infections such as *Plasmodium falciparum* as a result of capillary blockage due to sequestration of infected erythrocytes in the capillary bed.

The mechanisms of the host's defense against plasmodial parasites are not well understood, but there is a resistance to the consequences of infection in endemic populations which can exhibit high parasitemias without apparent ill effects. The development of immunity affects both parasites and host tissues. The parasites are killed more rapidly, and in the host there is hyperplasia of the reticuloendothelial system with stimulation of its phagocytic properites, especially in the spleen, liver, and bone marrow. The differences between pathological and physiological changes, such as those associated with the immune responses, are difficult to recognize. Conventionally, the morphological changes occurring during malarial infection have been described by pathologists, but attempts to correlate these changes with modern pathophysiological concepts of disease have not been made. In this chapter the prominent organ changes associated with *Plasmodium* infection will be described, and some of the physiopathological mechanisms involved will be presented.

II. SPLEEN PATHOLOGY

The spleen is the organ which shows the earliest changes in individuals with malaria. Spleen enlargement is a well-known physical sign of infection (Fig. 1), and its increase rate in human populations was used for the evaluation of malaria

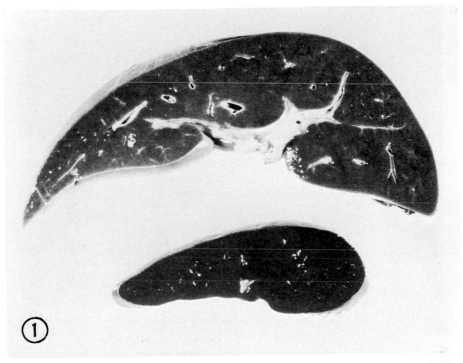

FIG. 1. Enlarged, dark liver and spleen characteristic of malaria. (Courtesy of D. Connor, AFIP #66-6163-1.)

prevalence within a region (Boyd, 1949). Changes in the spleen size in experimental nonhuman primates with malaria were evaluated by Coggeshall (1937) who demonstrated that *Macaca rhesus* infected with *P. knowlesi* and dying from 3 to 7 days after infection showed an average 57% organ size increase. If infections lasted longer because of treatment, the increase was 91%. In *P. inui*, a low-grade monkey pathogen, chronic infection in the rhesus produced an average spleen size increase of 171%.

Recently, Jervis *et al.* (1972), working with *P. falciparum*-infected *Aotus*, found the spleens of infected monkeys to be larger and heavier than those of uninfected control monkeys. Animals killed 2 weeks after the infection had larger spleens than monkeys killed earlier, but there was a poor correlation between infection time and spleen size. Variations were interpreted as being the result of several factors, such as cellular responses associated with acquired immunity, and degree of cullular destruction and hyperplasia.

On postmortem examination the spleen in patients who have died of acute malaria is dark red to chocolate color as a result of congestion and accumulation of malarial pigment (Fig. 2). The pulp's consistency is soft and friable, and the

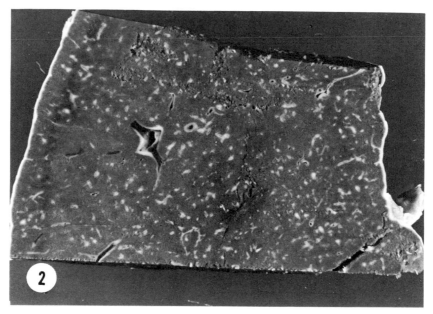

FIG. 2.   Dark spleen from a patient with *P. falciparum* infection. (Courtesy of D. Connor, AFIP #66-6870.)

spleen is easily ruptured. Microscopically, the white and red pulps show hyperplasia and hyperemia (Fig. 3). The sinuoids are dilated with numerous red blood cells, many of which have parasites in various stages of development. White pulp hyperplasia is due to the proliferation of endothelial cells, macrophages, and lymphoid elements which show many mitoses and large, immature cells. Neutrophil infiltration is abundant, especially in areas of necrosis (Taliaferro and Mulligan, 1937). Splenic hyperemia is severe, and it occurs in animals with high parasitemias during the first week of infection. Pigment is seen in macrophages, polymorphonuclear leukocytes, and parasitized red blood cells, and its presence is the histopathological hallmark of the infection (Fig. 4).

Following the changes which occur during acute infection there is a decrease in hyperemia and, as the infection becomes established, the white pulp may be markedly depleted in the chronic phase. Proliferative or hyperplastic changes take place in animals with malaria, although degenerative changes have been more commonly described. In chronic malaria the color of the organ becomes darker in proportion to the duration of the infection as a result of an increase in pigment present in the tissue. The spleen becomes firm, because hyperemia is less evident; the fibrous tissue of the trabeculae, follicles, and capsule are increased, and the reticuloendothelial system shows marked proliferation. In long-lasting infections, these changes are more pronounced, with diminution of the follicles,

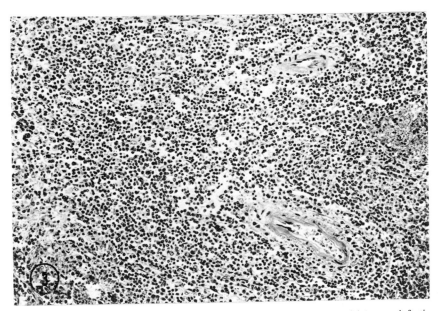

FIG. 3. Hyperplastic white pulp of the spleen from a patient with *P. falciparum* infection. ×150. (Tissue was supplied by V. Boonpucknavig.)

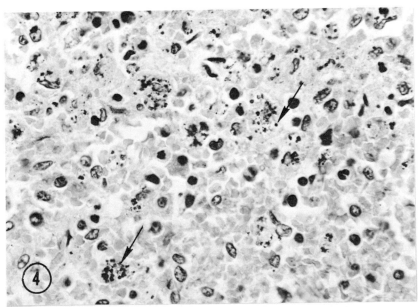

FIG. 4. Pigment (arrows) in macrophages and leukocytes of the spleen from a *P. falciparum*-infected patient. ×600. (Tissue was supplied by V. Boonpucknavig.)

and the pulp loses its normal character. Proliferative changes in the spleen are particularly prominent in humans, rodents, and some nonhuman primates, but in *Aotus* experimentally infected with *P. falciparum* the reticuloendothelial system is only moderately changed (Jervis *et al.*, 1972). The amount of neutrophil infiltration in the spleen is decreased, and neutrophils present are diffusely scattered throughout the spleen.

The degree of accumulation of malarial pigment in the spleen's phagocytic cells is directly proportional to both the parasitemia and the duration of the infection. Phagocytized pigment can be found in cells of the monocyte-macrophage series, neutrophils, and parasitized red blood cells, with pigment particles varying considerably in size and shape. The pigment occurs in small, discrete masses during the early acute stages of infection, while in animals with long-standing infections it is seen in clumps and large masses. If the infection is cured, the pigment will be processed by the host and will disappear ultimately, but it can be seen for at least 1 year. The malarial pigment, the altered and parasitized red blood cells, and the parasites stimulate the reticuloendothelial system throughout the body, with resultant marked hyperplasia and increased activity which in turn speeds up the rate of erythrocyte destruction by the spleen, leading to profound hemolysis. It is well known that after splenectomy of animals with experimentally induced malaria there is an increase in the parasitemia.

The presence of hemorrhagic areas in the splenic pulp has been attributed to partial or complete circulatory obstruction by thrombosis. The thrombosis is observed in the arterioles and capillaries of the spleen and can be due to both destruction of erythrocytes and sequestration of infected red blood cells in patients with *P. falciparum* infections. These thrombi cause hemorrhage, necroses, and infarctions. Schnitzer *et al.* (1973) reported that in the spleen of *M. mulatta* infected with *P. knowlesi* there was electron microscopic evidence of "pitting" of the portion of erythrocytes containing malarial parasites (Fig. 5). Cordal macrophages pit the parasite from the infected red blood cell, and this phenomenon may explain the presence of nonparasitized spherocytes in peripheral blood, as well as the discrepancy between the degree of hemolysis and the number of parasitized erythrocytes. Quinn and Wyler (1979) investigated the clearance of ^{51}Cr-labeled *P. berghei*-infected erythrocytes in rats in order to study the removal of parasitized erythrocytes by the spleen. Infected erythrocytes were removed more rapidly from the circulation than uninfected erythrocytes. The accelerated clearance appeared to result from greater splenic uptake in immune rats and to correlate with spleen size. They suggested that rheological alterations of parasitized erythrocytes might be more important determinants of clearance than antibody-dependent processes.

The anemia seen in malarial infections of humans and animals can sometimes be profound, and extramedullary erythropoiesis is often seen in the spleen.

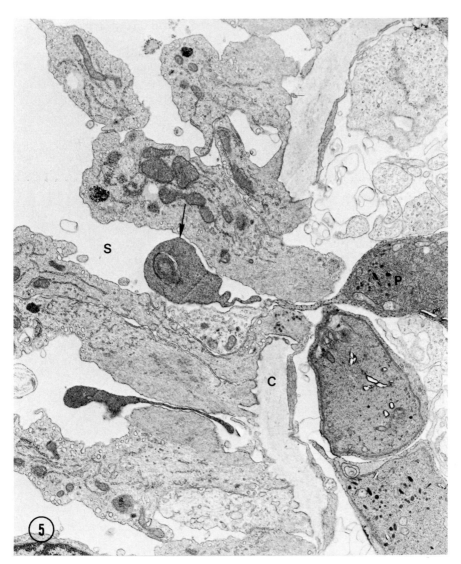

FIG. 5. Electron micrograph of the spleen of a rhesus monkey infected with *P. knowlesi*. A severed red cell, one part (arrow) having passed into a sinus (S) and the parasitized part (P) remaining trapped in cord (C) is seen. ×11,700. (Reproduced from Schnitzer, *et al.*, 1973, by permission of the author and publisher.)

Singer (1954) found that after the seventh day of *P. berghei* infection the chief activity of the spleen of mice was erythropoiesis.

The tropical splenomegaly syndrome (Pitney, 1968) may be a most important consequence of malaria. It occurs when malaria is endemic, and several lines of work have suggested a causal relationship between the malarial infection and the syndrome. Its incidence has decreased in endemic areas where massive chemoprophylaxis has been carried out. Moreoever, it is suggested that in Uganda 45% of patients with the tropical splenomegaly syndrome have been infected with *P. malariae*, a species capable of producing long-lasting infection in humans (Marsden *et al.*, 1965). However, similar studies in New Guinea failed to reveal an association between *P. malariae* infection and the tropical splenomegaly syndrome (Marsden *et al.*, 1967).

III. LIVER PATHOLOGY

Hepatomegaly is a common sign of malaria infection in humans, though variable in experimental animals (Fig. 1). Jervis *et al.* (1972) found that in *P. falciparum*-infected *Aotus* neither the wet nor the dry weight of the liver was significantly altered. However, the wet weight in experimental animals with *P. berghei* increased, while the dry weight remained unchanged, indicating that the increase was due to edema (Jervis *et al.*, 1968). *Plasmodium cathemerium* produces a marked liver enlargement in canaries, especially at the crisis and shortly thereafter (Taliaferro and Mulligan, 1937). Another significant liver abnormality is a progressive change in color from pink tan to dark brown. When the infection is prolonged, the liver becomes black, and this color is attributed to the deposition of the malarial pigment in the reticuloendothelial cells. In individuals with acute malaria, the organ becomes extremely friable and easily torn. In chronic infections the consistency of the liver is definitely increased, the color is dark, and the hepatic lobules are accentuated by the presence of pigment concentrated in large clumps in the portal areas (Fig. 6).

Light microscopy shows changes mainly involving the reticuloendothelial system. During the early infection, the perilobular Kupffer cells start to hypertrophy, and active phagocytosis of pigment and infected erythrocytes occurs (Figs. 7 and 8). As the infection progresses, midzonal and central lobular Kupffer cells hypertrophy. This distribution has been correlated in a human with the blood flow. MacCallum (1969a) has reported that the order of response of intrahepatic macrophages in guinea pigs infected with *P. berghei* is also a function of their spatial relationship to the portal blood flow. However, Maegraith (1954), working with the same parasite in rats, reported an initial midzonal activation of Kupffer cells. It is generally accepted that the endothelial cells lining the liver sinusoids are also phagocytic in nature and that they can transform into Kupffer

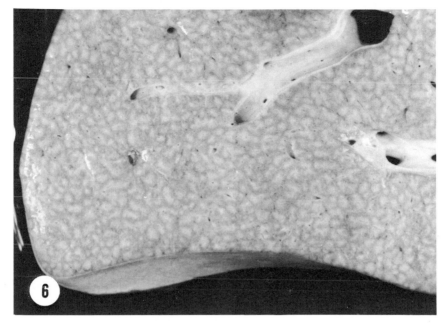

FIG. 6. Liver from a patient with chronic malaria. Malarial pigment accumulates in the portal areas in chronic malaria, accentuating the lobular architecture. (Courtesy of D. Connor, AFIP #69-3609.)

cells (Aikawa *et al.*, 1968). These transformed endothelial cells divide rapidly to increase the number of macrophages. Moreover, the macrophages containing pigment enter the sinusoids with the portal blood. There is an influx of splenic macrophages via the splenic vein. All these factors increase the number of phagocytic cells in the liver and their distribution within the lobule.

The sinusoidal spaces also contain parasitized red blood cells varying in amount in accordance with the parasite species. In *P. falciparum* of humans and experimental monkeys (Jervis *et al.*, 1972; Gutierrez *et al.*, 1976), large numbers of parasitized red cells are present, attached to the endothelial cells. The same phenomenon occurs in nonhuman primates infected with *P. knowlesi*. The increased number of cells in the sinusoids causes sluggish circulation in the organ, with resultant congestion and central necrosis due to portal hypertension. There are other factors in addition to attached parasitized erythrocytes which could affect the circulation through the liver. Skirrow *et al.* (1964) found that in monkeys with terminal *P. knowlesi* malaria there was marked constriction of the portal vein and its branches. This constriction is relieved by sympatholytic drugs, and liver necrosis can be definitely prevented if sympathectomy is performed before infection (Ray and Sharma, 1958). Finally, ultrastructural changes have been described in the sinusoidal endothelial cell lining in *P. falciparum*-infected

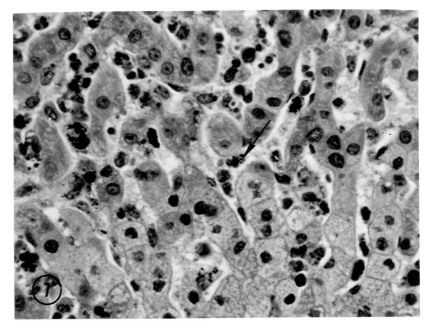

FIG. 7. Liver from an *Aotus* monkey with *P. falciparum* infection. Malarial pigment (arrow) is seen in the Kupffer cells and macrophages. (Courtesy of H. Jervis.)

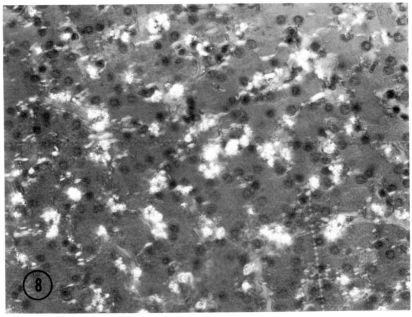

FIG. 8. Birefringent malarial pigment in the liver under polarized light. (Courtesy of D. Connor, AFIP #66-1426-2.)

Aotus, and these changes may alter permeability as well as circulation (Gutierrez *et al.,* 1976).

In animals in the acute phase of malaria, the malarial pigment is dispersed, as small globules and dividing macrophages are frequently observed. Later in the infection, the amount of ingested malarial pigment is increased, pigment becomes clumped, and phagocytes become rounded instead of elongated or stellate and are found lying free within the sinusoids. The nuclei of the phagocytes become irregular, and prominent nucleoli develop. As the disease progresses, the amount of pigment within the phagocytic Kupffer cells increases, and it clumps into even larger masses (Taliaferro and Mulligan, 1937).

Malarial pigment is an end product of the digestion of hemoglobin by the parasite. The pigment is a ferric ion containing porphyrin conjugated with a protein moiety derived from partial proteolysis of the globin portion of hemoglobin. The amino acid composition of this moiety varies in different batches of pigment. Although earlier investigators thought that pigment was toxic to the host and could produce cell changes, it is now regarded as inert. Clumping of malarial pigment can be produced by treatment with various drugs including sulfadiazine, pyrimethamine, chloroquine, and piperazine. Pigment-laden macrophages aggregate within the sinusoids, and eventually the macrophage cell membranes fuse, resulting in the formation of giant cells.

There is another pigment in animals with malaria—hemosiderin, produced as a result of red blood cell lysis. It is a yellow pigment seen in many other conditions where red blood cell destruction takes place. It is found in small granules in the central portion of the lobule, and its concentration diminishes toward the periphery. Hemosiderin is contained both in macrophages and hepatocytes. It is differentiated from malarial pigment because it does not give the prussian blue reaction.

Electron microscopy has shown that the Kupffer cells are vacuolated and contain electron-dense cytoplasmic bodies, large phagolysosomes containing infected erythrocytes (Figs. 9 and 10), and malarial pigment particles (Aikawa and Antonovych, 1964). There is no apparent digestion of the pigment particles, but digested parasitized red blood cells and acid phosphatase activity have been demonstrated in the phagolysosomes (Aikawa *et al.,* 1968).

The ultrastructural appearance of the pigment particles differs with the species. In animals with mammalian malaria it has a characteristic rectangular crystalloid shape, while in animals with avian and reptilian malaria it appears as a uniformly electron-dense material (Aikawa, 1971).

Electron microscopic studies of *P. falciparum*-infected *Aotus* show a direct relationship between the number of parasitized erythrocytes and liver changes. In heavily infected animals, there are structural alterations and a marked diminuation of hepatocyte mitochondria. The mitochondria become swollen, the cristae disappear, and the mitochondria matrix is replaced by an amorphous, electron-

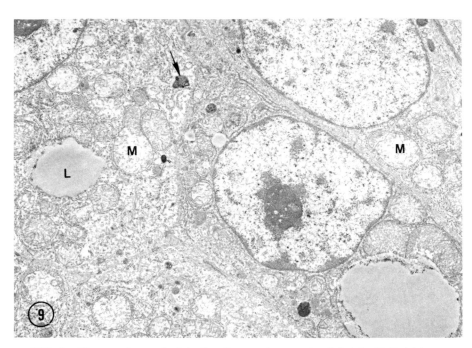

FIG. 9.   Electron micrograph of the liver from an *Aotus* monkey infected with *P. falciparum*. Note swelling and disorganization of mitochondria (M), lipid droplets (L), and lysosomes with malarial pigment (arrow). ×6500. (Reproduced from Gutierrez *et al.*, 1976, by permission of the author and publisher.)

dense, granular material (Fig. 9) (Gutierrez *et al.*, 1976). Structural changes in liver mitochondria of mice infected with *P. berghei* have been correlated with biochemical changes such as abnormal respiration and oxidative phosphorylation (Riley and Deegan, 1960; Riley and Maegraith, 1962). However, mitochondria from monkeys infected with *P. knowlesi* appear biochemically normal (Maegraith *et al.*, 1962), suggesting that rodent and monkey malaria have different pathophysiological mechanisms. Biochemical alterations in mitochondria are difficult to explain pathophysiologically. Animals with *P. knowlesi* and *P. berghei* infections have in their sera substances capable of producing biochemical disturbances in liver function *in vitro* (Riley and Maegraith, 1961; Maegraith *et al.*, 1963). Both the ultrastructural and the biochemical changes in the liver mitochondria in animals with experimental malaria infections are thought to be initiated by the parasite's erythrocytic phase directly or through mediators released into the animal's serum (Maegraith, 1966). Tissue anoxia produced either by an inadequate oxygen supply or by the cell's inability to use oxygen is the principal cause of shock and eventual death in animals and humans with malaria. The mitochondrial ultrastructural changes are a nonspecific response to various

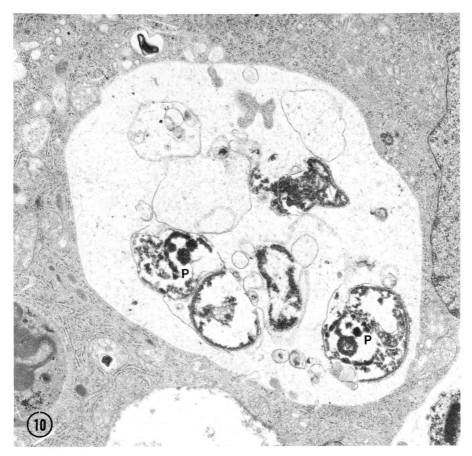

FIG. 10. Electron micrograph of Kupffer cells from a chicken infected with *P. gallinaceum* showing degenerating parasites (P) in a vacuole. ×22,000. (Reproduced from Aikawa *et al.*, 1968, by permission of the author and publisher.)

insults resulting in shock and eventually in death; however, it is not known which is the mechanism that initiates these changes in animals with experimental malaria.

The hepatocyte shows changes during malaria, also. The amount of fat augments and, as the infection progresses, there is a slight increase in the number of iron-containing granules. There is also glycogen loss. Bile canaliculi of monkey livers infected with *P. falciparum* show increases in alkaline phosphatase activity, but the increase is nonspecific since it may be observed in animals of several species subjected to various types of stress. Ultrastructurally, the hepatocytes in *Aotus* and humans infected with *P. falciparum* are swollen, with a loss of microvilli both in the space of Disse and in the bile canaliculi. Cytoplasmic

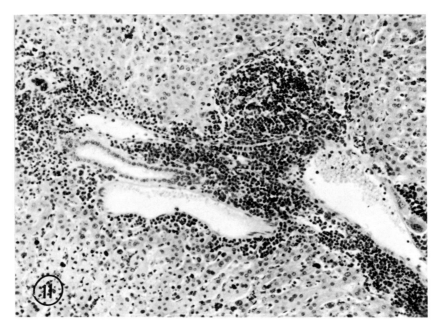

FIG. 11.   The liver of an *Aotus* monkey infected with *P. falciparum* showing cellular infiltration in the portal areas. ×150. (Courtesy of H. Jervis.)

glycogen is first depleted and disappears later, beginning in the central portion of the lobule, but the significance of these changes is not well understood (Jervis *et al.*, 1968). De Brito *et al.* (1969) speculated that alterations in bile canaliculi microvilli could be responsible for the hyperbilirubinemic state of some of his patients. Interestingly, in the six cases reported by de Brito *et al.* (1969) one had *P. falciparum* for 13 days and the rest had *P. vivax* for from days to months. Yet, the ultrastructural hepatocyte lesions were very similar. Bhamarapravati *et al.* (1973) attributed jaundice in malaria patients to impairment in bilirubin transport, either because of reticuloendothelial cell blockage or disturbance of the hepatocyte microvilli.

Finally, the liver shows cellular infiltration by lymphocytes and granulocytes of the portal triads (Fig. 11). Small nests of erythropoietic, granulocytopoietic, and megakaryopoietic cells can be seen within the liver sinusoids when there is severe anemia.

IV. HEART AND VASCULAR PATHOLOGY

There are no striking gross changes in the heart of patients dying of malaria. Microscopically (Fig. 12) there is fatty degeneration, focal fragmentation, and

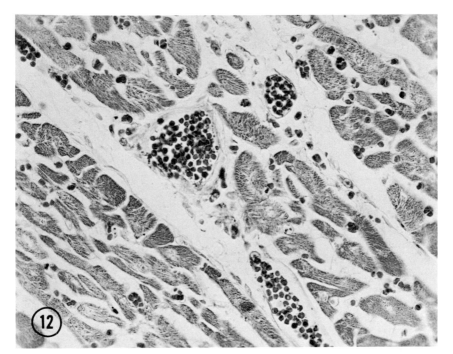

FIG. 12. Section of the heart from a patient with *P. falciparum* infection. The interstices are edematous and are infiltrated with mononuclear cells. The capillaries contain parasitized erythrocytes. ×200. (Courtesy of D. Connor, AFIP #69-1051.)

necrosis of the cardiac muscle due to capillary blockage by parasitized erythrocytes, especially in *P. falciparum* infection.

Ultrastructural changes in the heart have been studied recently in *Aotus* with experimental *P. falciparum* infections (Fig. 13). There is lipid droplet infiltration of muscle cells, usually next to the mitochondria. Mitochondria are swollen with loss of detail in the cristae, and the cardiac muscle is disorganized with fragmentation of the sarcomeres and A and I bands around the intercalated disk (Gutierrez *et al.*, 1976). These ultrastructural changes are nonspecific, because similar morphology has been described in animals dying of a variety of conditions such as hemorrhagic shock (Martin *et al.*, 1964; Hiott, 1969). However, *Aotus* dying of hemorrhagic shock have other cardiac lesions such as marked myofibrillar derangement with widening and fragmentation of muscle Z bands.

The vascular pathology associated with malaria consists mainly of capillary occlusions due to masses of agglutinated infected erythrocytes (Fig. 14). These capillary occlusions cause hemorrhage and necrosis in the perivascular areas of the brain, myocardium, intestinal mucosa, skin (seen as purpura), and other organs, especially in patients and animals dying of *P. falciparum* infection (Spitz, 1946).

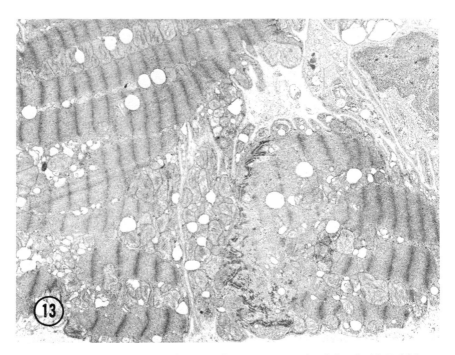

FIG. 13.   Electron micrograph of the heart from an *Aotus* monkey infected with *P. falciparum* showing alterations in muscle cells with disorganization of the sarcomeres. ×6500. (Reproduced from Gutierrez *et al.*, 1976, by permission of the author and publisher.)

There may be several causes of erythrocyte clumping in the small arterioles and capillaries. Erythrocytes infected with *P. falciparum* have membrane changes described as excrescences (Fig. 15). These excrescences play an important role in the attachment of infected red blood cells to the vascular endothelium (Fig. 16), resulting in the occurrence of the parasite's schizogony deep in the vasculature (Luse and Miller, 1971; Aikawa *et al.*, 1972). On the other hand, similar excrescences have been described in erythrocytes infected with both asexual forms and gametocytes of *P. coatneyi, P. malariae,* and *P. brasilianum,* but they must have a different function because they do not play an apparent role in deep vascular schizogony; however, they may contribute to erythrocyte agglutination (Aikawa *et al.*, 1975). The manner in which infected erythrocytes join together or to the endothelial membrane is not known. Kilejian *et al.* (1977) has demonstrated the presence of malarial parasite antigens on the excrescences. When erythrocytes infected with *P. falciparum* are incubated with homologous antibody, a prominent coat is formed on the excrescence surface (Fig. 17), supporting the idea that erythroagglutination is due to an antigen–antibody reaction (Chulay *et al.*, 1979). Other causes contributing to agglutination appear to

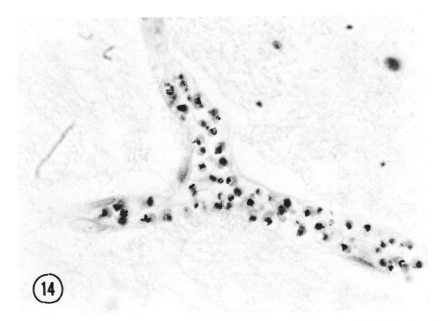

FIG. 14. Capillary containing many agglutinated, infected erythrocytes. ×1620. (Courtesy of D. Connor, AFIP #70-1051.)

be the escape of abnormal amounts of protein and fluid through the endothelial cell membrane which is rendered abnormally permeable by multiple factors of which anoxia may be the most important.

The end result of erythrocyte agglutination and especially of attachment to the endothelial wall is the formation of thrombi in the capillaries as described in the classic literature. Similarly the *P. berghei* 17X strain in rodents has been found to be capable of crossing the blood–brain barrier, of causing intravascular sequestration, and of producing multiple thrombi composed of infected erythrocytes and pigment (Yoeli and Hargreaves, 1974). The important consequence of thrombus formation in the host is vascular occlusion, with resultant hemorrhage and tissue necrosis. Local tissue anoxia, plus anoxia associated with anemia due to erythrocyte destruction, if widespread, can result in shock.

There are other hemodynamic changes which can follow the above events. Animals infected with *P. falciparum* show terminally a typical syndrome of disseminated intravascular coagulation (DIC) with a characteristic thrombocytopenia, decrease in blood coagulation factors, and increase in fibrin degradation products (Wellde *et al.*, 1972). The occurrence of hemorrhages and thrombosis in patients with malaria suggest that DIC plays an important role in the pathophysiology of death in this infection. Jervis *et al.* (1972) rarely observed thrombi during autopsies performed on *Aotus* with *P. falciparum* infec-

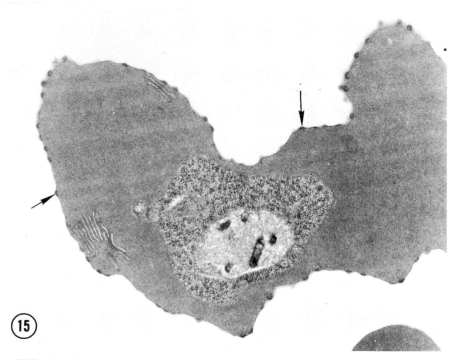

FIG. 15. Electron micrograph of erythrocyte infected with *P. falciparum* showing excrescences (arrows) on the plasma membrane. ×24,000.

tion, but fibrin strands were seen commonly in dilated capillaries and veins, suggesting that fibrinolysis was taking place. These findings are consistent with the DIC syndrome which occurs from various causes in animals.

Goodwin and Richards (1960) detected pharmacologically active peptides in the blood and urine of mice infected with *P. berghei*. One of these peptides, bradykinin, present in sera of rhesus monkeys with *P. inui* and *P. coatneyi* infection, increases vascular permeability. Desowitz and Pavanand (1967), working with monkeys infected with *P. coatneyi*, suggested that increased vascular permeability may be induced by antigen–antibody complexes. As a result of the increased vascular permeability there may be a rapid decrease in plasma volume, shock, and changes in the liver, such as centrilobular necrosis. Similarly, Maegraith and Onobanjo (1970) have demonstrated an increase in blood histamine of monkeys infected with *P. knowlesi*, which they believe contributes to increased vascular permeability and capillary damage.

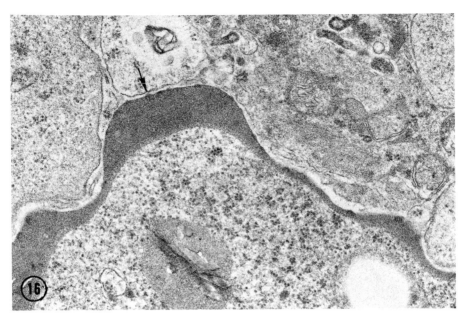

FIG. 16. Electron micrograph of an erythrocyte infected with *P. falciparum* in a capillary. Excrescences on the erythrocyte membrane form a junction (arrow) with the endothelial cells. ×27,000.

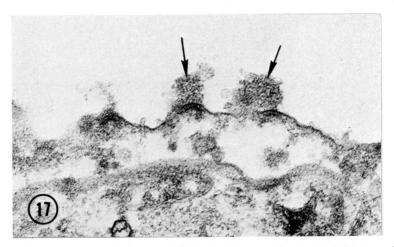

FIG. 17. Electron micrograph of a partially lysed erythrocyte infected with *P. falciparum* in the presence of immune monkey serum. Electron-dense surface coats (arrows) are seen over excrescences of the erythrocyte membrane. ×30,000.

V. HEMATOPATHOLOGY

Malarial parasites of rodent and avian-infecting species produce morphological changes in circulating infected and uninfected erythrocytes (Kreier *et al.*, 1972a). In humans *P. vivax* enlarges parasitized red blood cells greatly and changes their shape to angular when they are pressed by neighboring erythrocytes. In humans *P. falciparum*- parasitized cells tend to be smaller than normal, and there is some degree of crenation of infected and noninfected erythrocytes. In humans infected with *P. ovale* moderate enlargement and distortion of the red cell occur. A projection of the red cells with a fimbriated end, especially in quickly dried blood films, is common. *Plasmodium malarie* produces no changes in parasitized human red blood cells. The morphological alterations seen in red blood cells containing malaria parasites can be somewhat modified in chronic infections when there is some degree of anemia (Field and Shute, 1956; Seed and Kreier, 1972; Kreier *et al.*, 1972a,b).

Malarial parasites are also known for having preferences for certain red blood cell types. *Plasmodium falciparum* invades both young and old erythrocytes; *P. vivax*, young erythrocytes; and *P. malariae*, old erythrocytes. A similar phenomenon is seen in *P. berghei*, which is considered to be reticulotropic. The availability of these cells in peripheral blood is considered a limiting factor in the infection. In infected rodents reticulocytosis follows peak parasitemia, but in human malaria it is observed as a response to the anemia produced by the parasite.

Changes in the number of circulating red blood cells in malaria can be followed by hematocrit and erythrocyte counts (Wellde *et al.*, 1971a,b, 1972). The anemia in animals with natural or experimental malaria appears to be due to red blood cell destruction by several mechanisms: (1) erythrocyte rupture at the end of the parasite's erythrocytic phase, (2) increased erythrophagocytosis of parasitized and altered red blood cells, (Fig. 18), and (3) direct hemolysis due to an immune reaction against the red blood cell membrane. In relation to the third postulate, the presence of antigen on the membrane of infected erythrocytes has been described in *P. falciparum* (Kilejian *et al.*, 1977) and *P. vivax* (Aikawa *et al.*, 1975). Other autoimmune hemolytic mechanisms may also be operating, but they are not fully understood at present. (See this volume, Chapter 1 for a more complete treatment of this subject.)

Experimental *P. brasilianum* infections have been studied (Taliaferro and Kluver, 1940) from the hematological point of view. A mild anemia is observed, especially after the crisis near the end of fatal infections, or in the chronic phase. Changes in erythrocytes consisting of polychromatophilia and anisocytosis were also observed, as well as reticulocytosis. Similarly, in *P. coatneyi* infections, Desowitz *et al.* (1967) noted anemia, erythroid hyperplasia of the bone marrow, and increased numbers of normoblasts and reticulocytes in the peripheral blood.

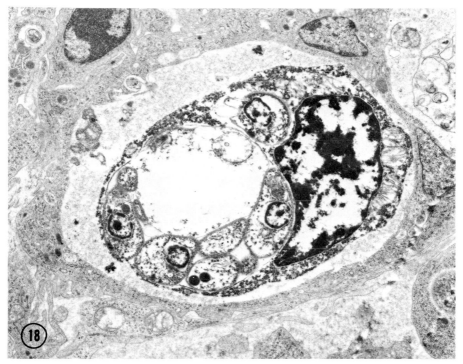

FIG. 18. Electron micrograph of an erythrocyte infected with *P. elongatum* within a phagolysosome of a macrophage in the bone marrow. ×11,000. (Reproduced from Aikawa and Sprinz, 1971, by permission of the author and publisher.)

The hemogram returned to normal as soon as the animals entered the chronic phase of the disease.

Schnitzer *et al.* (1973) demonstrated pitting of infected erythrocytes in the spleen, resulting in the production of small spherocytes which were more susceptible to hemolysis than normally shaped erythrocytes. Increased osmotic fragility has also been demonstrated in infected red blood cells. Red blood cell lysis has been studied in monkeys with experimental *P. knowlesi* infections where acute infection usually produces two types of lytic patterns. One is manifested by profound hemolysis following schizogony with a marked drop in red blood cell mass, hemoglobinuria, and death. The second pattern is that of infections with a moderate decrease in red cell count at the end of schizogony without hemoglobinuria (Devakul and Margraith, 1959). The red blood cells in animals belonging to the first group are most susceptible to lysis. The explanation of this phenomenon is not clear, but it is attributed to changes brought about by the parasite (Devakul and Maegraith, 1959). Similar studies (Seed *et al.*, 1976) have shown that erythrocytes from *P. berghei*-infected rodents have increased osmotic fragility.

In *P. gallinaceum* infections erythrocytes have shown a propensity to lysis even very early in the infection, returning to normal when the animal is placed under therapy and the parasites are cleared from the circulation (Swann and Kreier, 1973).

There are other phenomena produced by the red blood cell–parasite association. There is an apparent protection against infection with *P. falciparum* in individuals with sickle cell disease (Allison, 1954). Under laboratory conditions such protection has been documented by the use of *P. falciparum in vitro* cultures. Cultures of red cells containing sickle cell hemoglobin (HbS) from either homozygous (SS) or heterozygous (SA) trait carriers have been studied by electron microscopy. Parasites in SS cells appear to be disrupted by deoxy-HbS aggregates of needle-like form (Friedman, 1979). It is proposed that these ultra-structural alterations detected *in vitro* are the basis of the HbS gene carrier resistance (Friedman, 1979) against malaria infection.

Recently Miller *et al.* (1975) reported that initial recognition and attachment between *P. knowlesi* merozoites and erythrocytes probably involved specific determinants associated with Duffy blood group-related antigens. Duffy-negative erythrocytes were refractory to invasion by *P. knowlesi* and *P. vivax* (Miller *et al.*, 1976). Electron microscopic study (Miller *et al.*, 1979) demonstrated that there was no junction formation between Duffy-negative erythrocytes and *P. knowlesi* merozoites (see Chapter 4, Vol. 1).

Stippling is found in malaria-infected red blood cells. This stippling has different characteristics varying with the species of plasmodia and is sometimes useful for diagnosis. For example, in vivax- and ovale-type malaria, the red blood cell stippling is referred to as Schüffner's dots; in the falciparum type usually as Maurer's clefts, and in the malariae type as Ziemann's stippling. The electron microscopy of these structures and their relationship to the excrescences, caveolae, and caveola–vesicle complexes (Aikawa *et al.*, 1975) have been described in Chapter 4, Vol. 1.

The effects of malaria infections on the other blood cell elements have also been studied. Leukocytosis has been found in rats and mice with *P. berghei* infections, mainly because of an increase in peripheral monocytes (Singer, 1954). Wellde *et al.* (1971a,b, 1972) found leukopenia in *Aotus* infected with *P. falciparum* at the beginning, with moderate to marked leukocytosis if the infection lasted longer than 12 days. Leukocytosis was always accompanied by a rise in mononuclear cells. Monocytosis seen in malaria infections correlated with stimulation of the reticuloendothelial system to handle malarial pigment and the accelerated destruction of infected and noninfected red blood cells. In monkeys with *P. brasilianum* infections Taliaferro and Kluver (1940) found that the number of granulocytes decreased a few days after the malarial crisis and that the number of monocytes increased slightly to 3–8% for 1–2 weeks after the infection became patent. When the infection is prolonged and intense, monocyte counts will remain high but will return to normal if the infection becomes a chronic one with low parasitemia. In *P. falciparum*-infected *Aotus*, lymphocyte numbers vary erratically in the acute phase but can reach 50% during the chronic phase; numbers of eosinophils and basophils decrease gradually, and these cells almost disappear in chronic infections. Desowitz *et al.* (1967) found persistent leukocytosis beginning during the acute phase and continuing for a 5-month period in monkeys infected with *P. coatneyi*. A close relationship between malaria infection and Burkitt's lymphoma has been suggested on the basis of seroepidemiological data. Nkrumah *et al.* (1979) reported a link between *P. falciparum* infection and Burkitt's lymphoma in African children by studying immunoglobulin levels.

There are a few studies on platelets during malaria infections. In the patent period there is thrombocytopenia in all *Aotus* infected with *P. falciparum*. Thrombocytopenia increases with the parasitemia (Voller *et al.*, 1969). This thrombocytopenia has been studied in conjunction with other changes in coagulation factors. At least in one experimental animal it has been found that coagulation time is prolonged and factor VIII reduced, with no change in fibrinogen or factor V (Voller *et al.*, 1969). The thrombocytopenia, the long coagulation time, and the reduction in factor VIII have been interpreted as being consistent with disseminated intravascular coagulation. The normal fibrinogen values in falciparum-infected *Aotus* have been explained as being due to the unusually high levels of antithrombin normally present in *Aotus* (Voller *et al.*, 1969).

Dennis *et al.* (1966a,b, 1967) found that, in humans dying of acute falciparum malaria, there was thrombocytopenia, a prolonged prothrombin time, a decrease in multiple coagulation factors, a decrease in plasminogen, and an increase in fibrinogen degradation products. Devakul *et al.* (1966) have also demonstrated a precipitous decrease in fibrinogen and an increase in fibrinogen degradation products with the use of ^{131}I-labeled fibrinogen in patients with acute *P. falciparum* infections. Both Dennis *et al.* and Devakul *et al.* have concluded that in humans with acute falciparum infection disseminated intravascular coagulation is present.

Serum chemistry in malarial infections has been studied on a limited basis. Blood urea nitrogen levels are increased in rodents after the fourth day of infection with *P. berghei*, probably as a result of kidney changes (Sadun *et al.*, 1965). The same authors also found an increase in SGPT and SGOT as early as 2 days after infection, probably related to erythrocyte destruction and liver damage.

Low glucose levels have been seen in heavily infected animals starting on the fourth day of infection, returning to normal 2 days later. However, both in humans and animals glucose levels during malaria infections seem to depend on the stage of the disease and the severity of the infection. During *P. vivax* and *P. falciparum* infection, a fall in glucose levels has been observed, especially during the paroxysm due to increased metabolism during the fever or to hepatic cell damage. In monkeys with *P. knowlesi* infection hypoglycemia has been detected, especially in animals with low liver glucose storage (Fulton, 1939) or with terminal infections (Devakul and Maegraith, 1958). Similarly, hypoglycemia has been observed terminally in *P. lophurae*-infected ducks (Marvin and Rigdon, 1945). Devakul (1960) described a case of fatal *P. falciparum* in humans with 7.4 mg% glucose, but other patients did not show such drastic changes. The serum proteins are reduced in most individuals with malaria infections mainly because of a decrease in the albumin caused by liver damage (Sadun *et al.*, 1965).

VI. PULMONARY PATHOLOGY

The main pathological changes occurring in the lungs during malaria infection are pulmonary edema, congestion, and the accumulation of pigment-laden macrophages in the capillaries (Figs. 19 and 20). Taliaferro and Mulligan (1937) found no specific changes in lungs of animals dying of acute malaria, but acute congestion and hemorrhagic infarcts have been described. Animals with chronic malaria have pale, anemic lungs. MacCallum (1968, 1969b) reported that large numbers of macrophages with abundant malarial pigment accumulated in the pulmonary vascular bed of hamsters as early as 6 days after infection with *P. berghei*. These cells adhered to the capillary wall, giving the appearance of total occlusion (Fig. 21), but on the eighth and ninth days of the infection endothelial cells grew over to exclude them from the circulation.

MacCallum (1968, 1969b) also reported that hamsters with advanced *P. berghei* infection had dilated lymphatic vessels containing fibrin clots (Fig. 22), that the alveolar spaces contained a protein-rich granular exudate (Fig. 22), and that the alveolar spaces also contained a protein-rich granular exudate (Fig. 24). Based on these findings he postulated that alveolar capillary congestion and filling of pulmonary veins by macrophages (Fig. 23) resulted in increased blood pressure, altering fluid exchange across the capillary membranes. He considered that pulmonary edema was caused by this blood pressure increase and by the obstruction and dilation of the lymphatic system. Godard and Hansen (1971) demonstrated interstitial pulmonary edema without alveolar edema by x-ray examination. This edema was similar to that thought to occur in individuals with allergic hypersensitivity reactions. Suzuki (1975) studied ultrastructural lung changes in mice infected with *P. yoelii* and found many polymorphonuclear leukocytes present in the pulmonary capillary lumens and alveolar spaces (Figs. 25 and 26). In the later stages of infection, polymorphonuclear leukocytes were

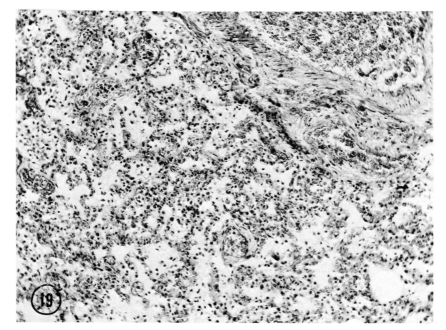

FIG. 19. Lung section from a patient with falciparum malaria showing congestion and pigment-laden macrophages. ×160. (Courtesy of D. Connor, AFIP #66-7207.)

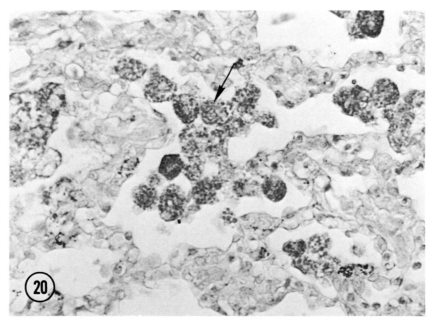

FIG. 20. Lung section for an *Aotus* monkey infected with *P. falciparum* showing many macrophages with malarial pigment (arrow). ×350. (Courtesy of H. Jervis.)

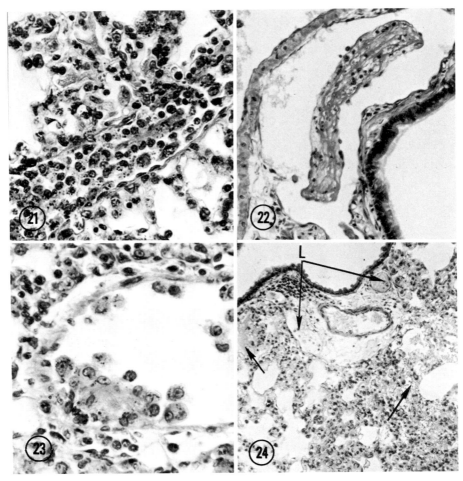

FIG. 21.   Lung section of a hamster infected with *P. berghei*. The pulmonary vein is occluded by a large number of macrophages. ×250. (Reproduced from MacCallum, 1968, permission of the author and publisher.)

FIG. 22.   Thrombus in a dilated lymphatic vessel from a lung section of a hamster infected with *P. berghei*. ×120. (Reproduced from MacCallum, 1968, by permission of the author and publisher.)

FIG. 23.   Mural thrombus with pigment-laden macrophages in a pulmonary vein of a hamster infected with *P. berghei*. ×275. (Reproduced from MacCallum, 1968, by permission of the author and publisher.)

FIG. 24.   Section of the lung from a hamster infected with *P. berghei*. The alveolar space contains a protein-rich granular exudate (arrows). Two dilated lymphatic vessels are seen adjacent to the bronchus (L.) ×75. (Reproduced from MacCallum, 1968, by permission of the author and publisher.)

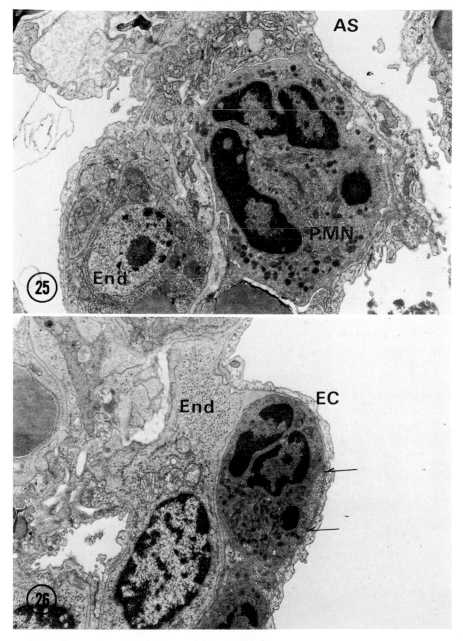

FIG. 25. Electron micrograph of the lung of a mouse infected with *P. berghei*. A neutrophil (PMN) obliterates a capillary space. AS, Alveolar space; End, endothelial cell. ×2000. (Reproduced from Suzuki and Waki, 1979, by permission of the author and publisher.)

FIG. 26. Another example of the lung from a mouse infected with *P. berghei* showing a neutrophil in direct contact with the basement membrane of the alveolar capillary (arrows). End, Endothelial cell; EC, epithelial cell. ×2000.

attached to the capillary basement membranes and cytoplasmic extensions of the endothelial cells which were piled one upon the other. Singer (1954), working with *P. berghei* in mice, also found an increase in granulocytes and lymphocytes early in the infection. Increases in the number of macrophages are seen in the lungs starting on the fifth day, and phagocytosis is most active on the eighth day of infection.

Patients with *P. falciparum* malaria, especially in southeast Asia, can have a syndrome of acute pulmonary insufficiency. Marks *et al.* (1977) studied a similar case in Rhodesia. The syndrome appears abruptly in patients with high parasitemia and is usually associated with cerebral or renal complications but not with heart failure. Hall (1976) suggested that impairment of the alveolar capillary microcirculation and excessive fluid therapy were the main causes of acute pulmonary insufficiency in malaria. Grossly, the lungs of these patients are markedly greater in weight than normal, congested, and edematous and also have hemorrhagic consolidation (Stone *et al.*, 1972). Microscopically, there are thickened alveolar septi (Fig. 27), diffuse alveolar edema, and focal or widespread hyaline membrane formation; pulmonary congestion and focal intra-alveolar

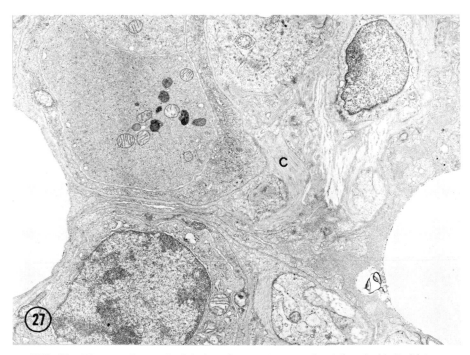

FIG. 27.   Electron micrograph of the lung from an *Aotus* monkey infected with *P. falciparum* showing a marked increase in septal collagen (C). ×9500. (Reproduced from Gutierrez *et al.,* 1976, by permission of the author and publisher.)

hemorrhages are present (Brooks *et al.*, 1978; Deaton, 1970; Punyagupta *et al.*, 1974). Sheehy and Reba (1967) suggested that aggregated parasitized erythrocytes or microthrombi in the hypothalamus might cause release of antidiuretic hormones and retention of fluid. Many investigators have noted that microcirculation dysfunction is followed by engorgement and accumulation of edema fluid and alveolar hyaline membrane formation.

Immunological reactions may be involved in the production of pulmonary injury in malaria. The pulmonary lesions in falciparum infection are often seen in individuals with immune complex deposits in the kidneys. The special immunological relationship which exists between the basement membranes of lungs and kidneys is apparent in diseases such as Goodpasture's syndrome, which provide a model for pulmonary lesions related to host immune reactions.

VII. THYMUS PATHOLOGY

Although T-lymphocyte functions and behavior have been extensively studied, information on thymus histopathology is very limited. Al-Dabag (1966) studied birds infected with *P. juxtanucleare, P. gallinaceum, P. rouxi, P. cathemerium,* and *P. elongatum* and observed that during the patent period the thymus was highly active and that a large number of mitotic figures were present. In the chronic stage lymphocytes were depleted, and increased lymphorrhexis was present; he also observed that Hassel's corpuscles were plentiful in infected animals as compared with controls. Taliaferro and Taliaferro (1955) also observed lymphoid depletion in the thymuses of chickens chronically infected with *P. gallinaceum.*

Eling *et al.* (1977) studied the relationship between thymus and body weight during *P. berghei* infection in mice and found a weight increase during the first week, but in general the thymus/body weight ratio decreased as the infection progressed. Gravely *et al.* (1976) observed that the thymus of healthy young rats atrophied during *P. berghei* infection. Tanabe *et al.* (1977) examined the thymuses from BALB/c mice infected with *P. berghei* and also reported a decrease in thymus size and weight (Fig. 28). Histopathological examination showed a depletion of thymocytes and a loss of distinction between the cortex and medulla (Fig. 29). *Plasmodium chabaudi* infections in mice cause thymus changes similar to those caused by *P. berghei,* and the thymuses return to normal on about the ninety-fourth day after the mice recover from the infection.

Several investigators have demonstrated that thymocytes may work adversely in malaria. Wright *et al.* (1971) implicated T lymphocytes in the development of cerebral lesions in golden hamsters infected with *P. berghei,* because antithymocyte serum prevented cerebral hemorrhages. Waki and Suzuki (1977) noted that athymic nude mice survived three times longer than phenotypically normal mice

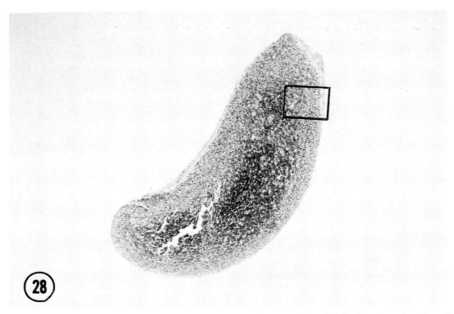

FIG. 28. Involuted thymus from a mouse 11 days after *P. chabaudi* infection. Lymphocytes of the cortex are depleted and are concentrated in the medulla. ×33. (Courtesy of K. Tanabe.)

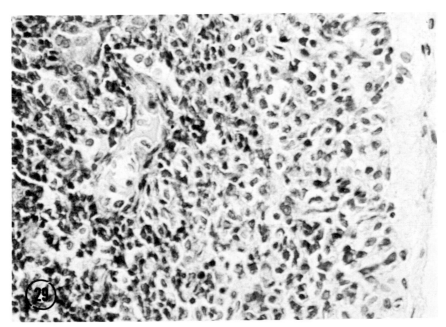

FIG. 29. Higher magnification of the micrograph in Fig. 28. The cortex consists mostly of connective tissue and reticular cells. ×330.

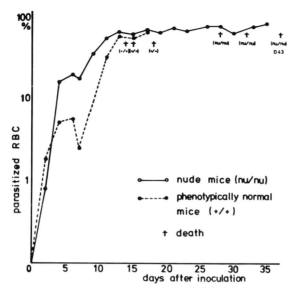

FIG. 30.   Relationship between parasitemia and survival time in *P. berghei*(NK65)-infected nude mice.

(Fig. 30), and this finding was confirmed by thymocyte replacement. Immunity to *P. berghei* blood forms is thymus-dependent and is transferred by cells more efficiently than by serum.

VIII. RENAL PATHOLOGY

A. *Plasmodium malariae*-Associated Renal Pathology

Since Watson in 1905 noted the presence of edema in a patient with malaria in Malaysia, the relationship between *P. malariae* infection and the nephrotic syndrome has been well documented. In 1940, Boyd observed albuminuria in 43 patients with quartan malaria, providing evidence for an etiological relationship between *P. malariae* and the nephrotic syndrome. Gilles and Hendrickse (1960, 1963) also demonstrated a relationship between *P. malariae* and the nephrotic syndrome in Nigerian patients. They found that in children the peak incidence of the nephrotic syndrome and *P. malariae* infection coincided. Kibukamusoke (1973) observed a relationship among rainfall, mosquito density, and frequency of hospital admissions for the nephrotic syndrome at Lagos University Hospital in Uganda.

Histologically, there is a proliferative glomerulonephropathy with increased endothelial and mesangial cells. Kibukamusoke and Hutt (1967) classified these changes into five subgroups based on 77 biopsies from nephrotic patients in

Uganda: (1) diffuse type with diffuse changes throughout the glomerular tufts, (2) lobular type with lesions in a lobular pattern, (3) focal type with abnormalities in less than 50% of the glomeruli, (4) chronic type with glomerular changes plus capsular adhesions, secondary membrane thickening, and sclerosis, and (5) minimal type with minor abnormalities in focal or segmental lesions. In 31 kidney biopsies from children, 28 corresponded to a type of proliferative glomerulonephropathy, and the rest were only minimally changed. In 46 biopsies from adults, 27 had proliferative glomerulonephropathy, and the rest showed only minimal abnormalities. In 9 biopsies, there was diffuse uniform thickening of the basement membrane with no evidence of proliferative changes, and in the remaining 10 there were other changes not related to malaria.

On the other hand, Gilles and Hendrickse (1963) described membranous glomerulonephritis in patients with quartan malaria and the nephrotic syndrome. Biopsies revealed subendothelial basement membrane lesions characterized either by a double-contoured or by a plexiform arrangement of periodic acid–Schiff (PAS)-positive material and argyrophilic fibrils (Hendrickse et al., 1972; White, 1973; Edington and Gilles, 1976; Figs. 31 and 32). In biopsies from patients with early lesions, glomerular changes were found only in occasional capillary loops, but in the more advanced cases there was diffuse capillary wall thickening and almost no mesangial cell proliferation. The name "quartan malaria nephropathy" was proposed for this condition, because of its unique characteristics (Hendrickse et al., 1972).

Allison et al. (1969) reported moderate basement membrane thickening and circumscribed subepithelial electron-dense deposits in kidney biopsies from Nigerian children. They concluded that the early stages of the nephrotic syndrome had lesions similar to those of immune complex glomerulonephritis of experimental animals (Feldman, 1963). Dixon (1966) and Allison et al. (1969) studied renal biopsies of Nigerian children by immunofluorescence and found irregular, beaded deposits of IgG and B1C globulin along the glomerular basement membrane, suggesting the deposition of antigen–antibody complexes at this site. Using a similar technique, Ward and Kibukamusoke (1969) found IgM, IgG, IgA, complement, fibrin, and malarial antigens in the glomeruli of East African patients who developed renal disease and the nephrotic syndrome following quartan malaria. They noted that IgM was the predominant immunoglobulin and that there were P. malariae antigens in the glomerular deposits in 3 of the 13 individuals studied. Ward and Conran (1969) examined 44 renal biopsies from patients with the nephrotic syndrome and found that IgM immunoglobulin was most abundant in the glomerular deposits.

There is little information available on the tubular changes which occur in quartan malaria nephropathy, but their extent appears to reflect the degree of glomerular damage. The epithelial cells of the proximal convoluted tubules may contain hyaline droplets (Kibukamusoke and Hutt, 1967; White, 1973) and develop fatty vacuolation (Allen, 1962). Marked glomerular sclerosis, tubular at-

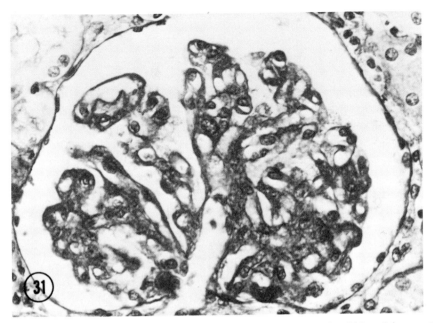

FIG. 31. A glomerulus in quartan malaria nephropathy showing the thickened basement membrane and mesangial expansion. ×500. (Reproduced from R. White, 1973, by permission of the author and publisher.)

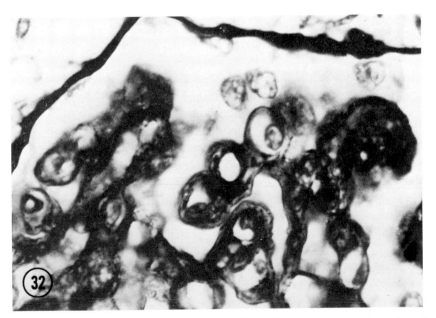

FIG. 32. High-magnification micrograph of a glomerulus in quartan malaria nephropathy showing the thickened basement membrane. ×1400. (Reproduced from R. White, 1973, by permission of the author and publisher.)

rophy, interstitial fibrosis, and, in severely affected kidneys, degenerative changes, including eosinophilic granular degeneration of the proximal tubular epithelium, were present (Gilles and Hendrickse, 1963).

Allison *et al.* (1969) detected well-defined fluorescent deposits between the lumen and the nuclei of tubular cells after staining with an anticomplement conjugate. Houba *et al.* (1971) reported that deposits of IgM and IgG were present in 17 out of 50 kidneys examined. One-fifth of the kidneys had complement deposits in the tubules, and *P. malariae* antigen was present in 11 out of the 36. In serial biopsies of patients with malaria, IgG and IgM staining was consistently positive in the tubules. Only three patients showed tubular staining with the anticomplement conjugate initially, but all became positive as the disease progressed.

Morel-Maroger *et al.* (1975) studied renal biopsies in Senegal where the prevalence of quartan malaria is low, but the nephrotic syndrome in children is common. Two distinct nephrotic syndrome types were seen. One was hypocomplementemic with extramembranous glomerulonephritis, termed "tropical extramembranous glomerulonephritis." The other showed features of progressive and segmental glomerulosclerosis similar to Ivory Coast and Nigerian quartan malaria nephropathy and termed "tropical nephropathy." Morphologically the tropical extramembranous glomerulonephritis was characterized by the proliferation of endothelial and mesangial cells with occasional subepithelial electron-dense deposits. Immunofluorescence studies showed diffuse granular IgG deposits along the peripheral capillary loops. IgA, properdin, Clq, and C4 were also detected in these kidneys. The etiology of these two nephropathies is unknown, although malaria may be involved. Viral, bacterial, and helminthic infection is prevalent among Sengalese children and may also be involved in this unique nephropathy.

Soothil and Hendrickse (1967) collected sera at random from children at the nephrosis clinic in Ibadan and found complement component B1C in a complex macromolecular form, indicating that it can be incorporated into circulating soluble antigen–antibody complexes. Epidemiological evidence has indicated that the nephrotic syndrome of Nigerian children is related to *P. malariae* infection. Therefore, it is probable that complement is incorporated into circulating immune complexes of individuals with quartan malaria nephrotic syndrome and that these complexes are similar to those deposited in the kidney.

B. *Plasmodium falciparum*-Associated Renal Pathology

It appears that the pathological changes in kidneys of patients with falciparum malaria vary from case to case depending on the stage of the disease and its severity.

Spitz (1946) observed glomerulonephritis with proliferative changes and basement membrane thickening in patients with falciparum malaria. Berger *et al.*

(1967) reported nephrotic syndrome associated with falciparum malaria in three patients. They described hypercellularity, adhesion of Bowman's capsule, and infiltration of polymorphonuclear leukocytes, but splitting and mild thickening of the glomerular basement membrane were also present in scattered glomeruli. Glomerular mesangial expansion, hypercellularity, and basement membrane thickening have been reported to be present in falciparum-infected patients by Hartenbower *et al.* (1972) and Bhamarapravati *et al.* (1973) (Fig. 33).

Using electron microscopy, Hartenbower *et al.* (1972) showed irregular basement membrane thickening with alterations in electron density, abnormal deposits of material in the subendothelial regions, large amounts of mesangial matrix, and focal endothelial cell proliferation. These changes were consistent with focal membranoproliferative glomerulonephritis. The authors also showed by immunofluorescence that the kidneys of patients with falciparum malaria contained focal small deposits of IgG, IgM, and BlC within the mesangium and along the basement membrane. Bhamarapravati *et al.* (1973), using immunofluorescence, studied 10 biopsies from Thai patients with acute falciparum infection and found fine, granular deposits in the mesangial areas and occasionally along the luminal sides of the glomerular capillaries. The granules consisted primarily of IgM (9/10 cases), B1C (8/10 cases), and IgG (3/10 cases).

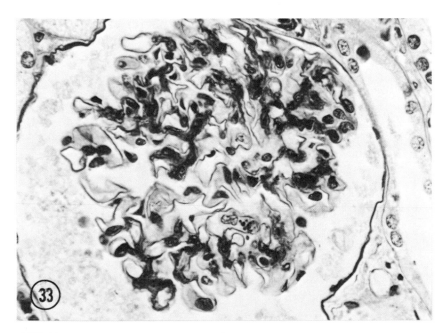

FIG. 33.   A glomerulus in falciparum malaria nephropathy showing mesangial expansion, focal thickening of the basement membrane, and hypercellularity. ×600. (The tissue was supplied by V. Boonpucknavig.)

IgA was identified only in one specimen from a patient who developed acute renal failure. *Plasmodium falciparum* antigen was detected in one patient.

Glomerular immune complexes disappear after patients have been treated and recover from malaria. Immunoglobulin deposits disappeared from kidneys of patients who responded to prednisone, cyclophosphamide, and azathioprine treatment (Adeniyi *et al.* 1970). On the other hand, IgG and B1C remained in patients refractory to treatment with these drugs. One micrograph in the paper of Adeniyi *et al.* shows linear immunoglobulin deposits in the kidney, a pattern which is characteristic of autoimmune nephritis. The patient with these linear deposits had a poor response to azathioprine. Moreover, in these individuals the distribution pattern appeared to change from granular to linear after treatment, implying that at some point in the course of the disease the pathogenic mechanism may have switched from antigen–antibody complex deposition to autoimmune damage. Hendrickse and Gilles (1963) suggested that untreated attacks of malaria in some patients may evoke an abnormal immunological response in which the glomerular basement membrane is damaged by antigen–antibody complexes. This damage then leads to an autoimmune response. A glomerular pattern changing from granular to linear may be a sign that damage mediated by immune complexes has become an autoimmune deterioration. Based on these reports it appears that immune complexes are involved in the genesis of glomerular lesions associated with falciparum infection in humans.

Pronounced renal tubular alterations have been reported in patients with falciparum malaria. There are hyaline droplets in the kidneys with cloudy swelling of the tubular epithelium and, in severely affected kidneys, fatty degeneration and necrosis. Changes are more pronounced in the distal convoluted tubules than in the proximal ones (Boonpuckavig and Sitprija, 1979). Biopsies taken after recovery showed abnormally large amounts of interstitial connective tissue and infiltration of lymphocytes, histiocytes, and eosinophils, and later focal interstitial scarring occurred (Berger *et al.*, 1967). Hemoglobin casts may be seen in the distal convoluted and collecting tubules (Winslow *et al.*, 1975).

Blackwater fever is an acute hemolytic condition associated with fever, anemia, jaundice, and hemoglobinuria, and it is generally considered to be a complication of *P. falciparum* infection (Edington and Gilles, 1976). There is usually a history of irregular chemosuppression or inadequate chemotherapy, especially with quinine. The diagnosis of blackwater fever can be made only in patients who do not have other drug-induced hemolysis (Gilles and Ikeme, 1960). For example, patients with erythrocytic glucose-6-phosphage dehydrogenase deficiency who manifest hemolytic anemia and "black urine" when treated with certain antimalarial drugs have a disorder different from classic blackwater fever (Edington and Gilles, 1976).

The incidence of blackwater fever has decreased; however, because of the reduction in immunity following treatment in individuals who live in endemic areas, it may be presently undergoing a surge. For example, Dukes *et al.* (1968) observed the syndrome in six Rhodesians (five of them Africans), mostly town dwellers, after 10 years without a case being seen. In addition to the danger of blackwater fever in individuals whose immunity has waned, the increased use of quinine, as a result of the appearance of chloroquine-resistant strains of *P. falciparum,* may also augment its incidence (World Health Organization, 1973).

Grossly, the kidneys of patients dying of blackwater fever are dark in color, enlarged, and edematous. The cut surface has a pale color, with evidence of cortical swelling and small hemorrhages, and congestion of the medulla (Fig. 34).

Microscopically, there are slightly abnormal glomeruli (Maegraith, 1948). Deposits of amorphous hyaline material are present in the capsular spaces (Edington and Giles, 1976). Rosen *et al.* (1968a) reported hyalinization and segmental fibrosis of glomeruli in a biopsy specimen. The principal histological changes are various degrees of degenerative change up to necrosis, mainly in the loops of Henle and in the distal convoluted tubules (Edington and Gilles, 1976). Epithelial, hyaline, or granular casts are often seen in the lumen. The number

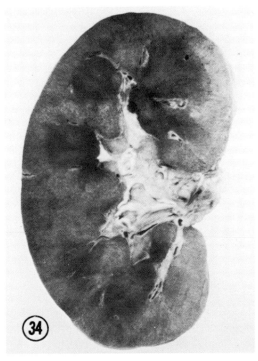

FIG. 34. Kidney from a patient with blackwater fever showing cortical swelling and congestion of the medulla. (Reproduced from A. Allen, 1962, by permission of the author and publisher.)

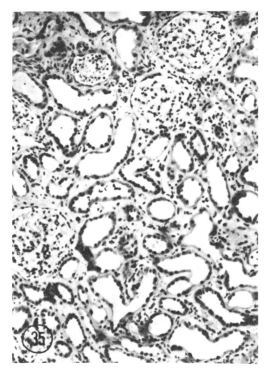

FIG. 35. Kidney biopsy from a patient with blackwater fever showing extensive tubular degeneration and diffuse interstitial increase. ×136. (Reproduced from Rosen *et al.*, 1968a, by permission of the authors and publisher.)

of hemoglobin casts in the kidneys of patients dying with falciparum-induced acute renal failure is less than in patients with clinical evidence of the blackwater syndrome (Winslow *et al.*, 1975). Moreover, patients with blackwater fever have a diffuse or focal stromal increase with interstitial lymphocytic infiltration (Fig. 35) (Rosen *et al.*, 1968a). Abnormal amounts of collagen and scattered fibroblasts are also found. Osmiophilic rectangularly shaped inclusion bodies which appear to be malarial pigment particles are seen within fibroblasts.

C. Renal Pathology in Experimental Animals

There has been work done in experimental animals to clarify the mechanisms of renal disease associated with malaria infection. Ward and Conran (1966) demonstrated malarial antigen, L globulin, and B1C globulin in the glomeruli of splenectomized monkeys infected with *P. cynomolgi*. In a later study, monkeys were splenectomized and unilaterally nephrectomized to increase the amount of circulating immune complexes passing through the kidneys. There were no histological alterations in these animals, though granular deposits of IgG, C2, and low amounts of malarial antigen were present over a 3- to 4-day period just after the primary peak of parasitemia (Ward and Conran, 1969). The deposits reappeared during a more sustained secondary parasitemia peak, and changes in their concentration paralleled changes in the parasitemia (Ward and Conran, 1969). Although there were circulating immune complexes in their experimental animals, Ward and Conran (1966, 1969) did not succeed in producing a picture of the nephrotic syndrome in monkeys. Geiman and Siddiqui (1969) infected *Aotus* with *P. malariae* to study quartan malaria nephropathy experimentally. Voller *et al.* (1971) used the same model and observed facial edema and proteinuria in these animals during recrudescences. In spite of antimalarial therapy, clinical deterioration occurred. There was generalized diffuse glomerulonephritis with proliferative and membranous changes. Prominent granular IgM deposits were seen in all glomeruli, but IgG, complement, and malarial antigen were not present. Degeneration of the proximal tubules and focal collections of lymphocytes, plasma cells, and occasional eosinophils in the interstitial tissue were also observed. Voller *et al.* (1973) also studied the kidneys of *Aotus* infected with *P. malariae* and *P. brasilianium*. In the acute phase there was an increase in mesangial matrix and a proliferation of endothelial and mesangial cells in some glomeruli. IgM deposits were found in the mesangial regions by immunofluorescence but not by electron microscopy. In chronic infections the animals showed segmental or diffuse changes in the glomeruli characterized by swelling and proliferation of mesangial cells with abnormally large amounts of mesangial matrix, sometimes extending to the peripheral capillary zone. IgM and B1C/B1A were identified by immunofluorescence. Electron microscopy showed variable thickening of the basement membrane, with areas of altered electron density and occasional small inclusions. No deposits were present in the basement membrane. The general features of *Aotus* nephrosis following *P. malariae* infection are similar to those described in patients with quartan malaria nephrotic syndrome (Voller *et al.*, 1971).

Histopathological studies of kidneys of rodents with malaria are scanty (Miller *et al.*, 1968). Greenwood and Voller (1970a,b) were the first workers to address the problem in New Zealand mice infected with *P. berghei*. Although several interesting findings were reported by these authors, unfortunately, because of spontaneous development of nephropathy and the possibility of a latent virus infection in this mouse strain, they are not suitable for study. Ehrich and Voller (1972) inoculated Swiss albino mice with *P. berghei yoelii* strain 17X. They observed that the deposition of glomerular immunoglobulin paralleled development of the parasitemia. One month after the disappearance of the parasitemia, the glomerular IgG deposits were no longer detected. Serum proteins did not appear in the urine until the sixth day after inoculation (Weise *et al.*, 1972), but on the eighth day there was a 10-fold increase and immune complexes were detected. Suzuki (1972) also reported glomerular IgM deposits in mice infected with virulent *P. berghei* (NK65 strain) for which they were treated. Boonpucknavig *et al.* (1972), in a study on mice infected with *P. berghei,* found antigen deposited along the glomerular capillary walls in a granular pattern and extending into the mesangial areas. Plasmodial antigen was detected on the third day after inoculation, and antibody and complement on the seventh day. Histologically, the glomerular lesion consisted of mesangial cell proliferation, endothelial cell hypertrophy, polymorphonuclear cell infiltrations, and thickening of the glomerular basement membrane. There was hemosiderin pigment in the proximal tubular cells.

Rhesus monkeys (*M. mulatta*) infected with *P. knowlesi* (Rosen *et al.*, 1968b) excreted large quantities of hemoglobin, became oliguric, and developed acute renal failure. They developed a condition resembling human blackwater fever. The rapid intravascular hemolysis was reflected by a progressive hematocrit decrease and a fall in total serum protein. Light microscopy revealed hyaline droplet degeneration and hemoglobin granules in the proximal tubules (Rosen *et al.*, 1968b; Boonpuckanavig, 1973). Suzuki (1974) produced immune complex disease in mice infected with *P. berghei* and treated with sulfamonomethoxine (DJ1550). In these mice the parasitemia persisted during a 60-day period, and in 15 mice studied there were generalized or localized diffuse or disseminated glomerular IgM deposits, but none had IgG deposits in their kidneys. In 7 out of 15 mice, focal antigen deposits were found in the glomeruli (Fig. 36). Histologi-

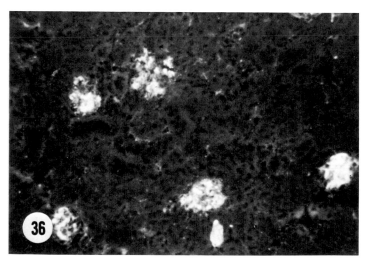

FIG. 36. Immunofluorescent micrograph of the kidney of a mouse infected with *P. berghei* showing diffuse staining for IgM in the glomeruli. ×360.

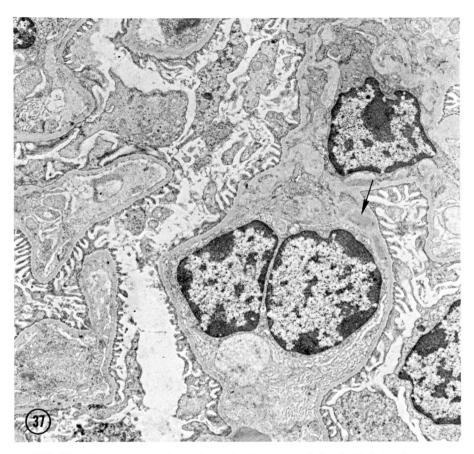

FIG. 37. Electron micrograph of a glomerulus from a mouse infected with *P. berghei* showing mesangial expansion and electron-dense deposits in the mesangial matrix (arrow). ×8000.

cally there was a massive mesangial matrix increase accompanied by glomerular hypercellularity (Figs. 37 and 38). George *et al.* (1976) studied malarial nephropathy in mice using several strain of mice infected with *P. berghei yoelii* 17X. They detected glomerular deposits of IgG and IgM; C3 persisted longer than the immunoglobulins, and malarial antigen was detected by the indirect fluorescent antibody technique.

All mice studied so far have developed acute glomerulonephritis during plasmodial infection, similar to acute falciparum glomerulonephritis, but none have developed lesions resembling those of the *P. malariae* nephrotic syndrome. The plasmodia antigens responsible for the malarial nephropathy observed in rodents have not been isolated yet. K. Waki (unpublished observation) inoculated nude mice with *P. berghei* (NK65) and detected IgG and IgM in low titers during the

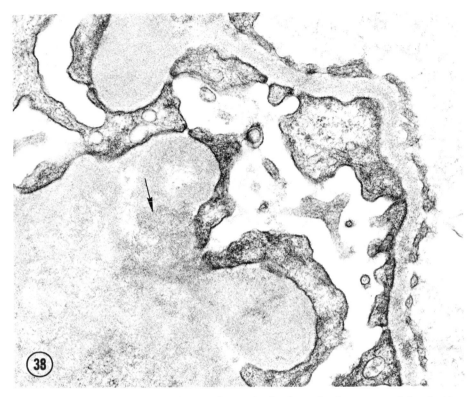

FIG. 38.   High-magnification electron micrograph of a glomerulus from a mouse infected with *P. berghei* showing electron-dense deposits (arrow) in the mesangium. ×36000.

primary attack. The IgG response indicates that T-cell-independent antigens occur in *Plasmodium* parasites. M. Suzuki (unpublished data) observed typical glomerular injuries in nude mice, suggesting that malarial glomerulonephritis is at least partly induced by a T-cell-independent antigen.

Kibukamusoke and Voller (1970), in Uganda, compared IgG, IgM, and malarial antibody levels in patients with active nephrotic syndrome to levels in individuals with the nephrotic syndrome in remission and to levels in individuals without the nephrotic syndrome. The first two groups had high levels of IgM and antiplasmodial antibody in their serum and immune complex deposits in renal biopsies, suggesting that IgM is related to malarial nephropathy. IgM immunoglobuin has also been observed in human glomeruli (Ward and Kibukamusoke, 1969; Ward and Conran, 1969; Bhamarapravati *et al.*, 1973), *Aotus* (Voller *et al.*, 1971, 1973), and mice (Suzuki, 1974). Dreesman and Germuth (1972) reported that rabbits injected with bovine serum albumin produced large immune

complexes whose major antibody class weakly bound antibody to 1
these animals the immune response is associated with a unique glot
lesion consisting of a focal glomerular necrosis without diffuse proliferative
changes. The nature of this IgM-induced lesion is reminiscent of glomerular
lesions seen in *P. malariae* where IgM is predominant and, moreover, it resembles nonproliferative glomerulosclerosis of the type described by White
(1973).

Lambert and Houba (1974) showed that ^{125}I-labeled anti-*P. malariae* IgG
persisted as a complex in *Aotus* monkeys infected with *P. malariae* but not in
control animals. Antimalarial antibodies were also demonstrated with labeled
IgG fractions in the infected monkeys. IgG specific for *P. malariae* is found in
greater amounts in glomeruli of monkeys infected with *P. malariae* than in those
infected with *P. falciparum*. Houba *et al.* (1976) examined the fate of [125]I-
labeled anti-*P. malariae* IgG in Nigerian nephrotics after intravenous administration and found a more rapid loss of anti-*P. malariae* IgG from the circulation
than of normal IgG. Subsequent biopsies from the patients injected with anti-*P.
malariae* IgG showed that much of the injected IgG was deposited in the kidneys.

Lambert and Houba (1974) measured levels of complement components C3,
C4, and C3 proactivator (C3PA) in the plasma of monkeys infected with *P.
brasilianum* and found these substances to decrease in association with the
parasitemia peak. This pattern of decreased complement component levels in the
plasma during parasitemia peaks may reflect complement absorption by circulating or deposited antigen–antibody complexes which are produced when the parasites are removed by the immune system.

IX. NEUROPATHOLOGY

There are many reviews of the literature on cerebral malaria (Spitz, 1940;
Thomas, 1971; Marsden and Bruce Chwatt, 1975), especially that dealing with
P. falciparum. Marked central nervous system changes occur with this parasite in
approximately 2% of patients with acute disease (Daroff *et al.*, 1967). Postmortem examination of patients who have died of cerebral malaria reveals an
edematous brain with broadened and flattened gyri (Fig. 39). The arachnoid
blood vessels are congested, giving the classic "pink brain" appearance (Fig.
39). The cortex is usually grayish-blue because of deposition of pigment, and
petechial hemorrhages are common.

Microscopically, capillaries are occluded by erythrocyte masses (Fig. 40)
(Connor *et al.*, 1976). Many red blood cells contain parasites, and in medium-
sized vessels they are seen marginated against the endothelial cells which are
often swollen, necrotic, or desquamated (Fig. 41). Malaria pigment is present,
and in good preparations schizonts are easily recognized. Medium-sized arteries

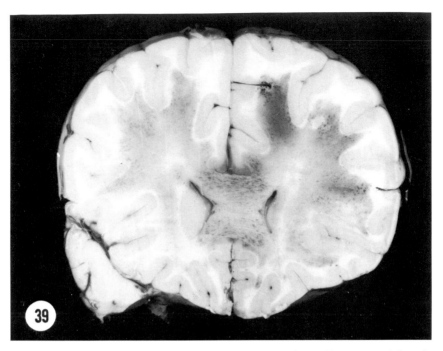

FIG. 39. Brain from a malaria patient showing congestion of the white matter and flattening gyri. (Courtesy of D. Connor, AFIP #76-2858.)

are not usually occluded, and chronic inflammatory cells are common, especially around the vessels.

After 10 days of infection, concomitant with thrombosis formation, ring-hemorrhages appear around the blood vessels (Figs. 42 and 43). The brain stroma, particularly around the neurons and the blood vessels, is vacuolated as a result of severe edema, with necrosis and demyelinization of nerve fibers. Later, these lesions will result in the formation of microgranulomata known as Dürck's granulomas (Dürck, 1917; Dhayagude and Purandare, 1943).

The final stages of the pathophysiology of cerebral falciparum malaria are not well-known. Anoxia plays an important role in the acute phase of the disease (Rigdon, 1944; Maegraith, 1965) and brain lesions are reversible, since treated patients recover and show no apparent sequelae later in life. There are studies on animals (Maegraith and Onabanjo, 1970; Onabanjo and Maegraith, 1970, 1971) suggesting that the clogging of brain capillaries produces an irreversible impedance of local blood flow. Kallikrein, an active blood peptide isolated from monkeys infected with *P. knowlesi,* has been found to produce increased brain capillary permeability. If the peptide plus protamine blue dye is injected into the brains of normal guinea pigs, staining of brain substance and the appearance of

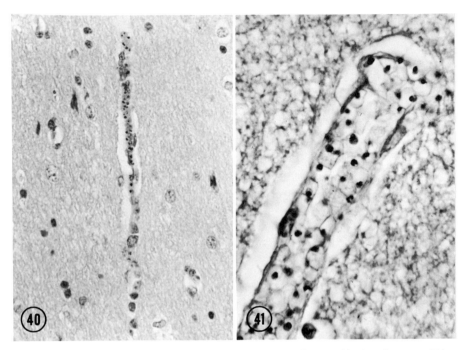

FIG. 40. Brain from a *P. falciparum*-infected monkey showing parasitized erythrocytes within the capillary. ×475. (Reproduced from Jervis *et al.,* 1972, by permission of the author and publisher.)

FIG. 41. Capillary showing infected erythrocytes and swollen endothelial cells. The space around the capillary may be due to edema. ×1500. (Courtesy of D. Connor, AFIP #66-6166-7.)

the dye in the cerebrospinal fluid are seen. Migasera and Maegraith (1965) have reported that a blood–brain barrier breakdown occurs in animals with acute *P. knowlesi* and *P. berghei* infections, suggesting that pharmacologically active substances are released when antibody and antigen react. The action of these substances on endothelial permeability could be one mechanism for the production of lesions in animal brains where parasitized erythrocytes are clumped in brain capillaries. Their experiments suggest that in malaria the endothelial lesion results from a combination of both mechanically and chemically mediated damage.

Yoeli and Hargreaves (1974) described a virulent (17X) strain of *P. berghei* (*P. berghei yoelii*) which produced infections in mice associated with prominent intravascular sequestration of parasitized and nonparasitized erythrocytes in the brain. The capillaries are blocked by sequestered erythrocytes, and ballooning of endothelial cells and fine petechial hemorrhages on the brain surface and in the stroma are seen. They suggested that the virulence of this strain is based on its

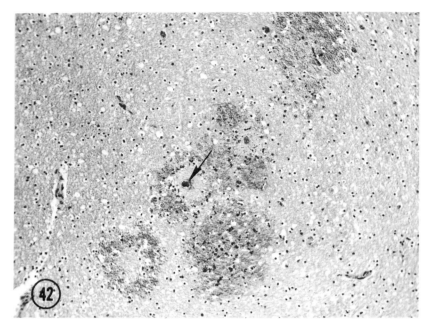

FIG. 42. Ring hemorrhages in the brain surrounding thrombosed vessels (arrow). ×100. (Courtesy of D. Connor, AFIP #56-21641.)

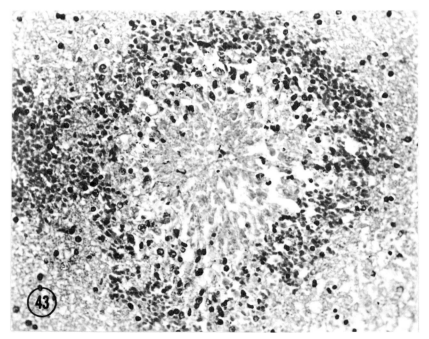

FIG 43. High-magnification micrograph showing a ring-hemorrhage in the brain. ×300. (Courtesy of D. Connor, AFIP #66-6870.)

ability to induce intravascular sequestration of infected erythrocytes with blockage of small and large brain capillaries. On the other hand, other virulent strains of *P. berghei* such as NK65 and KS61 do not produce vascular blockage in the brain, although they cause fatal infections. Mice infected with *P. vinckei* may also die, but only rarely are infected erythrocytes found in cerebral capillaries. Therefore, the 17X strain of *P. berghei* appears to be the only *Plasmodium* strain useful for studies on cerebral malaria.

Mercado (1965) described paralysis of rats infected with *P. berghei*. Their brains contained extensive focal cerebral hemorrhages. This paralysis apparently can be prevented by splenectomy prior to infection, suggesting an immunological mechanism in its development (Mercado, 1973).

X. PLACENTA PATHOLOGY

The placenta is involved in malaria infections. Grossly, there is enlargement, and the color is slate gray (Fig. 44). Microscopically, abundant parasites are seen in the maternal circulation in the intervillous spaces (Fig. 45). Pigment deposits are seen in macrophages located in the intervillous spaces and rarely in the parenchyme (Fig. 46). Lymphocytic infiltration may be focally present, with a picture of lymphocytic and histiocytic villitis. Placental infection by any or-

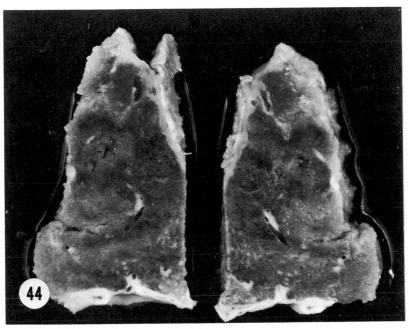

FIG. 44. Dark placenta from a malaria patient. (Courtesy of D. Connor, AFIP #76-2848.)

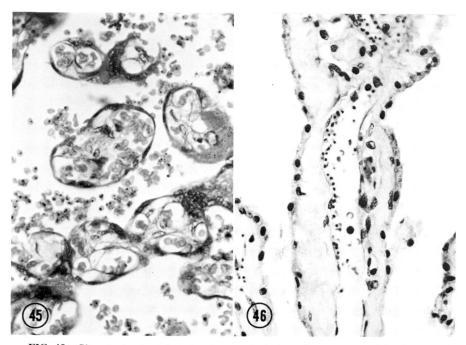

FIG. 45.   Placenta showing infected erythrocytes in the intervillous spaces. ×400. (Courtesy of D. Connor, AFIP #66-1636.)

FIG. 46.   Placenta showing pigmented cells in the intervillous spaces and rarely in the parenchyme. ×370. (Courtesy of D. Connor, AFIP #66-5892.)

ganism serves as a focus of fetal infections, and cases of intrauterine-acquired malaria are common in endemic areas. The effect of placental infection with *Plasmodium* on the fetus has been studied in Africa by Archibald (1956) who found that plasmodia caused at least 2% of all births in Africa to be premature. Tchakamakow (1954) reported postmortem findings in 20 stillborn infants from mothers with malaria in Macedonia and suggested that asphyxia was the cause of death.

It is known that the maternal circulation of the placenta retains erythrocytes infected with *P. falciparum*. Recently, Bray and Sinden (1979) examined, by electron microscopy, placentae of patients infected with *P. falciparum* and found no special concentration of infected erythrocytes attached to the syncitial trophoblast. They suggested that the surface irregularities seen in *P. falciparum* infected erythrocytes might delay the passage of these infected cells through the maternal circulation of the placenta. However, exact membranes causing retention of infected erythrocytes in the placenta are still not understood.

ACKNOWLEDGMENTS

This work was supported in part by research grants AI-10645 and AI-13366 from the U.S. Public Health Service, the U.S. Army R. and D. Command (DAMD17-79C-9029) and the WHO (M2/181/145).

The authors wish to thank Drs. A. Allen, D. Connor, H. Jervis, D. MacCallum, B. Schnitzer, and R. White for supplying micrographs, and Dr. V. Boonpucknavig for supplying autopsy material used in this chapter.

REFERENCES

Adeniyi, A., Hendrickse, R. G., and Houba, W. (1970). Selectivity of proteinuria and response to prednisolone or immunosuppressive drugs in children with malarial nephrosis. *Lancet* **1**, 644-648.

Aikawa, M. (1971). Parasitological review: *Plasmodium:* The fine structure of malarial parasites. *Exp. Parasitol.* **30**, 284-320.

Aikawa, M., and Antonovych, T. (1964). Electron microscopic observations of *Plasmodium berghei* and the Kupffer cell in the liver of rats. *J. Parasitol.* **50**, 620-629.

Aikawa, M., and Sprinz, H. (1971). Erythrophagocytosis in the bone marrow of canary infected with malaria: An electron microscopic observation. *Lab. Invest.* **24**, 45-54.

Aikawa, M., Huff, C. G., and Sprinz, H. (1968): Exoerythrocytic stages of *Plasmodium gallinaceum* in chick-embryo liver as observed electron microscopically. *Am. J. Trop. Med. Hyg.* **17**, 156-169.

Aikawa, M., Rabbege, J. R., and Wellde, B. T. (1972). Junctional apparatus in erythrocytes infected with malarial parasites. *Z. Zellforsch. Mikrosk. Anat.* **124**, 72-75.

Aikawa, M., Miller, L. H., and Rabbege, J. R. (1975). Caveola-vesicle complexes in the plasmalemma of erythrocytes infected by *Plasmodium vivax* and *P. cynomolgi. Am. J. Pathol.* **79**, 285-300.

Al-Dabagh, M. A., (1966). "Mechanism of Death and Tissue Injury in Malaria with Special Reference to Five Species of Avian Malaria," p. 240. Shafik Press, Bagdad.

Allen, A. C. (1962). "The Kidney," pp. 479-485. Grune & Stratton, New York.

Allison, A. C., (1954). Distribution of sickle cell trait in East Africa and elsewhere, and its apparent relationship to incidence of subtertian malaria. *Trans. Roy. Soc. Trop. Med. Hyg.* **48**, 312-318.

Allison, A. C., Hendrickse, R. G., Edington, G. M., Houba, V., de Petris, S., and Adeniyi, A. (1969). Immune complexes in the nephrotic syndrome of African children. *Lancet* **1**, 1232-1237.

Archibald, H. M., (1956). The influence of malarial infection of the placenta on the incidence of prematurity. *Bull. W.H.O.* **15**, 842-845.

Berger, M., Birch, L. M., and Conte, N. F., (1967). The nephrotic syndrome secondary to acute glomerulonephritis during falciparum malaria. *Ann. Intern. Med.* **67**, 1163-1171.

Bhamarapravati, N., Boonpucknavig, S., Boonpucknavig, V., and Yaemboonruang, C. (1973). Glomerular changes in acute *Plasmodium falciparum* infection. *Arch. Pathol.* **96**, 289-293.

Boonpucknavig, S., Boonpucknavig, V., and Bhamarapravati, N. (1972). Immunopathological studies of *Plasmodium berghei*-infected mice: Immune complex nephritis. *Arch. Pathol.* **94**, 322-330.

Boonpucknavig, V., and Sitprija, V. (1979). Renal disease in acute *Plasmodium falciparum* infection in man. *Kidney Int.* 16:44-52.

Boonpucknavig, V., Boonpucknavig, S., and Bhamarapravati, N. (1973). *Plasmodium berghei* infection in mice: An ultrastructural study of immune complex nephritis. *Am. J. Pathol.* **70**, 89–108.

Boyd, M. F. (1940). Observations on naturally and artifically induced quartan malaria. *Am. J. Trop. Med. Hyg.* **20**, 749–798.

Boyd, M. F. (1949). A comprehensive survey of all aspects of this group of diseases from a global standpoint. *In* "Malariology" (M. F. Boyd, ed.), Vol. 1, pp. 579–599. Saunders, Philadelphia, Pennsylvania.

Bray, R. S., and Sinden, R. E., (1979). The sequestration of *Plasmodium falciparum* infected erythrocytes in the placenta. *Trans. Roy. Soc. Trop. Med. Hyg.* **73**, 716–719.

Brooks, M. H., Kiel, F. W., Sheehy, T. W., and Barry, K. G. (1968). Acute pulmonary edema in falciparum malaria: A clinicopathological correlation. *N. Engl. J. Med.* **279**, 732–737.

Chulay, J., Aikawa, M., Diggs, C. L., and Haynes, J. D. (1979). Inhibition of *in vitro* growth of *Plasmodium falciparum* by immune monkey serum: A light and electron microscopic study. *In* "19th Inter-Science Conference on Antimicrobial Agents and Chemotherapy," Abstract #437 Boston, Massachusetts.

Coggeshall, L. T. (1937). Splenomegaly in experimental monkey malaria. *Am. J. Trop. Med. Hyg.* **17**, 605–617.

Connor, D. H., Neafie, R. C., and Hockmeyer, W. T. (1976). Malaria. *In* "Pathology of Tropical and Extraordinary Diseases" (C. H. Binford and D. Connor, eds.), pp. 273–283. Armed Forces Inst. Pathol., Washington, D.C.

Craig, C. F. (1909). "The Malarial Fevers, Haemoglobinuric Fever, and the Blood Protozoa of Man". Wood, New York.

Daroff, R. B., Deller, J. J., Jr., Kastl, A. J., Jr., and Blocker, W. W., Jr. (1967). Cerebral malaria. *J. Am. Med. Assoc.* **202**, 679–682.

Deaton, J. G. (1970). Fatal pulmonary edema as a complication of acute falciparum malaria. *Am. J. Trop. Med. Hyg.* **19**, 196–201.

de Brito, T., Barone, A. A., and Faria, R. M. (1969). Human liver biopsy in *P. falciparum* and *P. vivax:* A light and electron microscopy study. *Virchows Arch. A* **348**, 220–229.

Dennis, L. H., Eichelberger, J. W., and Conrad, M. E., (1966a). Depletion of coagulation factors in drug resistant *Plasmodium falciparum* malaria. *Clin. Res.* **14**, 338.

Dennis, L. H., Eichelberger, J. W., Doenhoft, A. E., and Conrad, M. E. (1966b). A coagulation defect and its treatment with heparin in *Plasmodium knowlesi* malaria in rhesus monkeys. *Mil. Med.* **131**, Suppl., 1107–1110.

Dennis, L. H., Eichelberger, J. W., Inman, M. M., and Conrad, M. E. (1967). Depletion of coagulation factors in drug-resistant *Plasmodium falciparum* malaria. *Blood* **29**, 713–721.

Desowitz, R. S., and Pavanand, K. (1967). A vascular permeability-increasing factor in the serum of monkeys infected with primate malarias. *Ann. Trop. Med. Parasitol.* **61**, 128–133.

Desowitz, R. S., Miller, L. H., Buchanan, R. D., Yuthasastrkosol, V., and Permpanich, B. (1967). Comparative studies on the pathology and host physiology of malarias. I. *Plasmodium coatneyi. Ann. Trop. Med. Parasitol.* **61**, 365–374.

Devakul, K. (1960). Sugar metabolism in malaria. *Trans. R. Soc. Trop. Med. Hyg.* **54**, 87.

Devakul, K., and Maegraith, B. G. (1958). Blood sugar and tissue glycogen in infections in *Macaca mulatta* with the Nuri strain of *Plasmodium knowlesi. Ann. Trop. Med. Parasitol.* **52**, 366–375.

Devakul, K., and Maegraith, B. G. (1959). Lysis and other circulatory phenomena in malaria (*Plasmodium knowlesi*). *Ann. Trop. Med. Parasitol.* **53**, 430–450.

Devakul, K., Harinasuta, T., and Reid, H. A. (1966). ^{125}I-labeled fibrinogen in cerebral malaria. *Lancet* **2**, 886–888.

Dhayagude, R. G., and Puranare, N. M. (1943). Autopsy study of cerebral malaria with special reference to malarial granuloma. *Arch. Pathol.* **36**, 550–558.

Dixon, F. J. (1966). Comments on immunopathology. *Mil. Med.* **131**, Suppl., 1233.

Dreesman, G. R., and Germuth, F. G., Jr. (1972). Immune complex disease, IV. The nature of the circulating complexes associated with glomerulonephritis in the acute BSA-rabbit system. *Johns Hopkins Med. J.* **130**, 335–343.

Dukes, D. C., Sealey, B. J., and Forbes, J. I. (1968). Oliguric renal failure in blackwater fevers. *Am. J. Med.* **45**, 889–903.

Dürck, H. (1917). Über die bei Malaria perniciosa comotosa auftretenden Veränderungen des Zentralnervensystems. *Arch. Schiffs- Trop. Hyg.* **21**, 117–132.

Edington, G. M., and Gilles, H. M. (1976). The urinary and Reproductive systems *In* "Pathology in the Tropics," pp. 616–652. Arnold, London.

Ehrich, J. H. H., and Voller, A. (1972). Studies on the kidneys of mice infected with rodent malaria. I. Deposition of gamma-globulin in glomeruli in the early stage of the disease. *Z. Tropenmed. Parasitol.* **23**, 147–152.

Eling, W., Van Zon, A. and Jerusalem, C., (1977) The course of a *Plasmodium berghei* infection in six different mouse strains. *Zeitschrift für Parasitenke*, **54**, 29–45.

Feldman, J. D. (1963). Pathogenesis of ultrastructural glomerular changes induced by immunologic means. *In* "Immunopathology" (P. Grabar and P. A. Miescher, eds.), pp. 263–281. Grune & Stratton, New York.

Field, J. W., and Shute, P. G. (1956). "The Microscopic Diagnosis of Human Malaria. II. A Morphological Study of the Erythrocytic Parasites," pp. 18–20. Government Press, Kuala Lumpur.

Friedman, M. J. (1979). Ultrastructural damage to the malaria parasite in sickled cell. *J. Protozool.* **26**, 195–199.

Fulton, J. D. (1939). Experiments on the utilization of sugars by malarial parasites (*Plasmodium knowlesi*). *Ann. Trop. Med. Parasitol.* **33**, 217–227.

Geiman, Q. M., and Siddiqui, W. (1969). Susceptibility of a New World monkey to *Plasmodium malariae*. *Am. J. Trop. Med. Hyg.* **18**, 351–354.

George, C. R. P., Parbtani, A., and Cameron, J. S. (1976). Mouse malaria nephropathy. *J. Pathol.* **120**, 235–249.

Gilles, H. M., and Hendrickse, R. G. (1960). Possible aetiological role of *Plasmodium malariae* in "nephrotic syndrome" in Nigerian children. *Lancet* **1**, 806–807.

Gilles, H. M., and Hendrickse, R. G. (1963). Nephrosis in Nigerian children: Role of *Plasmodium malariae*, and effect of antimalarial treatment. *Br. Med. J.* **2**, 27–31.

Gilles, H. M., and Ikeme, A. C. (1960). Haemoglobinuria among adult Nigerians due to glucose-6-phosphate dehydrogenase deficiency with drug sensitivity. *Lancet* **2**, 889–891.

Godard, J. E., and Hansen, R. A., (1971). Interstitial pulmonary edema in acute malaria. Report of a case. *Radiology* **101**, 523–524.

Goodwin, L. G., and Richards, W. H. G. (1960). Pharmacologically active peptides in the blood and urine of animals with *Babesia rodhaini* and other pathogenic organisms. *Br. J. Pharm. Chemother.* **15**, 152–159.

Gravely, S., Hamburger, J., and Kreier, J. P. (1976). T and B cell population changes in young and adult rats infected with *Plasmodium berghei*. *Infect. Immun.* **14**, 178–183.

Greenwood, B. M., and Voller, A. (1970a). Suppression of autoimmune disease in New Zealand mice associated with infection with malaria. I. (NZB X NZW) F_1 hybrid mice. *Clin. Exp. Immunol.* **7**, 793–803.

Greenwood, B. M., and Voller, A. (1970b). Suppression of autoimmune disease in New Zealand mice associated with infection with malaria. II. NZB mice. *Clin. Exp. Immunol.* **7**, 805–815.

Gutierrez, Y., Aikawa, M., Fremount, H. N., and Sterling, C. R. (1976). Experimental infection of *Aotus* monkeys with *Plasmodium falciparum:* Light and electron microscopic changes. *Ann. Trop. Med. Parasitol.* **70**, 25–44.

Hall, A. P., (1976). The treatment of malaria. *Br. Med. J.*, **1**, 323–328.

Hartenbower, D. L., Kantor, G. L., and Rosen, V. J. (1972). Renal failure due to acute glomerulonephritis during falciparum malaria: Case report. *Mil. Med.* **137,** 74–76.

Hendrickse, R. G., and Gilles, H. M. (1963). The nephrotic syndrome and other renal diseases in children in western Nigeria. *East Afr. Med. J.* **40,** 186–201.

Hendrickse, R. G., Adeniyi, A., Edington, G. M., Glascow, E. F., White, R. H. R., and Houba, V. (1972). Quartan malarial nephrotic syndrome: Collaborative clinicopathological study in Nigerian children. *Lancet* **1,** 1143–1148.

Hiott, D. W. (1969). Ultrastructural changes in heart muscle after hemorrhagic shock and isoproterenol infusions. *Arch. Int. Pharmacodyn. Ther.* **180,** 206–216.

Houba, V., Allison, A. C., Adeniyi, A., and Houba, J. E. (1971). Immunoglobulin classes and complement in biopsies of Nigerian children with the nephrotic syndrome. *Clin. Exp. Immunol.* **8,** 761–774.

Houba, V., Lambert, P. H., Voller, A., and Soyanwo, M. A. O. (1976). Clincal and experimental investigation of immune complexes in malaria. *Clin. Immunol. Pathol.* **6,** 1–12.

Jervis, H. R., MacCallum, D. K., and Sprinz, H. (1968). Experimental *Plasmodium berghei* infection in the hamster: Its effect on the liver. *Arch. Pathol.* **86,** 328–337.

Jervis, H. R., Sprinz, H., Johnson, A. J., and Wellde, B. T. (1972). Experimental infection with *Plasmodium falciparum* in *Aotus* monkeys. II. Observations on host pathology. *Am. J. Trop. Med. Hyg.* **21,** 272–281.

Kibukamusoke, J. W. (1973). Parasitology. Effect of rainfall on incidence of the nephrotic syndrome. *In* "Nephrotic Syndrome of Quartan Malaria," pp. 40–43. Arnold, London.

Kibukamusoke, J. W., and Hutt, M. S. R. (1967). Histological features of the nephrotic syndrome associated with quartan malaria. *J. Clin. Pathol.* **20,** 117–123.

Kibukamusoke, J. W., and Voller, A. (1970). Serological studies on the nephrotic syndrome of quartan malaria in Uganda. *Br. Med. J.* **1,** 406–407.

Kilejian, A., Abati, A., and Trager, W. (1977). *Plasmodium falciparum* and *Plasmodium coatneyi:* Immunogenicity of "knob-like protrusions" on infected erythrocyte membranes. *Exp. Parasitol.* **42,** 157–164.

Kreier, J. P., Seed, T., Mohan, R., and Pfister, R. (1972a). *Plasmodium* spp: The relationship between erythrocyte morphology and parasitization in chickens, rats, and mice. *Exp. Parasitol.* **31,** 19–28.

Kreier, J. P., Mohan, R., Seed, T., and Pfisten, R. (1972b). Studies of the morphology and survival characteristics of erythrocytes from mice and rats with *Plasmodium berghei* infection. *Z. Tropenmed. Parasitol.* **23,** 245–255.

Lambert, P. H., and Houba, V. (1974). Immune complexes in parasitic disease. *In* "Progress: Immunology" (B. Amos, ed.), pp. 57–67. Academic Press, New York.

Luse, S. A., and Miller, L. H. (1971). *Plasmodium falciparum* malaria: Ultrastructure of parasitized erythrocytes in cardiac vessels. *Am. J. Trop. Med. Hyg.* **20,** 655–660.

MacCallum, D. K. (1968). Pulmonary changes resulting from experimental malaria in hamsters. *Arch. Pathol.* **122,** 681–688.

MacCallum, D. K. (1969a). Time sequence study on the hepatic system of macrophages in malaria-infected hamsters. *RES, J. Reticuloendothel. Soc.* **6,** 232–252.

MacCallum, D. K. (1969b). A study of macrophage: Pulmonary vascular bed interactions in malaria-infected hamsters. *RES, J. Reticuloendothel. Soc.* **6,** 253–270.

Maegraith, B. G. (1948). "Pathological Process in Malaria and Blackwater Fever." Blackwell, Oxford.

Maegraith, B. G. (1954). Some physiological and pathological processes in *Plasmodium berghei* infections in white rats. *Indian J. Malariol.* **8,** 281–290.

Maegraith, B. G. (1965). Exotic diseases which may be encountered in temperate climates. *Bull. Soc. Pathol. Exot.* **57,** 738–744.

Maegraith, B. G. (1966). Pathogenic processes in malaria. *In* "The Pathology of Parasitic Diseases" (A. E. R. Taylor, ed.), pp. 15–32. Blackwell, Oxford.

Maegraith, B. G., and Onabanjo, A. O. (1970). The effects of histamine in malaria. *Br. J. Pharmacol.* **39,** 755–764.

Maegraith, B. G., Riley, M. V., and Deegan, T. (1962). Changes in the metabolism of liver mitochondria of monkeys infected with *Plasmodium knowlesi* and their importance in the pathogenesis of malaria. *Ann. Trop. Med. Parasitol.* **56,** 483–491.

Maegraith, B. G., Fletcher, K. A., Angus, M. G. N., and Thurnham, D. I. (1963). Further observations on the inhibition of tissue metabolism in malaria. *Trans. R. Soc. Trop. Med. Hyg.* **57,** 2.

Mannaberg, J. (1905). Malarial diseases. *In* "Nothnagel's Encyclopedia of Practical Medicine," pp. 17–517. Philadelphia, Pennsylvania.

Marchiafava, E., and Bignami, A. (1900). Malaria. *In* Twentieth Century Practice of Medicine. An International Encyclopedia of Modern Medical Science. *19*:227–252.

Marchoux, E. (1926). Paludisme. "Nouveau Traite de Medicine et de Therapeutique". Paris, Vol. **5,** 366.

Marks, S. M., Holland, S., and Gelfand, M. (1977). Malarial lung: Report of a case from Africa successfully treated with intermittent positive pressure ventilation. *Am. J. Trop. Med. Hyg.* **26,** 179–180.

Marsden, P. D., and Bruce-Chwatt, L. J. (1975). Cerebral malaria. *In* "Topics on Tropical Neurology" (R. W. Hornabrook, ed.), Vol. 12, pp. 29–44. Davis, Philadelphia, Pennsylvania.

Marsden, P. D., Hutt, M. S. R., Wilks, N. E., Voller, A., Blackman, V., Shah, K. K., Connor, D. H., Hamilton, P. J. S., Banwell, J. G., and Lunn, H. F. (1965). An investigation of tropical splenomegaly at Mulago Hospital, Kampala, Uganda. *Br. Med. J.* **1,** 89–92.

Marsden, P. D., Connor, D. H., Voller, A., Kelly, A., Schofield, F. D., and Hutt, M. S. R. (1967). Splenomegaly in New Guinea. *Bull. W.H.O.* **36,** 901–911.

Martin, A. M., Hackel, D., and Kurtz, S. M. (1964). The ultrastructure of zonal lesions of the myocardium in hemorrhagic shock. *Am. J. Pathol.* **44,** 127–140.

Marvin, H. N., and Rigdon, R. H. (1945). Terminal hypoglycemia in ducks with malaria. *Am. J. Hyg.* **42,** 174–178.

Mercado, T. I. (1965). Paralysis associated with *Plasmodium berghei* malaria in the rat. *J. Infect. Dis.* **115,** 465–472.

Mercado, T. I. (1973). *Plasmodium berghei:* Inhibition by splenectomy of a paralysing syndrome in infected rats. *Exp. Parasitol.* **58,** 1137–1142.

Migasera, P., and Maegraith, B. G., (1965). The blood brain barrier in *P. knowlesi* infection. *Trans. Roy. Soc. Trop. Med. Hyg.* **59,** 2.

Miller, L. H., Pavanand, K., Buchanan, R. D., Desowitz, R. S., and Athikulwongse, E. (1968). *Plasmodium berghei:* Renal function and pathology in mice. *Exp. Parasitol.* **23,** 134–142.

Miller, L. H., Mason, S. J., Dvorak, J. A., McGinniss, M. H., and Rothman, I. K. (1975). Erythrocyte receptors for (*Plasmodium knowlesi*) malaria: Duffy blood group determinants. *Science* **189,** 561–563.

Miller, L. H., Mason, S. J., Clyde, D. F., and McGinniss, M. H. (1976). The resistance factor to *Plasmodium vivax* in blacks: The Duffy blood group genotype, FyFy. *N. Engl. J. Med.* **295,** 302–304.

Miller, L. H., Aikawa, M., Johnson, J. G., and Shiroishi, T. (1979). Interaction between cytochalasin B-treated malarial parasites and red cells: Attachment and junction formation. *J. Exp. Med.* **149,** 172–184.

Morel-Maroger, L., Saimot, A. G., Sloper, J. C., Woodrow, D. F., Adam, C., Niang, I., and Payet, M. (1975). "Tropical nephropathy" and "tropical extramembranous glomerulonephritis" of unknown etiology in Senegal. *Br. Med. J.* **1,** 541–546.

Nkrumah, F. K., Sulzer, A. J., and Maddison, S. E. (1979). Serum immunoglobulin levels and malaria antibodies in Burkitt's lymphoma. *Trans. R. Soc. Trop. Med. Hyg.* **73**, 91–95.

Onabanjo, A. O., and Maegraith, B. G. (1970). Inflammatory changes in small blood vessels induced by kallikrein (*Kin nogenase*) in the blood of *Macaca mulatta* infected with *Plasmodium knowlesi. Ann. Trop. Med. Parasitol.* **64**, 227–236.

Onabanjo, A. O., and Maegraith, B. G. (1971). Pathological lesions produced in the brain by kallikrein (*Kin nogenase*) in *Macaca mulatta* infected with *Plasmodium knowlesi. Ann. Trop. Med. Parasitol.* **64**, 237–242.

Pitney, W. R. (1968). The tropcial splenomegaly syndrome. *Trans. R. Soc. Trop. Med. Hyg.* **62**, 717–728.

Punyagupta, S, Srichaikul, T., Nitiyanant, P., and Petchclai, B. (1974). Acute pulmonary insufficiency in *falciparum* malaria: Summary of 12 cases with evidence of disseminated intravascular coagulation. *Am. J. Trop. Med. Hyg.* **23**, 551–559.

Quinn, T. C., and Wyler, D. J. (1979). Intravascular clearance of parasitized erythrocytes in rodent malaria. *J. Clin. Invest.* **63**, 1187–1194.

Ray, A. P., and Sharma, G. K. (1958). Experimental studies on liver injury in malaria. II. Pathogenesis. *Indian J. Med. Res.* **46**, 367–376.

Rigdon, R. H. (1944). The pathological lesions in the brain in malaria. *South. Med. J.* **37**, 687–694.

Riley, M. V., and Deegan, T. (1960). The effect of *Plasmodium berghei* malaria on mouse-liver mitochondria. *Biochem. J.* **76**, 41–46.

Riley, M. V., and Maegraith, B. G. (1961). A factor in the serum of malaria-infected animals capable of inhibiting the *in vitro* oxidative metabolism of normal liver mitochondira. *Ann. Trop. Med. Parasitol.* **55**, 489–497.

Riley, M. V., and Maegraith B. G. (1962). Changes in the metabolism of liver mitochondria in mice infected with rapid acute *Plasmodium berghei* malaria. *Ann. Trop. Med. Parasitol.* **56**, 473–482.

Rosen, S., Hano, J. E., Inman, M. M., Gillilano, P. F., and Barry, K. G. (1968a). The kidney in blackwater fever: Light and electron microscopic observations. *Am. J.. Clin. Pathol.* **49**, 358–370.

Rosen, S., Hano, J. E., and Barry, K. G. (1968b). Malarial nephropathy in the *Rhesus* monkey. *Arch. Pathol.* **85**, 36–44.

Sadun, E. H., Williams, J. S., Meroney, F. C., and Hutt, G. (1965). Pathophysiology of *Plasmodium berghei* infection in mice. *Exp. Parasitol.* **17**, 277–286.

Schnitzer, B., Sodeman, T. M., Mead, M. L., and Contacos, P. G. (1973). An ultrastructural study of the red pulp of the spleen in malaria. *Blood* **41**, 207–217.

Seed, T. M., and Kreier, J. P. (1972). *Plasmodium gallinaceum:* Erythrocyte membrane alteration and associated plasma changes induced by experimental infections. *Proc. Helminthol. Soc. Wash.* **39**, 387–411.

Seed, T. M., Brindley, D., Aikawa, M., and Rabbege, J. R. (1976). *Plasmodium berghei:* Osmotic fragility of malaria parasites and mouse host erythrocytes. *Exp. Parasitol.* **40**, 380–390.

Sheehy, T. W., and Reba, R. C. (1967). Complications of falciparum malaria and their treatment. *Ann. Intern. Med.* **66**, 807–809.

Singer, I. (1954). The cellular reactions to infections with *Plasmodium berghei* in the white mouse. *J. Infect. Dis.* **94**, 241–261.

Skirrow, M. B., Chongsulphajaisiddhi, T., and Maegraith, B. G. (1964). The circulation in malaria. II. Portal angiography in monkeys (*Macaca mulatta*) with *P. knowlesi* and in shock following manipulation of the gut. *Ann. Trop. Med. Parasitol.* **58**, 502–510.

Soothill, J. F., and Hendrickse, R. G. (1967). Some immunological studies of the nephrotic syndrome in Nigerian children. *Lancet* **2**, 629–632.

Spitz, S. (1946). The pathology of acute *falciparum* malaria. *Mil. Surg.* **99**, 555–572.

Stone, W. J., Hanchett, J. E., and Knepshield, J. H. (1972). Acute renal insufficiency due to falciparum malaria: Review of 42 cases. *Arch. Intern. Med.* **129**, 620-628.

Suzuki, M. (1972). Chemotherapy and immunity in rodent malaria. I. Deposits of antigen and antilogous IgM in glomeruli in mice infected with *Plasmodium berghei* (NK65) following treatment by an antimalarial. Preliminary report. *WHO/MAL* **72**, 759.

Suzuki, M. (1974). *Plasmodium berghei:* Experimental rodent model for malarial renal immunopathology. *Exp. Parasitol.* **35**, 187-195.

Suzuki, M. (1975). Lung events in mice infected with rodent plasmodia. *Trans. R. Soc. Trop. Med. Hyg.* **69**, 20.

Suzuki, M., and Waki, K. (1979). Two aspects of immunity to malaria infection. *Proc. Jpn.-Ger. Coop. Symp. Protozoan Dis.* **1**, 181-194.

Swann, A. I., and Kreier, J. P. (1973). *Plasmodium gallinaceum:* Mechanisms of anemia in infected chickens. *Exp. Parasitol.* **33**, 79-88.

Taliaferro, W. H., and Kluver, C. (1940). The hematology of malaria (*Plasmodium brasilianum*) in Panamanian monkeys. I. Numerical changes in leukocytes. *J. Infect. Dis.* **67**, 121-161.

Taliaferro, W. H., and Mulligan, H. W. (1937). The histopathology of malaria with special reference to the function and origin of the macrophages in defense. *Indian Med. Res. Mem.* **29**, 1-138.

Taliaferro, W. H., and Taliaferro, L. G., (1955). Reactions of the connective tissue in chickens to *Plasmodium gallinaceum* and *Plasmodium lophurae*. I. Histopathology during initial infection and superinfections. *J. Infect. Dis.* **97**, 99-136.

Tanabe, K., Waki, S., Takada, S., and Suzuki, M., (1977). *Plasmodium berghei:* Suppressed response to antibody-forming cells in infected mice. Exp. Parasitol. **43**, 143-152.

Tchakmakov, A. (1954). Le paludisme comme cause de la mortalité foetale et des accouchements prématurés. *Acta Fac. Med. Shophiensis* **1**, 55-62.

Thayer, W. S. (1897). "Lectures on the Malarial Fevers". Appleton, New York.

Thomas, J. D. (1971). Cerebral malaria: Clinical and histopathological correlation. *Trop. Geogr. Med.* **23**, 232-238.

Voller, A., Richards, W. H. G., Hawkey, C. M., and Ridley, D. S. (1969). Human malaria (*Plasmodium falciparum*) in owl monkeys (*Aotus trivirgatus*). *Am. J. Trop. Med. Hyg.* **72**, 153-160.

Voller, A., Draper, C. C., Shwe, T., and Hutt, M. S. R. (1971). Nephrotic syndrome in a monkey infected with human quartan malaria. *Br. Med. J.* **4**, 208-210.

Voller, A., Davies, D. R., and Hutt, M. S. R. (1973). Quartan malarial infections in *Aotus trivirgatus* with special reference to renal pathology. *Br. J. Exp. Pathol.* **54**, 457-468.

Waki, S. and Suzuki, M., (1977). A study of malaria immunobiology using nude mice. "Proc. II. Internat. Workshop on Nude Mice," pp. 37-44, Univ. Tokyo Press, Tokyo.

Ward, P. A., and Conran, P. B. (1966). Immunopathological studies of simian malaria. *Mil. Med.* **131**, Suppl., 1225.

Ward, P. A., and Conran, P. B. (1969). Immunopathology of renal complication in simian malaria and human quartan malaria. *Mil. Med.* **134**, 1228-1236.

Ward, P. A., and Kibukamusoke, J. W. (1969). Evidence for soluble immune complexes in the pathogenesis of the glomerulonephritis of quartan malaria. *Lancet* **1**, 283-285.

Watson, M. (1905). Some clinical features of quartan malaria. *Indiana Med. Gaz.* **40**, 49-52.

Weise, M., Ehrich, J. C. H., and Weise, R. (1972). Studies on the kidneys of mice infected with rodent malaria. II. Characterization of urinary proteins by microdisc electrophoresis. *Z. Tropenmed. Parasitol.* **23**, 399-405.

Wellde, B. T., Johnson, A. J., Williams, J. S., Langbehn, H. R., and Sadun, E. H. (1971a). Hematologic, biochemical and parasitologic parameters of the night monkey (*Aotus trivirgatus*). *Lab. Anim. Sci.* **21**, 575-580.

Wellde, B. T., Johnson, M. R., and Zimmerman, M. R. (1971b). Parasitologic, biochemical, hematologic, and pathologic investigations of *Aotus* monkeys infected with *Plasmodium falciparum*. *J. Parasitol.* **56**, 364.

Wellde, B. T., Johnson, A. J., Williams, J. S., Diggs, C. L., and Sadun, E. H. (1972). Experimental infection with *Plasmodium falciparum* in *Aotus* monkeys: I. Observations on host parasitology, hematology, and serology. *Am. J. Trop. Med. Hyg.* **21**, 260–271.

White, R. H. R. (1973). Quartan malarial nephrotic syndrome. *Nephron* **11**, 147–162.

Winslow, D. J., Connor, D. H., and Sprinz, H. (1975). Malaria. *In* "Pathology of Protozoal and Helminthic Diseases" (R. A. Marcial-Rojas, ed.), pp. 195–224. Williams & Wilkins Co. Baltimore.

World Health Organization (1973). Chemotherapy of malaria and resistance to antimalarials. *W.H.O., Tech. Rep. Ser.* **529**, 121.

Wright, D. H., Masembre, R. E., and Bazira, E. R., (1971). The effect of antithymocyte serum on golden hamsters and rats infected with *Plasmodium berghei*. *Bri. J. Exp. Path.* **52**, 465–477.

Yoeli, M. and Hargreaves, B. J. (1974). Brain capillary blockage produced by a virulent strain of rodent malaria. *Science.* **184**, 572–573.

Colonization and Maintenance of Mosquitoes in the Laboratory

Woodbridge A. Foster

I. INTRODUCTION

The colonization and maintenance of mosquito colonies is, at present, prerequisite to any laboratory work with malaria requiring completion of the sporogonic cycle. This applies first to studies on the extrinsic cycle of *Plasmodium* and the mechanisms of its transmission. It also includes studies on vaccines in which a natural or seminatural challenge is preferred, or in which sporozoites are the immunogenic material. Furthermore, laboratory transmission by mosquitoes is necessary in the maintenance of *Plasmodium* strains if they are to retain the ability to infect mosquitoes (see Killick-Kendrick, 1971). Mosquitoes also act as vectors of a great many other pathogens and parasites of vertebrates, and they are in themselves a nuisance to humans and sometimes cause economic loss through their attacks on livestock. All these concerns have contributed to an ever-growing effort to colonize more species of mosquitoes, to refine the techniques for doing so, and to develop methods of mass production. The colonies are then used to study mosquito–disease relationships and the bionomics, physiology, genetics, and toxicology of individual species and local varieties in order to find more effective means of mosquito control. Mass production methods have been heavily emphasized in recent years because of the imminent possibility of controlling mosquitoes through the massive release of sterilized or genetically different laboratory-reared mosquitoes into natural populations (see Smith, 1966; Chambers, 1977). The result of these efforts in mosquito rearing has been a voluminous and continually expanding literature on technique, covering a wide range of mosquito species under a variety of laboratory conditions.

The literature on mosquito rearing is diffuse and often redundant. Fortunately, the older literature has been reviewed or summarized several times (e.g., Bates, 1949; Bradley *et al.*, 1949; Trembley, 1955; Russell *et al.*, 1963); the most recent review (Gerberg, 1970) is quite comprehensive and covers the majority of techniques currently in use; it includes specific procedures for maintaining colonies of various species in 18 mosquito genera. Though techniques for many more mosquitoes have been developed since that time, an account of them is beyond the scope of the present chapter. Aside from the fact that most of the mosquitoes are of little concern to malariologists, published rearing techniques seldom represent the final product of an intensive and systematic effort to find the most efficient and productive methods; more often they are simply methods that are successful. The formulas of success are continually evolving, and there are also probably many highly successful sets of rearing procedures currently in use which have never been published. Most of the substantial developments in rearing technique have been made with species which have already been colonized and which are being mass-produced. It is only then worthwhile to invest considerable effort to increase efficiency by determining which procedures are unnecessary or detrimental. In view of these points, this chapter will attempt to deal as much as possible with generalizations that have broad applicability and to emphasize major recent contributions. Even among the recent literature, however, only representative citations will be given—and then mainly from major journals in the English language. For easy access to the great majority of literature on mosquito-rearing methods which has been published since the review of Gerberg (1970), the reader is referred to "Literature References to Mosquitoes and Mosquito-Borne Diseases," by Sollers-Riedel (1963–present) which occurs in each issue of *Mosquito News*.

Mosquito collecting and colony founding are seldom part of the activities of malaria laboratories these days. Yet they are integral parts of the entire process of colony maintenance, because they are partly responsible for the relevance of laboratory strains to actual field populations that transmit malaria. Therefore, a brief summary of collecting methods is included in this chapter.

II. BASIC MOSQUITO BIOLOGY

Before examining the details of collecting mosquitoes and establishing and maintaining colonies, it is necessary to review their characteristics and natural history. The efficiency with which all these tasks are performed is greatly enhanced when the natural animal is borne in mind. It is also appropriate at this point to introduce the terminology and fundamental knowledge used in the discussions which follow. Major recent references on mosquito biology include Christophers (1960), Clements (1963), Mattingly (1969), and Gillett (1971).

A. Systematic Arrangement

Mosquitoes comprise the dipteran family Culicidae. Some authors include dixid and chaoborid midges in this family as well, but they are more commonly placed separately. The family is divided into three subfamilies, and numerous genera, as follows (Knight and Stone, 1977; Knight, 1978):

Subfamily Anophelinae
    Genus *Anopheles*
        Bironella
        Chagasia
Subfamily Culicinae
    Tribe Aedeomyiini
        Genus *Aedeomyia*
    Tribe Aedini
        Genus *Aedes*
            Armigeres
            Eretmapodites
            Haemagogus
            Heizmannia
            Opifex
            Psorophora

                 Udaya
                 Zeugnomyia
Tribe Culicinae
  Genus *Culex*
          Deinocerites
          Galindomyia
Tribe Culisetini
  Genus *Culiseta*
Tribe Ficalbiini
  Genus *Ficalbia*
          Mimomyia
Tribe Hodgesiini
  Genus *Hodgesia*
Tribe Mansoniini
  Genus *Coquillettidia*
          Mansonia
Tribe Orthopodomyiini
  Genus *Orthopodomyia*
Tribe Sabethini
  Genus *Limatus*
          Malaya
          Maorigoeldia
          Phoniomyia
          Sebethes
          Topomyia
          Trichoprosopon
          Tripteroides
          Wyeomyia
Tribe Uranotaeniini
  Genus *Uranotaenia*
Subfamily Toxorhynchitinae
  Genus *Toxorhynchites*

B. Life Cycle

The mosquito life cycle consists of four stages: egg, larva, pupa, and adult. These stages are always divided between two different habitats, an aquatic and a terrestrial one; the larva and pupa are always aquatic, and the adult always terrestrial. The egg and pupa may conveniently be considered transitional forms between two separate organisms, the larva and the adult, each occupying a totally different ecological niche. This is made possible by complete metamorphosis during pupation, and as a consequence natural selection has acted rather independently on the two phenotypes arising from the single genotype. This has resulted in divergent evolution, as each form is continually modified to optimize its survival or reproductive output. Yet the two life forms must integrate their tactics to provide the most advantageous life history strategy.

Understanding the balance between divergent evolution and coevolution of the larva and the adult helps to explain much of the diversity apparent among mosquito biologies. Larvae in general are specialized for growth and the storage of nutrients, whereas adults are specialized for dispersal and reproduction. The former have special adaptations for moving, breathing, and feeding in an aquatic environment, while the latter have the more conservative features of flying terrestrial insects. But there also has been adaptive radiation of each stage. Larvae of different species are suited for occupying different kinds of water, different sites in the water, and different foods; different species of adults have different mating habits, different foods, and different ways of utilizing the food. Nevertheless, the adaptations of the larva and adult are clearly integrated. For example, larvae which can store large amounts of protein turn into adults which do not need blood; adults which take blood can produce more eggs and can therefore afford to lay them in habitats with more larval enemies or scatter them in riskier environments. Both adult oviposition behavior (including general habitat preference) and egg physiology are directly connected to the larva's chances of survival in a particular habitat, given the adaptations possessed by the larva.

C. Characteristics of Life Stages

1. Eggs

Mosquito eggs are basically of two types (1) those which are laid on the water surface or underwater and hatch spontaneously after embryonation (most *Anopheles, Culex, Culiseta, Mansonia, Sabethes, Toxorhynchites, Wyeomyia,* etc.), and (2) those which are laid on damp substrates likely to be inundated later and which remain quiescent until that time (most *Aedes, Psorophora, Haemagogus,* etc.). Embryonation usually is completed in 2–3 days at 25°–27°C in either egg type, but sometimes takes more than 1 week. The substrate of eggs of the quiescent type must be kept damp until they have embryonated, after which some will survive for months or years on a dry substrate and at low temperatures so long as the ambient humidity is high. Most probably survive longer if the substrate is damp, at least periodically. Hatching of these eggs occurs in response to low oxygen tension, a condition which develops in standing water as microorganisms begin to flourish in it. In some species hatching will not occur even then, because of a short photoperiod, a low temperature, or both. A short photoperiod may maintain a state of egg diapause even if the temperature is optimal for larval growth. Eggs which are in diapause or have been exposed to a period of cold must be conditioned for a few days in a warm, damp, long-day environment before they will hatch when inundated, and, even then, often only a portion of the eggs will hatch. In many species, within a single clutch eggs vary in the number of inundations necessary before hatching occurs. There are also species which undergo an obligatory egg diapause so that they will not hatch under ideal conditions until they have first experienced a cold period.

2. Larvae

Mosquito larvae of all species pass through four larval instars or intermolt developmental stages, each one followed by a molting of the cuticle to allow for growth. The fourth instar is the largest and takes the longest time before molting. The duration of total larval development depends greatly on the species, temperature, and availability of food. At 25°–27°C and optimum feeding conditions the larval period lasts about 5–10 days in commonly colonized species. Under some field conditions mosquitoes may spend most of a year in the larval stage (e.g., temperate *Coquillettidia*). It may also serve as the overwintering stage, diapausing in response to a short photoperiod and a lowering temperature.

Larvae feed in a variety of ways, and each species is somewhat flexible in its techniques, depending on circumstances. The most common method is filter feeding, by creating water currents that draw small particles (floating or suspended organic matter and microorganisms) to the mouthparts; anophelines most frequently do this right at the water surface, whereas culicines usually do it with the head well below the surface. Other feeding methods include swallowing dissolved nutrients, grazing microbial growth from the surface of submerged objects, gnawing on submerged solid organic objects, swallowing small swimming aquatic invertebrates, and preying on other mosquito larvae including those as large as themselves. Chemically defined diets for *Culex pipiens* and *Aedes aegypti* larvae indicate that, while there are no unusual requirements, the nutritional demands of the growing stage are characteristically complex compared to those of the adult.

At "rest," most larvae are attached to the surface film of water, either by the air tube near the end of the abdomen (culicines and toxorhynchitines) or by palmate hairs along the entire length of the body (anophelines), and they often filter-feed intermittently in this position. If food is insufficient at the surface, they may dive in order to browse on deeply submerged food, returning to the surface periodically for oxygen. They will also dive if disturbed by vibrations or a sudden reduction in light intensity, and usually swim toward darkness. They often aggregate in darker areas even when at the water surface. Culicines generally are more prone to dive and to choose dark places than are anophelines. Some mosquitoes never come to the surface; *Mansonia* and *Coquillettidia*, for example, remain attached to the submerged parts of aquatic plants, obtaining oxygen from tissue air spaces. Other species may temporarily leave the aquatic environment and crawl about on damp vegetation or mud.

3. Pupae

The pupal stage occupies a single instar. Pupae have much of the external form of adults, in which antennae, proboscis, legs, and wings are already distinct, while internal changes continue. Functionally they remain aquatic, with air tubes arising from the thorax and special swimming paddles at the end of the abdomen. Mosquito pupae do not feed, but they are unusual among insect pupae in being actively mobile when disturbed; their diving response is similar to that of larvae, though they are more buoyant and quickly rise to the water surface if they do not continue to swim. The duration of the pupal stage at 25°–27°C is about 2–3 days in commonly colonized species. The molts to the pupal stage and to the adult often tend to occur at a particular time of the day or night. The pupal stage is not used for hibernation or estivation and does not undergo diapause.

4. Adults

The time of emergence of adults from the pupal cuticle is set by the time of pupation, which is in turn set by the light cycle. Males pupate earlier than females and therefore tend to emerge first. They may mate at the breeding site soon after emergence, but males of most species cannot mate for at least 1 day and females for at least 2–3 days. Most mosquitoes mate in a special aerial swarm which the males form in particular places and at a certain time of day. Swarms most commonly occur above prominent or contrasting objects. Males of some species swarm around the host to which females are attracted for blood meals. Females entering this swarm are seized by one or more males who are attracted to the female flight sound at close range, and copulation and insemination occur as the pair leaves the swarm and settles nearby. In mixed swarms and other aggregations, species recognition during contact appears to serve as the species-isolating mechanism (Nijhout and Craig, 1971; Lang and Foster, 1976). Females are thought to be inseminated only once in a lifetime. Species capable of mating in small cages are said to be stenogamous, whether or not flight or a swarm is necessary. Probably the majority of species is eurygamous, in captivity either requiring a very large cage for mating or refusing to mate at all. There could be many reasons why a mosquito in confinement will refuse to mate; the most common are probably (1) inability to form swarms because of insufficient space, lack of swarm sites or "markers," or inappropriate lighting conditions, and (2) insufficient space for copulation as a pair falls from the swarm. Besides mating, another important event in the adult lives of many mosquitoes is migration and dispersal. In laboratory colonies this activity is at most reflected in a general period of intense flight activity.

Adult females of most species utilize three kinds of natural foods: water, sugar, and blood; males utilize only the first two. The extent to which water is taken, independently of sugar and blood, is not known. Both sexes first take sugar within the first few days after emergence, probably usually before mating and migration. This sugar comes from floral and extrafloral nectaries of plants, from the honeydew of homopterous insects, from fruit, and from other more unusual sites. It is usually principally a mixture of aqueous solutions of sucrose, fructose, and glucose, varying widely in concentration according to source and air saturation deficit; it often ranges above 50% in nectaries and approaches solid sugar in dried honeydew. It may temporarily be stored in the ventral diverticulum (crop) in its raw form, or absorbed and converted to trahalose, lipid, and glycogen, serving as an energy store in the hemolymph or fat body. Females of a few species, such as *A. aegypti* and *Anopheles gambiae,* can survive for long periods on blood alone, but most species must supplement their blood intake with sugar in order to live very long or realize their full reproductive potential. Some species do not mate as readily or as soon if they have not received substantial amounts of sugar, and others will not take blood until they have had sugar (Nayar and Sauerman, 1975). It is likely that in nature sugar is taken as frequently as blood. Females maintained in the laboratory without blood but with access to sugar and water live just as long, and often longer, than females given repeated blood meals as well.

Sugar, however, is essentially a nonreproductive nutrient. In autogenous mosquitoes, which produce eggs without a blood meal either during the first gonadic cycle or throughout adult life, sugar may either enhance egg production or be a necessary prerequisite to it. Expression of the autogenous trait is also affected by larval nutrition. Typically egg development is anautogenous, being initiated by a large blood meal taken some time after mating. Each species has a characteristic biting time during the daily light cycle, and it can be categorized generally as diurnal, nocturnal, or crepuscular. *Anopheles* and *Culex* are generally nocturnal; in *Aedes* it depends on the subgenus or species, and some *Aedes* are entirely diurnal. Host preference shows even greater variability, some species having broad preferences and others quite narrow ones. The blood protein is converted primarily into mosquito egg protein and to some extent into lipid and glycogen which can be used for energy as well as egg development. Eggs become mature at 24°–27°C in as little as 2 days after the blood meal in some *Anopheles* and three or more days in *Aedes* and *Culex* species. As soon as they are chorionated, the eggs can be laid and a new gonotrophic cycle begun. Some mosquitoes will take more than one blood meal per cycle; this is particularly common among *Aedes* species. If such environmental conditions as a short photoperiod, low temperature and humidity, and lack of oviposition sites simulate a season of reproductive inactivity (winter or dry season), the females may refuse to feed or may take repeated blood meals without laying any eggs or without developing any eggs. The last situation will also occur if blood meals are below the critical size. Above the critical size (which varies with the size and species of female) the number of eggs produced increases, up to a point, with the size of the blood meal and also the kind of blood taken (see Nayar and Sauerman, 1977).

Oviposition, like biting, often has a characteristic time in the daily light cycle, as well as a characteristic site. Gravid females often will refuse to oviposit under optimal conditions if they have not been inseminated. The choice of an appropriate oviposition site is determined by a combination of chemical, visual, and tactile stimuli. Some of these stimuli may be less important than others, depending on the species. Eggs may be laid either singly or in clusters. Of those laying clusters, *Mansonia* lay them underwater on the undersides of leaves of aquatic plants, whereas *Culex, Coquillettidia,* and most *Culiseta* females form a raft of eggs which floats on the surface. The egg cluster generally represents the entire batch of eggs produced during one gonotrophic cycle. Of those laying eggs singly, *Anopheles, Sabethes,* and *Toxorhynchites* typically drop them on the water surface, where in *Anopheles* they are held with the aid of special floats. *Aedes, Psorophora,* and *Haemagogus* lay them on damp substrates such as under dead leaves or on the sides of tree holes and other water containers above the waterline. Rather than being laid all in one place, the singly laid eggs are often scattered over several different sites or over a fairly broad area during a prolonged period of time. The species that lay single eggs on the water surface may do so during a special hovering or dancing flight.

III. COLLECTION OF FIELD MATERIAL

A. Habitats

Since mosquitoes breed in almost every conceivable type of aquatic habitat outside the open marine environment, they are collected almost everywhere. Each of the approximately 3000 species has a relatively restricted distribution, however, based primarily upon the specificity of its breeding site. Most mosquito species are confined to particular geographic regions, usually a single biome within a single continent. Wider geographic distribution is probably prevented as often by the absence of specific breeding sites, specific hosts, other biotic factors, and competitive exclusion, as it is by physical barriers to dispersal. Even cosmopolitan species are fairly specific about habitat; the fact that the species with the widest distributions (e.g., *A. aegypti, C. pipiens* complex) are domestic is probably due both to the ease of dispersal by human transport and to the general uniformity of habitat provided by humans throughout the world.

1. Immatures

Larval habitats have been classified in various ways in an attempt to reveal ecological affinities of various species while also categorizing fundamental types of environments themselves. The classification shown in the tabulation below was adapted from the ones presented by Bates (1949) and Mattingly (1969) and illustrates the diversity of mosquito breeding sites. These habitats are further subdivided according to whether the breeding sites are shaded or exposed to sun, are associated with vegetation or not, and contain particular dissolved chemicals. Even then, further subdivisions are necessary to delineate the habitats of particular species, whereas less fastidious species may be found in more than one of the above categories.

Larval habitats are generally determined by the oviposition site preferences of adult females, and these are consistent with larval adaptations for the occupation of particular niches. However, larvae may be reared successfully in the laboratory under a much wider variety of aquatic conditions than they are found in nature. This is because a species' unique combination of biological characteristics (such as rate of development, ability to undergo quiescence or diapause, feeding efficiency, predator evasion, and pathogen protection) is not challenged in the laboratory by competitors, natural enemies, or a severe and capricious physical environment. Nevertheless, many specific conditions must be met in rearing procedures; among the more obvious are water salinity for salt marsh mosquitoes and certain aquatic plants for the submerged larvae and pupae of *Mansonia* and *Coquillettidia* species. It is, therefore, necessary to know as much as possible about the breeding habitats of mosquito species destined for laboratory colonization, both in order to collect them in large numbers and to design

Ground water habitats	Container habitats
Temporary pools	Tree holes
Brackish water	Bamboos
Rainwater	Leaf axils
Floodwater	Pitcher plants
Permanent water	Miscellaneous ground containers
Running water	Rock holes
Forest streams	Crab holes
Open gravel bed streams	
Open vegetated streams	
Standing water	
Pools	
Lakes	
Marshes	
Swamps	
Subterranean water	

effective rearing procedures. A general guide to the earlier natural history and bionomical literature of individual species on a worldwide basis is given by Horsfall (1955).

2. Adults

Adult habitats are not so clearly defined as larval ones. Although adults of some species may be found in greatest density near the breeding sites, they forage over much broader areas for blood and nectar sources. Distinct but undirected migrations sometimes occur after emergence, as in *A. taeniorhynchus* (Provost, 1957), so that females travel up to at least 40 km; similarly long dispersal flights occur in *A. vexans* (Horsfall *et al.,* 1973). The direction of these migrations seems to be determined mainly by wind direction. Even among mosquitoes without a distinct migratory phase, circumstances often require that females seek blood meals several kilometers from breeding sites and then return to oviposit. Nevertheless, adults have habitat preferences, both during times in the diel rhythm when they are active and when they are at rest. For example, Bidlingmayer (1971) found that in Florida some species preferred open grassy areas both day and night, others rested in woods during the day but foraged in open areas at night, and still others remained in woods for both resting and foraging. Mosquito species differ in the time of flying activity, and it is difficult to draw generalizations about genera; *Anopheles* and *Culex* are most often nocturnally active, whereas in *Aedes* and certain other genera it depends very much upon the species. When adults are active, they are involved in seeking mates, sugar, hosts, and oviposition sites. Females in the middle of a gonotrophic cycle (i.e., those that have taken a blood meal but whose eggs are not fully developed) are also active to some extent (Edman and Bidlingmayer, 1969). Resting adults comprise both sexes, all ages, and all physiological states of females, and their microhabitats during this phase of the diel rhythm are fairly distinctive. In general, resting sites tend to be protected from wind and direct sunlight and are usually in relatively dark, humid locations. However, the actual resting site of a species is usually restricted to one of the following microhabitats: ground foliage, shrub and tree foliage, leaf litter, earth cavities, tree cavities, and tree trunks; and each of these categories actually consists of several subcategories which a given mosquito species may prefer. For example, earth cavities include abandoned animal burrows, caves, culverts, and human dwellings, which are not used equally by any one species even when physical conditions seem to be about the same in all. Females of some species of mosquitoes are attracted to hosts and take blood if the hosts happen to intrude upon a resting site during the inactive phase of the diel rhythm; others will ignore hosts until the appropriate biting time. Whether collections of adults are made when the population is active or inactive, a knowledge of both activity rhythms and preferred habitats is extremely helpful in making large catches to establish laboratory colonies and in maintaining them.

B. Collecting Methods

Effective mosquito collecting requires that efforts be concentrated in the preferred larval and adult habitats of the species sought. In addition, the correct technique is necessary. Reliable methods are not yet available for many relatively important species, though a huge variety of methods has been developed. Existing techniques are continually being modified, and new ones are being developed in an attempt to broaden a collector's abilities and increase collecting efficiency. An extensive and detailed description of methods for collecting anophelines has been given by Bradley *et al.* (1949). A further description of techniques and equipment is available from the World Health Organization (1975). The most comprehensive review of general mosquito-collecting techniques has been made by Service (1976), who included not only descriptions but also sample results. A summary of available methods is given here.

1. Eggs

Eggs laid on the surface of standing water are usually collected by skimming the water in likely places. To collect *Anopheles* eggs, the water may be scooped with a dipper and then poured through a fine sieve to concentrate the eggs, or the dipper may contain a sieve in the bottom. In either case the eggs are washed from the sieve into a container. *Culex* and *Coquillettidia* eggs are laid in rafts on the water and may be lifted individually with a spatula. Eggs laid on damp soil or leaf litter, such as those of *Aedes* and *Psorophora* that breed on temporary pools, can be obtained by a variety of extraction procedures or by soaking substrate samples in water to induce hatching; in the latter case the larvae are collected from the water surface. Eggs laid in container habitats are placed either on the water surface (e.g., *Anopheles, Sabethes, Toxorhynchites,* and *Culex*) or on substrates surrounding the water (e.g., *Aedes* and *Haemagogus*), and in either case they can be difficult to obtain from natural sites. This is done by scraping the sides and bottoms of tree holes, soaking mud from rock pools, etc. It is much simpler to make artificial oviposition sites with removable paper linings or sticks on which the eggs are laid. Artificial sites can also be used to collect the eggs of pool breeders.

2. Larvae and Pupae

Larvae and pupae are easier to collect than eggs, because they are almost always in water and are readily visible (against a light background) as soon as they have been collected. In large bodies of water, dippers and various types of sieves and nets are most commonly used; after being caught, the larvae and pupae may be concentrated with various devices to facilitate handling. Aquatic traps of several designs can be used in collecting, but they are more often used for sampling. Specialized larval habitats require special collecting techniques:

Coquillettidia and *Mansonia,* whose larvae and pupae remain submerged and attached to aquatic vegetation, require digging and sieving operations; container breeders are most easily withdrawn with suction devices, such as pipets for leaf axils and large siphon tubes for deep tree holes. Larvae in loose containers (coconut husks, snail shells, and water jugs) can simply be poured into a collecting vessel. As in egg collections, artificial breeding sites make good sources of larvae and pupae because they are easy to find and to manipulate.

3. Adults

Mosquito adults may be collected in two basic ways: active collecting and trapping. Active collecting involves either gathering mosquitoes from resting sites, catching them in the air, or attracting them to a host. The advantage of collecting from resting sites is that it is possible to collect both males and females in large numbers and to collect females that are blood-fed or gravid. They are caught in a variety of ways, depending on the type of resting site and on how numerous the mosquitoes are. Small numbers can be collected in glass tubes, various types of small mouth-operated or battery-powered aspirators, sweep nets, drop nets, and aerial nets swept over disturbed resting sites. Larger collections can be made with large hand-held or vehicle-mounted power sweepers. Artificial resting shelters are used to increase and facilitate manual resting catches. Mosquitoes may be caught while they are active in the air—either in mating swarms, general migrations, or appetential flights to find hosts, etc.—by using aerial nets; these are most productive when mounted on vehicles moving at moderate speed. Collecting mosquitoes at a host is advantageous if resting sites are unknown or inaccessible, or if the adults are thinly distributed. The host (a human or a confined or tethered animal, or host stimuli, e.g., slow carbon dioxide release) serves essentially as an aggregation point for females, allowing the collector to gather them with an aerial net as they approach, or with tubes or aspirators after they alight on the host and after they engorge on blood. Drop nets often facilitate capture at a host. Allowing females to feed before they are captured is advantageous for the many species less likely to bite in confinement. Males will be collected by this method only in species using hosts as mating sites, which include species of *Aedes, Haemagogus,* and *Mansonia.*

Trapping is more convenient than active collecting because many traps can be set up and left to operate unattended. Nonattractive traps depend upon the normal flight activity of mosquitoes to bring them to the trap, and they fly into the trap of their own accord (e.g., ramp traps, emergence traps, malaise traps), are drawn in by an air current (e.g., suction traps), are blown in by wind (e.g., stationary nets), or are captured in a moving net (e.g., rotary traps). There are many designs of nonattractive traps, but most utilize the principle of a funnel trap, in which the wide end of the funnel is exterior and the narrow end projects into the trap cage, making entry much easier than exit. Attractive traps often operate on this principle also, but they possess one or more stimulus characteristics which cause mosquitoes to enter them in greater numbers than if the stimuli were absent. Some such traps simply make use of suitable artificial resting sites with a one-way entry. They may employ bold designs and dark-colored surfaces for attraction. Light traps work by somehow attracting mosquitoes (or at least causing them to aggregate) at artificial light sources at night; they are most successfully employed in combination with a fan to provide suction into the trap net. Most other attractive traps depend on one or more host stimuli. Dark and strongly contrasting colors and designs offer visually attractive properties that appear to be host-related. Carbon dioxide is commonly used, either by itself or in combination with other attractive features; it greatly enhances light trap catches, for instance. In traps baited with live hosts, a combination of odors, carbon dioxide, heat, and visual stimuli attract the mosquitoes. They enter through either a funnel device or through a louver (baffle); the latter works on the principle that an insect will fly upward through a crack to reach a host but will seldom fly downward to escape from confinement. (Louver and funnel principles are often combined.) The trapped mosquitoes can be prevented from feeding on the host by particular trap designs that screen off the host from the mosquitoes; an extreme example would be cone traps which are placed in the windows of houses. As mentioned above, though, it is often advantageous to allow mosquitoes to take blood before they "realize" they are trapped or are manipulated in an aspirator, since they may refuse to feed after capture. However, recently blood-fed mosquitoes must be handled more carefully to avoid injury. Most kinds of traps must be visited at least daily to collect the trapped mosquitoes and maintain the attractant, and also to check for problems (improper function, ant invasion, etc.).

Like other methods of collection, trapping is selective. A trap and its use often have to be modified or specifically designed for certain mosquitoes, for reasons that are usually obscure. Light traps are effective for some species, but not others; choice of bait is often crucial to bait trap productivity. Furthermore, the location and time of operation may be critical. Finally, it should be remembered that most attractant traps, including those using light, catch primarily unfed (hungry), inseminated females.

C. Tentative Identification

When a particular mosquito species is being sought for colonization in the laboratory, it is very useful to make a tentative identification in the field. It allows the collector to direct and concentrate his or her efforts. To be able to do this, the collector should be familiar with the characteristics which distinguish the target species from other species in the area. Live specimens can often be identified by such features as behavior, general shape, and body markings—features not necessarily used in formal taxonomic descriptions or in identification keys. Adults are the easiest of live specimens to identify in the field. If the specimens must be viewed under magnification to be identified, they are generally killed (adults in poisonous vapors, and larvae and pupae in hot water or ethyl alcohol) and examined with a hand lens or microscope and a portable light source. Identification keys to the mosquitoes of the region can then be used, although it is always simpler to have the differentiating characters already firmly in mind. Once identification of killed material is made, it is still necessary to make live collections for colonies on the basis of appearance to the unaided eye unless there is a simple way of separating live look-alikes under a lens. It is easier to take care of this problem in the laboratory.

IV. TRANSPORT OF LIVING MATERIAL

A. Transport Conditions

Whether mosquitoes are transported to a laboratory from field sites only an hour away, from remote localities several days distant by land over rugged terrain, or from other continents by air, they may incur heavy mortality. The main causes of this are mechanical agitation and improper physical conditions. For long trips, nutrition may also be a problem.

1. Eggs

These must be protected from extremes of temperature. They must not be held below freezing unless they have previously been exposed to conditions that induce winter diapause, and they must not exceed a certain upper temperature, depending on the species and especially the duration of exposure (see Clements, 1963). Even tropical species succumb quickly above 40°C. Eggs must also be kept in a high humidity, at least 70% RH and preferably higher. *Aedes* eggs may rest on a dry substrate; *Culex* and *Anopheles* should be kept on a damp or wet substrate. If the eggs of *Anopheles* and *Culex* are kept cool, they do not hatch as soon, allowing a longer transportation time.

2. Larvae and Pupae

These must be likewise protected from freezing and lethally high temperatures, usually between 34° and 45°C. Temperatures in this range may be sustained for short periods (see Clements, 1963), but survival is greatest in the 20°–30° range over long periods (Shelton, 1973). Since they must also be kept wet at all times, the water acts as a convenient temperature buffer to a small extent. Even sublethal temperatures may cause abnormalities which appear later in the adults. They may be kept in a large volume of water, offering greater temperature stability, and an open water surface gives evaporative cooling; but if there is much agitation of the water during transport immatures sometimes drown from spending little or no time at the water surface. If transportation takes more than 1 day, natural organic matter from the breeding site or artificial larval food should be added to the water or wet substrate. Pupae are not usually suitable for long transports, because of their short duration (as short as 1.5 days), but a low temperature (as low as 4°C) greatly prolongs the pupal stage and slows larval development, thus reducing adult emergence and increasing survival.

3. Adults

Water and large, wet surfaces are detrimental to adults in confined spaces because they may become mired. Nevertheless, moderately high humidity is essential for survival, especially at the higher end of the temperature range (30°–35°C) (see Clements, 1963). Even at high humidity and moderate temperature, however, adults traveling for more than a few hours should have a source of drinking water; at high temperatures the demand for water is increased. A source of sugar is also necessary on long trips. The need for sugar depends on the energy reserves of the captured mosquitoes and the rate at which reserves are depleted, depending on temperature and activity. At temperatures below 25°C most field-caught adults can survive at least 1 day without sugar if they are kept quiet; but agitation, crowding, and the presence of host stimuli reduce this time. Some workers (e.g., Davies, 1969; Kardatzke, 1976) reduce mortality by giving females a blood meal before transport. Certainly a requisite of all forms of adult transport is a suitable vertical substrate for standing in the normal resting position; highly polished surfaces such as glass and plastic do not provide a grip.

B. Containers

Bradley *et al.* (1949), Macdonald (1971), and the World Health Organization (1967) have suggested some methods for mosquito transport. There are no prescribed procedures for fulfilling all the conditions necessary for successful transport of the various stages. The needs are quite variable, depending on the species, the length of transport, and the prevailing weather conditions; the available materials may also be severely limited. There is, however, one general technique now widely used to protect all stages from mechanical damage and from extremes of temperature or to maintain low temperature—insulation in the form of foam plastics, such as inflated polystyrene (styrofoam) and urethane, which are molded into boxes and cylinders (e.g., Burton, 1971). These containers are in wide use for packing, so they can be used second-hand at no expense, or they can be especially designed to meet special requirements (cf. Smittle and Patterson, 1974). It must be emphasized that even well-insulated containers become ineffective when subjected to long periods of excessive heat or cold. They should be kept out of direct sunlight whenever possible and covered with aluminum foil when this is unavoidable. A second item which is also ubiquitous and highly versatile in mosquito transport is the plastic (polyethylene, etc.) bag; it is widely used to maintain high relative humidity for eggs and adults, to prevent water leakage, and to hold larvae and pupae.

1. Eggs

The eggs of *Aedes, Psorophora,* etc., which are collected from damp surfaces, are undoubtedly the easiest mosquito forms to transport. Once embryonated, they will remain quiescent and survive for months or years without hatching, as long as the atmospheric humidity is sufficiently high and they are not submerged. The World Health Organization (1967) recommends placing the eggs on a filter paper and sealing it inside a small plastic bag. The paper itself need not be wet as long as the air inside the bag is humid. The bag may then be transported in a cardboard mailing tube or insulated container.

The eggs of *Culex, Anopheles,* etc., collected from water surfaces, are more awkward to handle because they hatch spontaneously when embryonation is completed. They may be transported in the same manner as the quiescent eggs mentioned above, except that the filter paper should be wet. Egg hatching can be retarded if the temperature is kept low by ice or precooled materials packed inside the container (Mouchet, 1967). Although some embryos may die from this treatment, survival can still be greater than if the eggs hatch and have nothing to eat. This problem can be circumvented in a different way, as long as the shipment arrives in the laboratory within a day or two, by sprinkling powdered larval food onto the wet egg paper; in many species first-instar larvae can feed and grow on the surface film of water. The obvious alternative to shipping these eggs on filter paper is to place them on a water surface in a plastic bottle or tightly sealed plastic bag. This may be successful if agitation is slight. Usually, even small movements in a car will cause splashing, so that eggs may either become lodged above the water or sink and drown. At least in this fluid environment hatched larvae can swim about and feed normally if food has been added to the water in advance.

2. Larvae and Pupae

The same basic options available for transporting nonquiescent eggs also apply to larvae and pupae. They may be transported in a vessel of water (bottle or bag) containing also a large pocket of air or an air vent (see Russell *et al.,* 1963). They can withstand agitation as long as there are frequent calm periods that allow them to remain at the surface for awhile and to feed normally. The amount of agitation they can withstand seems to vary widely with the species. Small amounts of food are necessary if more than 1 or 2 days are spent in the vessel; it may be less for early first-instar larvae. The alternative method, which avoids the agitation problems, is to place the immatures on a wet surface, such as water-soaked paper. This paper is then placed inside a watertight container (plastic bag, plastic cup, etc.) to prevent evaporation, and this is placed within the insulated container. Larvae may survive for several days on this substrate, especially if a tiny amount of powdered larval food is added to the water film; pupae will survive to emergence, and the adults can emerge normally, even though they are resting on their sides. The survival of immatures, transported by either method, is increased if the temperature is reduced by packing the insulated containers with ice or cold materials.

3. Adults

Successful transport of mosquito adults is generally the most difficult, since they are mobile and are not protected by a water buffer from mechanical damage, temperature extremes, and low humidity. They should be handled gently during transfer to transport containers, using an aspirator with very light suction and transferring only a few at a time. In some cases it may be necessary to immobilize them in a collecting container and then transfer them by pouring them or picking them up individually (by the wings or legs) with forceps; diethyl ether is the best and most convenient anesthetic, but a low temperature and nitrogen also result in good survival.

Transport containers vary greatly in type and size, from stoppered test tubes to 1-m^3 cages. Small containers of glass or plastic should be scratched or etched on the sides to allow mosquitoes to rest; plaster on the bottom and one side is even better. Cardboard cartons should have rough paper walls. Cages with screened sides offer good resting surfaces. High humidity is maintained in containers by applying a water wick through the stopper of small vessels, soaking the plaster bottom of jars with water, or draping soaked towels around the outside of screened cages. If one or more containers with screened openings are placed inside a larger airtight container (e.g., a plastic bag within an insulated box), water-soaked cotton may merely be placed at the bottom of the larger container. If the container is airtight, it must be kept cool, since the mosquitoes themselves and the water sources have no evaporative cooling power in a saturated atmosphere. In most instances, the water source used to maintain humidity also serves as a drinking water source; otherwise, damp or wet material, such as a soaked cotton wool pad or water wick made of cotton wool protruding from a secured water vial, should be available to the adults if they must be transported for more than a few hours. Alternatively, if drinking water is always available, adults are able to tolerate lower atmospheric humidities. In either case the water must be confined to the cotton wool or porous material provided; loose water may cause heavy mortality if the container is agitated or if the mosquitoes are very active.

Sugar may be available either as a solid or in solution. Many workers find it most convenient to offer sugar and water together in a 5–10% solution of sucrose or honey on a cotton wool pad or wick. Higher concentrations are apt to become sticky if there is much evaporation. Solid sucrose (as a cube) is easier to handle and may be fastened firmly inside the container during the entire transport period without maintenance. A possible disadvantage might be that solid sugar can be consumed less rapidly than dissolved sugar. The same applies to the common use of dried fruit (usually raisins) as a sugar source. A separate water supply is necessary if solid sugar is to be utilized successfully. The advantage of using natural (honey or fruit) sugar sources, whether solid or in solution, is that they provide attractants. This may not be important in small containers, in which chance encounter probably ensures that all adults will feed on the sugar; but in large cages they may be unable to find it unless it is widely distributed or has an odor, or is at least wet (water being the attractant in this case).

As already noted, blood-feeding enhances the survival of some mosquitoes in transport. Kardatzke (1976) found that both survival and subsequent oviposition were far better among transported *Aedes* spp. which took blood after collection. In this case the mosquitoes were also offered blood meals daily while in transit. The blood meal makes the females more vulnerable to damage if they are violently agitated, but it also makes them more quiescent and offers at least some nutrients for maintenance.

A last consideration is adult density. The more likely the mosquitoes are to interact with each other, the more active they become. This increases their mortality, either by reducing the intrinsic life span in some way or by increasing physical damage to wings and other parts. There are no available guidelines for computing the survival probability as density increases, but Gerberg (1970) has reported that 1.8 cm^2 of vertical resting surface area per mosquito gives good results in colony cages. If the mosquitoes will be agitated in transport, which is nearly always the case to some extent, then the recommended density might well be less than this.

C. Export–Import Regulations

Transport of living organisms from the collection site to the laboratory, or from one laboratory to another, may require crossing boundaries between nations and their various regional subdivisions. Such transport is often restricted, either because certain organisms present a threat to a particular geographic or political region, or because valuable organisms in a region are being excessively depleted. Thus, government import and export regulations may require prior authorization for the transport of live mosquitoes. Although in the case of mosquitoes it seems that import is the major concern, nevertheless some national governments insist that exporters of any kind of living organism apply for a permit. Since regulations vary so much according to place and time, they cannot be detailed here. It is up to the persons responsible for the transfer of mosquitoes to be informed of current regulations and to comply with them. Generally, this involves applying for an import permit, stating which species and strain will be imported, what it will be used for, and how it will be destroyed. It is usually necessary to describe the qualifications of the investigators, the procedures to be followed, and the facilities available to prevent escape from the laboratory. These formalities are often necessary, whether the species is exotic or already native, since local biotypes of the same species may be quite different. The decision to grant an importation permit is presumably based upon the likelihood of accidental release and its probable consequences, weighed against the importance of the research in that location.

V. REARING

A. Colony Establishment

The methods one uses in initiating a colony of mosquitoes are generally the same as the standard rearing procedures described below. The exact methods depend very much upon what is already known of the genus and species, particularly its natural environment and behavior. If it has been colonized before, one obviously starts with a similar rearing system. If it has not, one uses methods and conditions used in rearing related species, but perhaps modified in ways that seem appropriate to the species to be cultivated. Below are some general guidelines. In addition, there are three special problems that should be considered at this stage (1) How does one minimize the chances of introducing pathogens into the laboratory? (2) How many individuals are necessary to start a healthy colony? (3) How does one confirm the identity and purity of the colony?

1. General Guidelines

Russell *et al.* (1963) have outlined a few basic principles that apply to all attempts at colonization (1) The natural aquatic medium and food are most effective for rearing larvae; (2) desirable temperatures should be maintained; (3) humidity should be high; (4) excessive larval feeding should be avoided; (5) all stages should be protected from air currents, vibrations, soap, and insecticides; (6) cages should be large enough to allow mating. Repeated attempts at colonization may be necessary before even the minimal requirements have been met. Bates (1949) recommends the following steps: First, one should develop an adequate method for rearing the larvae, which may require considerable experimentation with various containers, water sources, types and amounts of food, and temperatures. Then large numbers of adults are reared, either from larvae collected in the field or from eggs laid by field-collected adult females. These newly emerged adults are used to determine the conditions for mating. The first mating trial should be made in a small cage, such as 50 cm^3; females are dissected and their spermathecae checked for sperm during the first week. If insemination has not occurred, the second trial should be made in a room-sized cage, and tests should be made to determine how the light cycle, photoperiod, light intensity and color, and contrasting surfaces on the floor of the cage can be used to induce swarm formation (see Section II). Once the necessary conditions have been determined, it may be possible to reduce the size of the cage by simply recreating the conditions on a smaller scale or by gradually reducing the cage size over a number of generations—thus selecting for stenogamy. Otherwise, it is advisable to resort to the forced copulation technique (see Section V, C). Subsequent obstacles include getting the females to blood-feed, by offering various vertebrate hosts, and to oviposit, by offering various likely oviposition sites with or without organic matter. It is necessary, in accomplishing all these steps with adults, to provide conditions for maximum survival. Cages should be provided with good resting surfaces, high humidity, and attractive sugar sources; there should be no air flow and no predators (e.g., spiders or ants), and disturbances should be minimized. The optimum temperature, which is often a trade-off between maximum longevity and maximum reproductive output, has to be determined by experiment.

2. Isolation and Decontamination

A commonly recommended way of rearing larvae in the laboratory for the first time is to use their natural aquatic medium. This may include live plants, decaying plant matter, and all the microorganisms associated with them at the breeding site. Since both the medium and the mosquitoes may contain mosquito pathogens, this places other colonies already in the laboratory in jeopardy. For this reason it is wisest to hold field-collected material in a separate room for at least one generation, using a completely separate set of equipment and supplies. The danger is somewhat reduced if one can avoid using the natural larval medium by rinsing and transferring eggs and larvae to clean water before or soon after bringing them to the laboratory and giving them artificial food. If the mineral content of the natural water seems important, it can be used after boiling or coarse filtering, which at least eliminates most nematodes, protozoa, and fungi. Although pathogens generally invade larvae, they may be associated with any stage. Field-caught adults are best handled by simply removing dead ones from cages frequently and providing oviposition sites that minimize the chances of adults dying on or in them. If there is pathogen-associated mortality within the first generation, it is often self-limiting so long as each stage (eggs, larvae, pupae, and adults) is transferred to a new, clean container, the dead individuals are quickly disposed of, and the first three stages are rinsed during transfer. The most effective way to clean a colony of all but some transovarially transmitted pathogens is briefly to wash the eggs with various chemicals such as ethyl alcohol, sodium hypochlorite, hexylresorcinol, benzalkonium chloride, and

White's solution (mercuric chloride, sodium chloride, hydrochloric acid, and ethyl alcohol). These methods have been summarized by Gerberg (1970). Some have been used to start axenic mosquito cultures. Only after the mosquitoes show no pathogen-related disease or death should they be moved to the main rearing rooms containing other colonies.

3. Starting Size

A colony should be started with as many individuals as possible. This is partly to offset mortality caused by various nongenetic factors, but more importantly it is to draw upon a maximum amount of genetic variability. In this way the sample is more likely to include genotypes suitable for laboratory conditions. It is also recommended that the founder colony be established from stock taken from central populations or central portions of large populations, where genetic diversity is greatest, rather than more homogeneous marginal ones; this centrality is determined more precisely by average population size and by persistence in the environment than by geographic centers of distribution or numerical abundance (Mackauer, 1976). Genetic variability may also be increased by pooling colonies that have different origins or by supplementing existing colonies with new field material. This may improve the likelihood of successful colonization, but it can also disrupt coadapted gene complexes and create an unnatural gene pool (Whitten and Foster, 1975; Mackauer, 1976). On the basis of studies on genetic variability of natural populations, Mackauer (1976) suggests that a founder colony, started from about 500 individuals collected over a large central area, will give adequate diversity to characterize the parental population.

It is usually necessary to choose the parental population not only on the basis of its diversity but also on the existence of particular traits. Within the range of a species there may be a continuous or discontinuous array of biotypes which differ with regard to important biological characteristics—susceptibility to *Plasmodium* infection, for example. Thus, the sample should be taken from central portions of a large population or group of populations of the appropriate biotype. However, if the preferred biotype consists of a relatively small population, or if the desired characteristics are not common in the central portion of a large population, it may be necessary to compromise between sampling for diversity and for particular genotypes. The alternatives is either to introduce the appropriate trait by hybridization after the colony is established or, if the desirable trait occurs at low frequency, to select for it in the laboratory.

4. Positive Identification

It is necessary, at some stage during the establishment of a colony, to confirm the identification of the species, or even the biotype. There are several rather obvious reasons for doing this, such as to make sure that the research on the colony will be relevant to a particular problem in nature, to make use of previously published information, and to ensure that information derived from the colony is "biologically indexed" for future reference. A corollary reason is to check that the colony is pure rather than a mixture of two or more species.

If one is colonizing a species which presents no taxonomic problems—that is, it is known to be distinctly different from others in the same area—then positive identification can usually be made by any competent biologist using up-to-date keys and descriptions of the mosquito fauna of the region. A large random sample of individuals from the colony, both larvae and adults, is killed and prepared according to standard methods; the larvae are mounted on microscope slides, the adults on double-mount pins—either with *minuten nadeln* or paper points (see Bradley *et al.,* 1949; Belkin, 1962). The male genitalia may also have to be mounted and examined, and eggs and pupal cuticles are also useful when keys are available for them. Even if the identification seems certain, it is wise to send a large series of specimens to authorities on particular mosquito groups or geographic regions to obtain a confirmation; such authorities are usually associated with national museums and universities. In the more difficult taxonomic situations, where complexes of sibling species make identification difficult, special differentiating characters are sometimes used; these include the banding patterns of polytene chromosomes, enzyme electrophoretic patterns, hybrid sterility with sibling species already identified, and variations in mating, host preference, and oviposition behaviors.

When it has been determined that a colony is a mixture of species, all the individuals must be sorted one at a time. This is time-consuming but not difficult if morphological characters, however subtle, can be used to differentiate the species under a microscope when the individuals are confined or lightly anesthetized. If, on the other hand, the specimens must be killed to be identified (for example, to make measurements, to examine larval and genitalic characters, or to examine choromsomes), then one must kill and identify some of the offspring of each isolated female in the population before appropriately pooling the remaining offspring.

B. Facilities and Environment

A thorough discussion of how to design and equip a modern mosquito insectary is given by Gerberg (1970), and ideas for creating smaller and more primitive mosquito housings—including those without access to electricity—are provided by Bates (1949). Both are briefly reviewed and appended here.

1. Housing

Very small colonies may be kept in incubators and temperature-control cabinets. Larger ones are kept in walk-in environmental chambers or specially designed rooms. The ability to maintain the desired temperature and humidity is the main requisite of a good rearing area. Therefore, they operate most efficiently when they are heavily insulated and watertight. Heating units, cooling units, or both are necessary to maintain appropriate temperature, depending on the climate, and some sort of humidification system is usually required. These may be controlled by simple thermostats and humidistats. If there is sufficient space, it should be subdivided into autonomous controlled compartments, so that the entire rearing facility is not dependent upon one large environmental control unit. Other useful features include a controlled lighting system, hot and cold running water, and a single entrance preceded by an anteroom; the doors at either end of the anteroom should be protected by overlapping curtains of netting. For large-scale rearings, pans of larvae and cages of adults are conveniently kept on movable racks.

2. Temperature and Humidity

The optimum temperature varies with the mosquito species and also with the stage. For most *Anopheles* species the optimum range is 21°–32°C (Bradley *et al.*, 1949). Adults tolerate higher temperatures when the humidity is also higher (see Clements, 1963). Earlier larval instars seem to thrive at higher temperatures (Huffaker, 1944; Bar-Zeev, 1958). Olson and Horsfall (1972) found that 26°C and above prevented testicular development in *Aedes stimulans,* a northern mosquito, and even 23°C had suppressive effects. On the other hand, *A. aegypti* grows most rapidly at 32°C, and only above 36°C is it incapable of completing development (Bar-Zeev, 1958). A temperature of 24°–27°C is often considered an adequate compromise for many species (Russell *et al.,* 1963; see Shelton, 1973). The water temperature within the larval rearing vessels is lower than the ambient air in a rearing room unless the vessel is covered; this may be compensated for by seating the vessels on a heating tape (Dame *et al.,* 1978). Also, the air temperature will not be the same in all parts of the room unless it is constantly being circulated (see Klassen and Gentz, 1971); and since air movement may seriously reduce adult survival (McCray *et al.,* 1972), cages should be designed or positioned to reduce direct airflow through them. In most mosquito-rearing efforts there is every attempt to keep the temperature constant, for three reasons: first, it is easy to monitor deviations from the prescribed setting; second, it is easy to repeat experiments and utilize previous experimental results from the same and other laboratories; and third, standard rearing methods at constant temperatures have, for many species, already been worked out. Yet, constant temperature is a laboratory artifact which may give an erroneous view of mosquito bionomics and mosquito-borne pathogen development (see Hagstrum and Hagstrum, 1970). For example, Huffaker (1944) showed that *Anopheles quadrimaculatus* larvae developed more rapidly at temperatures that fluctuated daily than at a constant mean temperature, especially if the high-temperature period lasted only 6-9 hours out of each diel cycle. Fluctuating temperatures can also have effects on adult longevity (e.g., Nayar, 1972). There are numerous devices now available for giving cyclically variable temperature control (e.g., Hagstrum and Hagstrum, 1970; Walker and Rogers, 1971), but they are not yet widely used in mosquito rearing. To provide the necessary heat, light-free or concealed heaters are recommended so that there is no possibility of interfering with the photoperiod during scotophase. Cooling is provided by air conditioners connected to the outside of the building or, in the case of small cabinets, by a self-contained refrigeration unit.

The exact humidity is not so important to mosquitos, so long as it is high, although adult longevity may be reduced if humidity is too high (e.g., 90% RH) (see Clements, 1963). Some species are capable of withstanding much lower humidities than others, but 80% RH at 25°-27°C is a rough guideline of adequacy for most adults. Crude humidification may be achieved by blowing air over or through wet materials or by boiling water. Precise humidities can be obtained in small spaces by using aqueous solutions of chemicals. But the best humidifiers for long-term use in most situations are mist generators that break water into fine droplets, using centrifugal force or air pressure, and steam nozzles connected to a central steam system in a steam-heated building.

3. Lighting

The simplest lighting is natural indirect sunlight allowed into the insectary through large windows or skylights (e.g., Ising, 1972). This source is reliable and gives natural crepuscular periods, but it is disadvantageous because it reduces insulation and because the photoperiod cannot be controlled. Rearing rooms usually have artificial lighting from fluorescent or incandescent lamps which are automatically turned on and off during each 24-hour cycle by a time switch. The best photoperiod for colony production depends on the species and often also on the local biotype. A 12-hour photophase (light period) is usually sufficient for mosquitoes from tropical latitudes, whereas longer photophases— 14 or 16 hours—are used to prevent diapause in those from temperate regions. Longer photophases are more convenient to work with because they allow longer access to the rearing area each day. Very bright light sometimes inhibits feeding and mating behavior and should therefore not be used except when procedures require it. However, there are no clear guidelines on optimum light intensity; it should probably approximate the amount of light at natural resting and breeding sites. Crepuscular periods at the beginning and end of photophase are sometimes either helpful or necessary for mating (see Foster and Lea, 1975). Light-dimming devices may be connected to the time switches that control the photoperiod (e.g., Moody et al., 1973) and may operate with either incandescent lamps or specially adapted fluorescent fixtures.

C. Rearing Procedures

The details of mosquito rearing described below are only generalizations about some of the techniques which have been successfully used. As Bates (1949) has pointed out, the culture of each species is a separate problem, and success depends a great deal on an intangible factor of experience that cannot be communicated with printed words.

1. Egg Handling

Eggs laid on the water surface hatch spontaneously after a few days, and no special stimuli are required. *Culex* eggs may be concentrated by transferring the egg rafts with a spatula from the oviposition dish to a convenient hatching dish. If the average number of eggs in a raft is known, these rafts can be distributed among hatching dishes according to the number of larvae desired in one container. *Anopheles* eggs may be concentrated by rinsing them onto a fine screen and then rinsing them off the screen into a fresh container with a little water; alternatively, the water may simply be siphoned off, leaving the eggs stranded. The eggs may first be passed through a coarse screen to remove dead adults from the oviposition water (Ford and Green, 1972). To measure large numbers of *Anopheles* eggs, they may be poured onto a screen and dried, and then poured into a small cylinder and measured volumetrically (Dame *et al.*, 1978). They must then be returned rapidly to the water surface of a hatching container. A floating ring may be used to prevent the eggs from becoming stranded on the sides of the container before they hatch (see Bradley *et al.*, 1949).

Eggs laid on damp substrates are often easier to handle. Container-breeding *Aedes* will place their eggs on damp paper or cloth kept damp at least until the eggs have been "conditioned" or embryonated (at least 2–3 days) and then stored in an airtight container in a saturated atmosphere. Since eggs are easily damaged when removed from the paper, their numbers cannot be measured volumetrically unless a more flexible substrate, such as nylon organdy, is used for oviposition. Temporary pool breeders often prefer to lay eggs on a porous material, such as gauze pads. Eggs may be harvested by shaking the pads or other material in ice water (to prevent hatching) and concentrating them on a screen. They can be measured volumetrically and then spread out on a damp substrate in aliquots of appropriate size. They may also be measured in a modified colorimeter (Bentley *et al.*, 1974). Quiescent eggs kept at normal rearing temperatures can be hatched at any time by simply immersing them in water. Since hatching is usually a response to low oxygen tension, a larger percentage of eggs may hatch at one time if the hatching water is preboiled, held in a vacuum or perfused with nitrogen gas during the hatching process, or contains reducing agents or larval food to encourage growth of microbes. Repeated submersions and dryings may be necessary to hatch all eggs. Barbosa and Peters (1969) found that the vacuum method gives the fastest, highest, and most uniform hatch of *A. aegypti*, whereas Novak and Shroyer (1978) obtained almost complete hatches of *Aedes triseriatus* using biotic deoxygenation in small vials, as described by Horsfall *et al.* (1973).

2. Egg Storage

Quiescent eggs laid on solid materials can be conveniently stored for months or even years on damp or dry substrates. If the substrate is dry, the atmosphere of the egg container should be 100% RH for maximum longevity (Meola, 1964). Fungal growth on and around the eggs can be prevented by keeping them on an inert substrate (such as a synthetic fiber material), treating the paper substrate with a fungal retardant, e.g., Roccal (Greenberg, 1970), or holding the container at a low above-freezing temperature (e.g., 4°C) if the species is cold-adapted. Even a moderately low temperature (16°C) appears to improve the survival of *A. aegypti* eggs (Meola, 1964). When eggs have been held in cold storage, they should be exposed to the normal rearing temperature and photoperiod for several days before being submerged for hatching (Horsfall, 1955). Eggs of most *Culex* and *Anopheles* species cannot be stored for long periods; they usually hatch on damp-to-wet substrates and survive for relatively short periods on dry substrates. Exceptional *Anopheles* species will survive unhatched for 2–14 days on moist substrates (Bates, 1949). A low temperature prolongs the embryonation period, hence allows short-term storage (3–6 days) of a variety of *Culex* and *Anopheles* eggs (e.g., Asman, 1975; Tubergen *et al.*, 1978). Dried eggs stored in bottles are still 50% viable at 10°C after 12 days in *Anopheles quadrimaculatus* and after 14 days in *A. albimanus* (Bailey *et al.*, 1979).

3. Larval Handling

It is often wise to add a very small amount of larval food (see below) to the water in an oviposition container before or soon after the eggs begin to hatch. This is especially important if the eggs will be hatching over an extended period of time, so that the early ones do not starve before the last have hatched. It may also be necessary to give food to newly hatched larvae if more than a few hours are necessary to count larvae and distribute them in rearing vessels. Larvae are easily manipulated in water; they may be handled individually or in groups with pipets and droppers, or handled in bulk by pouring them with water. They may be concentrated on fine screens just as eggs can. Various methods have been devised for counting larvae so that a uniform number can be placed on each vessel. The most precise method is to make an exact count—as they are drawn into a pipet or dropper from a wide pan, or after they are dispensed a few at a time from a pipet into beads of water on a dry pan. Faster approximate methods are useful in mass rearing. Relatively accurate counts may be made by maintaining uniform dispersal of larvae in a water container and determining the number of larvae in samples of a certain volume of water drawn from the container; subsequent samples of appropriate volume will then contain known numbers of larvae (Morlan *et al.*, 1963; Gerberg *et al.*, 1968). Larvae can also be estimated volumetrically by packed volume in sintered-glass filters (Bar-Zeev, 1962) or graduated hematocrit tubes (Rutledge *et al.*, 1976). More qualitative methods include counts of approximately equal subsamples (Ford and Green, 1972) and eye comparison of the density of the sample with photographs of samples of known density (Rutledge *et al.*, 1976).

4. Larval Development

Larvae may be reared in a wide variety of containers, the most commonly used of which are shallow pans and trays—even for container breeders. The pans may be of glass, plastic, enamel, aluminum, and paraffin-coated galvanized iron; however, some species seem to fare better in one type than in another. Broad, shallow pans offer good visibility, a large surface/volume ratio, and an even distribution of food. Strongly negatively phototactic larvae tend to clump at one end of the pan during daylight hours, but this has not been shown to affect development. There appears to be no limit to pan size, although larger ones are more unwieldy. If the pans have lids, there is little or no problem of water surface cooling and water loss from evaporation. Lids are seldom used on large pans, and temperature reduction in these circumstances can be prevented without overheating the ambient air by resting the pans on heating tapes (Dame *et al.*, 1978). Large pans should also have a drain outlet to draw off water and larvae or pupae. Usually the source of water for rearing is not critical, but some species do poorly in certain groundwaters, perhaps because of large amounts of inorganic impurities (Bates, 1949). City water treated with chlorine may be detrimental to young larvae, so it is usually allowed to stand for a few days before being used in rearing. Nevertheless, tap water is often recommended in preference to rainwater or distilled water because inorganic ions are necessary for development, though they are available in abundance in most larval foods anyway. For example, El-Gayar *et al.* (1972) found that *Anopheles pharoensis* did better in a solution of sodium bicarbonate, calcium chloride, and potassium sulfate than in river water, tap water, or distilled water. In the special case of rearing brackish-water species, small amounts of salt are added to the rearing water—either sodium chloride or balanced sea salts. For example, Ford and Green (1976) recommended rearing *Aedes taenioryhrhus* in water containing 0.19% (small pans) or 0.28% (large pans) of salt.

Special conditions may have to be met in rearing unusual mosquitoes. For example, predaceous larvae such as those of *Toxorhynchites* must be reared in isolation in small containers to prevent cannibalism (Trpis and Gerberg, 1973; Trimble and Corbet, 1975; Holzapfel and Bradshaw, 1976; Crans and Slaff, 1977; Furumizo *et al.*, 1977), although holding pooled larvae in the dark with excess prey minimizes this (Focks *et al.*, 1977). For *Mansonia* and *Coquillettidia*, which normally remain attached to plants, either suitable plants themselves must be present or various kinds of porous paper must serve as substitutes (see Gerberg, 1970).

A wide variety of foods has been used to rear mosquito larvae successfully; these diets have been briefly reviewed by Asahina (1964). Infusions containing large bacterial or protozoan populations have been widely used and often provide the best growth rates (e.g., Hazard *et al.*, 1967), though they are inconvenient to prepare and difficult to standardize. Chemically defined media are also successfully used for rearing larvae in axenic cultures (e.g., Rosales-Ronquillo *et al.*, 1973; Dadd and Kleinjan, 1976; Sneller and Dadd, 1977); these are expensive and require special equipment and precautions to maintain sterility (e.g., Hamilton and Bradley, 1977). Most standard rearing operations use a finely powdered form of a complex balanced diet intended for laboratory or domestic animals such as dogs, pigs, rats, mice, or fish. This is often mixed with yeast, liver powder, dried blood, lactalbumin or other protein-rich substances, or one of these substances is used by itself or in combination with others. The food is added to the pan of water containing larvae, in some prescribed amount at specified intervals, as determined by experiment. For culicine larvae the food is mixed thoroughly with the water, while for anophelines it is administered as an evenly distributed surface deposit, owing to their different feeding behaviors. The larvae feed not only on the supplied food but also upon the microorganisms that begin growing in the pan. Axenic cultures amply demonstrate that microbes are not necessary to development, as long as all essential nutrients are supplied, and their absence can improve adult longevity (Lang *et al.*, 1972). But they are a necessary part of most crude diets (see Wallis and Lite, 1970, for brief review). Furthermore, they affect the rate at which food can be supplied. This is because an excess of food results in excess microbial growth, thus reducing water oxygen, creating a surface scum through which the larval air tubes cannot penetrate, and perhaps producing enough toxic materials to harm the larvae directly. There are two ways to cope with this problem (1) A system of hoses connected to a pressurized air source can supply each pan with a nozzle that continuously bubbles air through the rearing water (e.g., Chapman and Barr, 1969); this is convenient in that the larvae can be given food in larger amounts and less often. (2) The larvae are fed small amounts of food rather more frequently (e.g., daily)—either precise amounts known to give rapid and uniform development without excess microbial growth (administered in various-sized scoops known to hold certain weights of food) or irregular amounts according to the apparent need (judging from water turbidity); this approach requires more personal attention but obviates the cumbersome aeration system. The use of tropical fish food to some extent bypasses the problems of each approach, because fish food flakes decompose in water much more slowly than other animal foods; excess can be added without producing a scum (Pappas, 1973). Reisen (1975) and Reisen and Emory (1977) attempted to solve the microbial growth problem by adding antibiotics to the rearing water; this resulted in a net increase in microbes in the water and increased larval mortality. (See Section VII.) *Toxorhynchites* and species of other genera with predaceous larvae are periodically fed the larvae of other, more rapidly developing mosquito species such as *A. aegypti*. They will develop slowly, however, on a nonliving diet (Focks *et al.*, 1978).

The last major problem to consider in larval development is larval density, which is to some extent related to feeding, since the number of larvae determines the amount of food that must be supplied. It is complicated, however, by the fact that increased density also enhances the concentration of both autophagostimulants (Dadd, 1973; Dadd and Kleinjan, 1974) and waste products and induces the elaboration of growth-retardant substances (Moore and Whitacre, 1972). This general topic has been reviewed by Peters and Barbosa (1977). The main effect of overcrowding is either retarded growth and prolonged development, leading to small adults emerging over a broad span of time, or high mortality. Peters *et al.* (1969) and Barbosa *et al.* (1972) considered 0.5 larvae/ml of water to be the optimum rearing density for *A. aegypti* in terms of development rate, mortality, and adult weight. Mortality was lowest under conditions of moderate stress (2 larvae/ml), but development rate and adult weight were adversely affected (Barbosa *et al.*, 1972). Since the shape of the rearing vessel seems to be crucial to the degree of stress from crowding, other workers have expressed density in terms of surface area of the rearing water. For example, Reisen and Emory (1977) consider 0.5 larvae/cm² surface area to be an uncrowded situation, but 3.0 or 6.0 larvae/cm² to be overcrowded and to cause severe mortality in *Anopheles stephensi*. As a demonstration of the effects of crowding on *Culex pipiens quinquefasciatus* larvae, independent of the number of larvae per volume of water, Ikeshoji and Mulla (1970a) showed that the water from larvae reared in a jar (at 5.7 larvae/ml but 20–27 larvae/cm²) was much more toxic than water from a pan containing the same number of larvae and amount of water (but 2.9–3.8 larvae/cm²). These results could be interpreted to mean that crowding is "measured" by the larvae in terms of interindividual distance at the water surface. However, the surface/volume ratio might also affect food availability (cf. Moore and Whitacre, 1972), bacterial growth (Ikeshoji and Mulla, 1970b), and chemical changes in the water; so conclusions about the stimulus which induces the release of the growth retardant factor must be drawn with care. Moore and Whitacre (1972) found no relation between growth retardant production and density in *A. aegypti,* but a negative correlation between the retardant and food availability. At least some of the growth retardant effects are independent of microbial action, since they occur in axenic cultures (Kuno and Moore, 1975) and have been chemically identified (Ikeshoji and Mulla, 1970a, 1974a,b).

5. Pupal Handling

After the fourth-instar larvae pupate, the pupae should be transferred from the larval vessels to a separate container placed in a cage where adult emergence can occur. The pupal container should have clean water—not the larval rearing water—to improve the percentage of successful emergence. The greater surface tension of the clean water provides better support for the emerging adults of some species. It is also important not to overcrowd the pupae, since too much activity at the water surface and too many cast pupal skins interfere with emergence, causing adults to become mired. Maximum suitable pupal densities have not been determined, but it is probably best to have no more than 5 pupae/cm^2 of water surface. The pupal container may be any type of bowl, cup, or dish; some workers prefer it to have floating debris or roughened sloping sides (or else to be full of water to the brim) to aid in adult emergence and dispersal into the cage. If there are already many adults in the cage, a screen cone with a small hole at the top should be inverted over the container. This prevents older adults from ovipositing or drowning, while allowing newly emerged adults to crawl out the top.

When the larvae are well synchronized in development (which is attainable if the eggs all hatch together, if the developmental conditions are relatively uniform, and if the development time is short), the pupae may all be harvested at once. A few may remain larvae in any circumstances, but these can be ignored in large rearing operations. The entire contents of a rearing vessel are poured through a sieve, washed free of debris from the rearing medium, and then rinsed or knocked into the water of the pupal container.

However, since the pupal period is considerably shorter than the larval period, quite commonly the mosquitoes cannot be sufficiently synchronized to prevent emergence of the first adults before the majority of the larvae have pupated. In this case it is necessary to separate the pupae from the larvae every 1–2 days. This is done either by picking out the pupae individually or separating them from the larvae with some process that handles large numbers. Pupae are picked out individually with a wide-mouthed pipet, a small lifting screen, or a wire loop. The pipetting procedure goes much faster if the tube is connected by a small hose to a flask which is in turn connected to a vacuum pump; the pupae may then be picked continuously and collected in the flask. Various methods for the mass separation of pupae from larvae have been devised. Ice water may be used effectively for a variety of species, since in cold water larvae tend to sink, whereas pupae remain afloat (Weathersby, 1963; Hazard, 1967) and can be poured off; alternatively the cold larvae can be drawn through a port at the bottom of a flask. Bar-Zeev and Galun (1961) magnetically separated larvae from pupae by mixing iron dust with the larval food. Mechanical pupal

separators operate to catch mosquitoes in prescribed size ranges and can sometimes be used to separate male from female pupae as well (Sharma *et al.,* 1972,
1974). There are several designs for separators (see Gerberg, 1970; Ansari *et al.,*
1977), which usually operate by sifting the mixture of larvae and pupae through a
trough or pan containing openings, screens, or slits of a particular size for
retaining pupae but allowing larvae (or male pupae) to be flushed out or to crawl
through.

Pupae may be counted volumetrically in a manner similar to counting large
numbers of eggs or larvae. Known numbers are accumulated in a length of tubing
with one screened end, and the level of pupae is then marked on the tube; pupae
are easily removed from this calibrated tube by inverting it and flushing it with
water (Gerberg, 1970).

6. Adult Handling and Maintenance

Adults may be allowed to emerge in small, clear, plastic cages to facilitate
sorting by sex, in large mating cages, or in regular colony cages from which they
never have to be transferred. If transferring is required, adults are handled with
some type of aspirator which draws them into a tube or container using suction
provided by mouth or by an electric fan or compressed air (see Gerberg, 1970).
The suction should be the minimum amount necessary to catch and hold them, so
that they are not damaged. Some of the larger mechanical models can collect
several hundred mosquitoes in a few minutes, but excessive crowding and prolonged aspiration cause more damage. Adults caught in aspirators should be
gently blown upward into the new cage.

Many types of mosquito cages have been successful, and several of the most
widely used ones are described and illustrated by Gerberg (1970). The best
construction materials are metal and plastic, because they can be easily cleaned.
Most types have a cloth-sleeved entrance, so that the floor of the cage can be
cleaned, mosquitoes collected, etc. Most also have one or more screened sides to
allow air conditions similar to the environment in which the cage is held and to
prevent accumulation of moisture. Screening also provides a good vertical resting surface; if most of the cage is plastic, the sides should be scratched with
horizontal lines to provide more resting sites. Some cages have built-in compartments for holding hosts within access of the mosquitoes—such as a hammock
of netting on the top or a screened tunnel from the side. Others allow the addition
of pupae and removal of eggs, as well, without the need to enter the cage (Gillett,
1976). Still others, such as those of McCray (1963) and of French (1970), are
even more elaborate, containing rearing trays and oviposition sites that are acces-
sible from the outside. The size of the cage depends entirely upon the requirements of a particular mosquito species—particularly for mating, as already mentioned in Section V, A—and on the numbers of adults to be maintained. The

optimum adult density in relation to the resting surface (vertical sides) may depend on the species, but it is clear that overcrowding decreases the efficiency of colony productivity. Most workers have used densities of no less than 1 cm² of vertical surface per mosquito and usually 3–4 cm² (see Gerberg, 1970). It has also been recommended that fewer males than females be kept in a colony cage, both because it increases female density without a drop in fecundity (since one male can inseminate several females) and because repeated male attacks upon mated females may reduce the latter's longevity.

Sources of sugar and water should be made available in the cage within a day after emergence, and this may be provided in a number of ways. A 5 or 10% solution of sucrose is commonly used to provide sugar and water at the same time, either from a wick inserted in a bottle of the solution or from a soaked pad placed on the cage screen. Pads must be replaced daily, and wick bottles must be replaced every few days to avoid microbial growth; replacement of bottles is easiest if they protrude into the cages from the outside. Higher sugar concentrations (25 or 50%) will induce greater sugar intake, but the pads or wicks become sticky rapidly because of water evaporation, and it may take a longer period of fasting before the females are willing to take blood. A less time-consuming method is to provide solid sugar (as cubes) and a separate water source (see Polk, 1978), because water and sugar then need to be replaced only at very infrequent intervals. The mosquitoes apparently discover the sugar by chance, so in a large cage sugar cubes should be available in several places. One advantage of this method may be that the females take relatively small amounts of sugar, so that it does not interfere with blood feeding. A third source of sugar commonly used is fruit, which may be either relatively dry (e.g., raisins, giving the properties of sugar cubes) or wet (e.g., preserved apple slices, giving the properties of strong sugar solutions); the special advantage of these natural sugar sources is that they apparently contain attractants, making them easier for the mosquitoes to find. This advantage is also gained if honey, rather than sucrose, is used to make sugar solutions.

7. Mating

If the appropriate conditions for mating are known (see Section V, A), they must be maintained until all females are inseminated (which may be only 1–2 days or as much as 1–2 weeks after emergence). Afterward, they may be separated from males and used as breeding stock or experimental subjects under a variety of conditions. Normally, however, a breeding colony is designed so that all phases of adult life take place within a single cage. And rather than being all of the same age, a caged population usually consists of all ages, because new adults are periodically added to replace dead ones and maintain a standard density. This is much more efficient in the use of space and rearing effort than either discarding discrete middle-aged adult populations or maintaining them until most are dead, though it is not possible to keep track of the number of generations completed.

One major complication of handling adults during reproductive maturation is the inability of many mosquito species to mate in captivity, no matter how large the cage and even when swarm markers and gradual light dimming are provided. This problem has been circumvented by a technique known as induced or forced copulation, by which individual females are mated to males manually. There are many variations of the method, and most of them have been summarized by Gerberg (1970) and McCuiston and White (1976). Essentially, females are lightly anesthetized and then held upside down with a suction pipet or nontoxic glue; males are lightly anesthetized, often decapitated, and held upside down or vertically with a suction pipet, nontoxic glue, or a needle that pierces the thorax. The bodies of male and female are oriented end-to-end at an angle between 45° and 180° (depending on the species), so that they are positioned somewhere between venter facing venter and both with ventral sides up. Then the genitalia are brought into contact, the male's genitalia clasp the female's, and insemination ensues. Some workers find that success is enhanced if the males are cooled in advance (e.g., Bryan and Southgate, 1978), and nitrogen seems to be a better anesthetic than carbon dioxide or chloroform (Fowler, 1972; Horsfall *et al.,* 1973). Variable success has also depended on temperature, on how often the male is used before it is discarded, on the ages of the male and female (which should be at least 3 days old), and on whether a meal of sugar or blood was given prior to mating. With one method or another, a large number of species in at least five genera have been successfully induced to mate, and through assembly-line procedures it has been possible to mate females at a rate of 40/hour (Gerberg, 1970). Nevertheless, even under the best of conditions not all males attempt to copulate, not all copulations result in insemination, and the percentage of insemination success varies widely with the species and the practitioner.

8. Blood Feeding

Females may be willing to blood-feed within 1 day of emergence, especially if not supplied with water or sugar, but it is best to wait until mating is completed. The greatest percentage of blood feedings at one time is obtained if (1) the mosquitoes have been kept on a low-sugar diet (or have been deprived of sugar until their energy reserves are low, (2) appropriate environmental conditions have been created (e.g., high humidity, darkness, appropriate time in the light–dark cycle) and (3) a suitable host is used. The usual laboratory animals serving as hosts are rats, rabbits, guinea pigs, and chickens, and in some laboratories a human forearm is routinely used. The choice of host used for feeding a particular species of mosquito is often based upon a compromise between the mosquito's host preference and the ease of maintaining and handling the host animal. Many species have preferences sufficiently broad that only the latter consideration is necessary. Before exposing the host to the mosquitoes, it must be either anesthetized with pentabarbitol (or a similar drug) by intraperitoneal injection or restrained in some way. The simplest method of restraining is to strap the animal's legs together or to strap the animal onto a rack, and there are many variations of this, some quite elaborate. Another basic principle involves confinement, either in a box that allows exposure of certain body parts or a very cramped wire cage. The animal is usually first clipped or shaved on a part of the body to allow easier access of the mosquitoes to skin. The anesthetized or restrained animal may then be placed inside a large cage of mosquitoes. The disadvantages of doing this are that mosquitoes may escape or be damaged when the host is removed from the cage, an incompletely restrained host may attack the mosquitoes (bird's beaks should be muzzled), and the host can foul the cage with excrement and urine. It is much simpler to apply the host against the cage from the outside, either in a screened tunnel from the side or a hammock of netting on top. A variation of this is the application of very small mosquito cages (e.g., screened-top plastic cups) to the shaved sides of the host; they are held there by straps or by integral parts of the animal restraining apparatus. In this way chickens and rabbits, but also very much larger animals, can be utilized effectively. A list of references describing some of these feeding methods has been given by Gerberg (1970). Most females going to take blood do so within the first hour of exposure, but it is sometimes necessary to leave a restrained host exposed overnight. There appear to be no established guidelines on the number of mosquitoes that can be allowed to bite an animal, either at any one time or over extended periods, without causing ill effects. Using rats, I generally allow no more than 50 engorgements per female per month.

An alternative to using live hosts is to provide pooled blood, either soaked onto a pad or contained beneath a membrane. These are referred to as artificial feeding methods, and guides to the literature are given by Gerberg (1970) and Wade (1976). For mass rearing, there are obvious advantages of dispensing with the maintenance and handling of live animals; these advantages are discussed by Bailey *et al.* (1978). The blood is defibrinated, heparinized, or citrated after collection to prevent coagulation and is stored at a temperature slightly above freezing until it is used. If blood is to be offered on pads of netting, gauze, or cotton wool, it must be heated to the host body temperature to be attractive. Otherwise, it may be left exposed for a long period, containing sucrose to serve as a phagostimulant or honey to serve additionally as an attractant. The blood–sugar mixture may go first to the crop instead of directly to the midgut, but the blood is eventually utilized for egg production anyway. Membranes are often considered superior for artificial feeding, because they confine the blood and help maintain the host temperatures to which the blood is warmed; they may also be responsible for inducing the mosquitoes to take larger blood meals. The membranes may be either artificial (e.g., Parafilm) or derived from animal skin, mesentery, or intestine. The membrane feeding system may be quite simple, such as an inverted test tube filled with warm citrated bovine blood and capped with a Baudruche (intestinal) membrane (Wills *et al.*, 1974; Carroll *et al.*, 1976); or it may involve large membranes, circulating warm-water baths (Rutledge *et al.*, 1964), and stirring devices to prevent sedimentation (Wade, 1975, 1976). Citrated blood and defibrinated blood do not give as many eggs per female as fresh whole blood, and the overall productivity of *A. albimanus* colonies fed on this blood through membranes is only about one-half that observed when they are given live hosts (Bailey *et al.*, 1978). Wade (1975) has found that the addition of heparin and antibiotics causes increased egg production as compared to membrane feedings without them, although in excessive amounts these additives reduced egg production, and excess antibiotics reduced longevity as well. Adenosine triphosphate serves as a phagostimulant and facilitates engorgement when added to preserved blood in minute amounts (see Friend and Smith, 1977), but it has not been widely used for the membrane feeding of mosquitoes.

9. Oviposition

Eggs are usually ready to be laid about 2–3 days after blood feeding in commonly colonized mosquito species held at 25°–27°C. In autogenous mosquitoes, which do not need blood during at least the first gonotrophic cycle, the eggs are ready about 5 days after emergence. During this period after blood feeding and during egg maturation, the females should be handled as little as possible, because they are more vulnerable to physical damage when they are heavy. The time of oviposition may be somewhat specific, so that eggs will not be laid after egg maturation until the appropriate time in the light–dark cycle is reached. Among *Aedes* species the eggs may be laid over an extended period if they normally distribute their eggs among several sites (e.g., Rozeboom *et al.*, 1973; Shroyer and Sanders, 1977). If the oviposition site provided is not sufficiently suitable, gravid females will retain their eggs for many days and perhaps not lay them until nearly dead. This, however, can be sufficient to start a colony which will automatically select for individuals less particular about the oviposition site.

The usual oviposition sites for colonies of mosquitoes which lay their eggs on the water surface (e.g., *Culex* and *Anopheles*) are shallow dishes and cups containing a small amount of water. Some workers line these containers with paper so that *Anopheles* eggs will not stick to the sides, and others support a piece of filter paper just beneath the surface of the water (Gerberg *et al.*, 1968), add floating objects to the water (Yoeli and Boné, 1967), or simply use wet filter paper as the laying substrate (Osgood, 1971a). Also, gravid females can be isolated in tubes containing a little water in the bottom (Jupp and Brown, 1967).

Mosquitoes which lay their eggs on damp substrates (e.g., *Aedes* and *Psorophora*) may be induced to lay them on damp materials presented in various ways. Container breeders will lay their eggs on the inside of a dark cup, in the 2–3 cm above the waterline, on a wet paper or cloth lining; those which have been under cultivation for long periods will lay on almost any damp surface, including water or sugar wicks. Temporary pool breeders will lay their eggs on damp, porous materials, such as sponges and pads of cotton wool wrapped in cheesecloth.

The color, or at least light reflectance, of the oviposition site sometimes influences its suitability (see Trembley, 1955; Williams, 1962; Wilton, 1968), and chemicals often have a very significant effect. Salts, decaying organic materials, and ripe infusions are frequently used to make the oviposition site more attractive or stimulating (see Bates, 1949); water from rearing vessels also sometimes acts as an oviposition stimulant (e.g., Hudson and McLintock, 1967; Soman and Reuben, 1970; Kalpage and Brust, 1973; Bentley *et al.*, 1976; Reisen and Siddiqui, 1978), as do the eggs themselves (Osgood, 1971b; Starratt and Osgood, 1972).

VI. SELECTION PROCEDURES

A. Genetic Drift

When founding a colony, one attempts to include as much variability as possible by taking a large sample or several large subsamples from a central portion of the natural population (see Section V, A). This provides a more realistic representation of the natural gene pool and allows a greater chance that a colony can become established in the rather different environmental conditions of the laboratory. Even a relatively large founder colony, however, is subject to founder effects, so that it may not contain the same genetic diversity inherent in the natural population. Furthermore, the colony size influences the rate of random change in gene frequency and the rate at which it approaches homozygosity. Heterozygosity appears to be important to the fitness of mosquito populations, because of heterotic effects enhancing fecundity, longevity, and rapid development (Asman *et al.*, 1963; Craig and Hickey, 1967). Therefore, to maintain diversity and vigor it is important not to allow stocks to dwindle temporarily, as this enhances the rate of loss of alleles through random sampling errors (Mackauer, 1976).

B. Inbreeding

In well-established colonies it may be useful to develop inbred lines to provide genetic uniformity for basic research. This may be done by single-pair brother–

sister matings for successive generations, so that about 95% of gene loci are homozygous by the F_{10} generation and approximately 99% by the F_{20}. Using this procedure, Craig and co-workers (Craig and Hickey, 1967) found that inbreeding was most difficult in the F_4–F_7 generations, when recessive deleterious factors appeared, but not after that. Nevertheless, the inbred lines have reduced vigor, fecundity, and longevity. The F_1 hybrid cross between two inbred lines is generally more fit than either parental stock, however, and is often more fit than a random-bred strain. The heterosis (which is lost in later generations) provides not only high fitness and general hardiness, but also uniformity and synchronized development. This method could therefore be used to provide standardized strains for general laboratory use (Craig, 1964). Guidelines for the development of standardized strains have been presented by the World Health Organization (1967).

C. Selection

The frequency of mutations in some mosquito populations is surprisingly high. Genetic load has been found to be variable and often heavy in *A. aegypti*, both in laboratory colonies (VandeHey, 1964) and in field populations (Craig and Hickey, 1967), with frequencies of up to three visible morphological mutations per individual, concealed in the heterozygous state. If this sort of load can occur in other species of mosquitoes, there is ample opportunity for the rapid evolution of laboratory ecotypes in mosquito colonies.

The environment and procedures used to maintain a laboratory colony exert strong selection pressures for traits that maximize fitness under those particular conditions. It has been shown that gene frequencies vary widely with the rearing conditions in the same laboratory (Adhami, 1962; see Craig and Hickey, 1967) and in many different laboratories (Craig *et al.*, 1961; Craig, 1964). As Craig and Hickey (1967) have pointed out, there is no such thing as a typical laboratory strain, since laboratory strains are very different from field populations and each laboratory strain is both distinctive and constantly changing. However, a colony which is adapting by natural selection to a rearing regime in a laboratory does not necessarily become more efficient. The relaxation of selective pressures normally maintained in the field can lead in the opposite direction. For instance, if restrained hosts are left exposed to mosquitoes for long periods, the mosquitoes might, by random sampling error, become less responsive to host stimuli, less wary, and engorge more slowly, as shown by Gillett (1967). Similarly, if all larvae are reared to adulthood, including those that develop very slowly, the development time might become prolonged and less uniform. The heritability of observed variation in a colony is not always high, but there is substantial evidence that a variety of useful breeding characteristics can be established, maintained, or enhanced through prudent selection. These include aspects of egg hatching, mating behavior, host preference, oviposition behavior, and insecticide resistance (see Mattingly, 1967; Spielman and Kitzmiller, 1967; Craig and Hickey, 1967). In some cases, selection may only lead to a trade-off that gives no net advantage. For example, an increased reproductive output early in adult life may be accompanied by a shorter life span and lower total fecundity (Schlosser and Buffington, 1977).

Apart from increased colony efficiency, artificial selection can also be used to develop particular traits useful for research. Of particular importance is susceptibility to vertebrate pathogens, so that laboratory-reared mosquitoes may serve as intermediate hosts and vectors. This aspect has been reviewed by Macdonald (1967, 1971). Mosquito populations in nature vary widely in their susceptibility to malaria and filarial infections. Through selection, dramatic increases in the susceptibility of strains of *Anopheles, Culex,* and *Aedes* species to bird malaria, and of *Aedes* and *Culex* to several filarial nematodes, have been achieved. The susceptibility of *A. aegypti* to *Plasmodium gallinaceum* appears to be based on a single pair of genes or a group of closely linked genes (Ward, 1963); its susceptibility to *Brugia malayi* appears to be monofactorial, recessive, and sex-linked (Macdonald, 1962). Care must be taken to maintain the susceptibility of laboratory populations by selective breeding of susceptible individuals, since they may evolve to become relatively refractory (see Macdonald, 1971).

D. Genetic Markers

Marker genes are extremely useful in providing rapid identification of individuals belonging to particular strains or colonies when more than one strain is being maintained in the same laboratory. Markers prevent the possible misidentification or cross-contamination of stocks. Identification may also be useful in tracing the source of escaped mosquitoes and of differentiating them from field material. Easily visible markers are currently available for *A. aegypti* (Craig and Hickey, 1967) and for *Culex* (Laven, 1967; see also World Health Organization, 1967). Genes that affect flight or vision without altering other characteristics of a laboratory colony may also be useful to deter escape and prevent establishment of the species or strain in the field (Craig and Hickey, 1967).

VII. PATHOGEN AND PESTICIDE PROBLEMS

A. Pathogens

A wide variety of parasites occurs in mosquitoes, and many of them are pathogenic, invading the hemocoel and destroying the cells of various tissues (Kramer, 1964). The most widely studied mosquito pathogens are viruses, bacteria, fungi, ciliate and microsporidian protozoa, and mermithid nematodes.

Most of the research on them has concerned their natural occurrence, descriptive biology, and potential as biological control agents of mosquitoes. Extensive literature surveys of the pathogens have been made by Jenkins (1964), Laird (1971), and Roberts and Strand (1977). Chapman (1974) has reviewed the subject from the viewpoint of biological control.

1. Effects

Most of the pathogens are found as natural infections in the field and seldom invade laboratory colonies, although experimental transmission is often easily achieved and pathogen cultures may be maintained. Infection usually occurs in the larval stage, and mortality is usually highest then; mild infections may persist into the adult stage. The principal agents responsible for epizootics in mosquito colonies appear to be viruses and microsporidians, particularly the latter. Since both of these pathogens may be transmitted transovarially from female mosquito to offspring, they are easily able to maintain themselves in the laboratory. Some species of microsporidia have decimated *Anopheles* colonies, principally *Nosema stegomyiae, N. algerae,* and *Plistophora culicis* (e.g., Fox and Weiser, 1959; Hazard, 1970; Vavra and Undeen, 1970). Other species appear not to cause much pathology and mortality, or only male larvae succumb to them (Chapman *et al.,* 1966; Kellen *et al.,* 1965). Relatively low infective inocula of even the virulent *N. algerae* do not have much effect on larval or pupal survival, but they severely reduce adult longevity and egg production (Reynolds, 1971; Anthony *et al.,* 1972; Undeen and Alger, 1975). Infections which endure into the adult have been found to have confounding effects on experimental malaria infections in colonized *Anopheles* species. Garnham (1956) noted that microsporidia make it more difficult to identify developing oocysts and suggested that oocyst development was affected by the infection. Other workers have since shown that *Nosema* causes retardation or degeneration of oocysts (Bano, 1958; Bray, 1958; Ward and Savage, 1972) and reduced sporozoite production (Savage *et al.,* 1971). Similar phenomena were observed when experimental *Plasmodium* infections were concomitant with virus infections (Bertram, 1965; Davies *et al.,* 1971), but midgut bacteria may be beneficial to oocyst development (see Killick-Kendrick, 1971). It may be noted here that the cytoplasmic incompatability phenomenon, in which certain crossing types of mosquitoes from different geographic regions possess a maternally inherited factor making them reproductively incompatible (Laven, 1967; McClelland, 1967; World Health Organization, 1967, Appendix A), has been attributed to rickettsia-like organisms (Yen and Barr, 1973).

2. Prevention and Treatment

To prevent epizootics of pathogens in a mosquito colony, it is necessary to use the precautions already described when bringing new material into a laboratory and then to follow certain procedures, either to minimize other sources of contamination or to keep existing contamination at a tolerable level. These routine procedures are many and varied, depending greatly on the threats to a particular rearing facility. In general, it is important to clean all rearing materials after each use, either by physical or chemical means; this applies particularly to vessels used for oviposition, rearing, pupal holding and emergence, and adult maintenance. Larval food and rearing water should also be at least clean, if not heat-treated. Greenberg (1970) has reviewed and evaluated the principal methods for sterilizing insect-rearing materials: moist heat (autoclaving), boiling, dry heat, ultraviolet radiation, disinfectants, oxidizing agents, ethylene oxide, alcohol, heavy-metal salts, and antibiotics. The appropriate use of the method depends not only on the materials to be treated (plastic versus metal) and the nature of the pathogen (spores, etc.) but also on the balance between cost and risk. If the risks are not great, it is probably sufficient to use very hot tap water to wash equipment and also to provide the rearing water (after cooling and standing to allow dechlorination).

Chemicals which have proved effective in sterilizing the surfaces of mosquito eggs were mentioned in Section V,A. A review of these chemicals and methods of treatment is given by Gerberg (1970). In addition, Alger and Undeen (1970) and Ford and Green (1972) have described simple and effective *Anopheles* egg-rinsing techniques with water, to keep microsporidian infections low (average of 2%) and light; the infection is apparently transmitted on the outside of the egg, at least in *N. algerae* (Canning and Hulls, 1970). Alger and Undeen (1970) found that 1% hydrochloric acid and 1% sodium hydroxide did not kill *Nosema* spores but that they were killed by 0.1% Formalin overnight, 95% ethyl alcohol, or 5 days of drying. For the storage of *Aedes* eggs, Greenberg (1970) recommends a 1:1000 solution of Roccal disinfectant applied to the paper the eggs are laid on, to inhibit the growth of mold. For larvae with heavy infestations of external ciliate protozoa, a 30- to 45-second dip in 70% ethyl alcohol has saved a colony (Horsfall, in Greenberg, 1970). Some workers have attempted to improve the survival of larvae reared under crowded conditions, or in an excess of food, by adding antibiotics to reduce populations of free-living bacteria. Williams (1953) reported that terramycin and streptomycin treatment yielded larger larvae, and this effect has been generally confirmed by other workers (Bar-Zeev, 1957; De St. Jeor and Nielsen, 1964; Reisen, 1975). However, Reisen and Emory (1977) showed that, although antibiotics (penicillin G, chloramphenicol, and amphotericin B combined) produced larger larvae (and also caused more rapid development when they were not overcrowded), there was also significantly higher larval mortality—which could account for the larger larvae because more food would have been available for survivors. It is interesting also that in the antibiotic-treated medium the total microbe count actually went up, because of an increase in a resistant *Pseudomonas* group bacterial population.

B. Pesticides

Perhaps it is superfluous to mention the danger of insecticides to mosquito colonies. Their use anywhere close to rearing facilities or host animal quarters can have disastrous effects. Contact and internal poisons may contaminate rearing materials, larval food, rearing water, host animals, or the clothing and bodies of laboratory personnel who move between insecticide-treated areas and rearing rooms. Insecticides with a fumigant action may enter rearing rooms through doors, drains, and ventilation systems from other rooms or even nearby buildings where pest insects are being controlled. Construction materials for the rearing facility itself may contain insecticides that prevent colony maintenance. Examples of contamination are seldom published, but Service (1970) gives an account of the failure to rear *A. gambiae* in rearing rooms later found to have been constructed from insulation board and paint treated with organochlorine insecticides.

Despite the risks, it is sometimes necessary to apply insecticides in or near rearing facilities, to control cockroaches and ants, for example, when it is not possible to exclude them or to eliminate them in any other way. In such cases, the poisons should have a very low volatility and be confined in small containers with a bait; thus, they will not have to be widely distributed, and contamination of rearing materials can be prevented.

REFERENCES

Adhami, U. M. (1962). Changing gene frequencies for yellow larva in populations of *Aedes aegypti*. *Bull. Entomol. Soc. Am.* **8**, 103 (Abst.).

Alger, N. E., and Undeen, A. H. (1970). The control of a microsporidian, *Nosema* sp., in an anopheline colony by an egg-rinsing technique. *J. Invertebr. Pathol.* **15**, 321–327.

Ansari, M. A., Singh, K.R.P., Brooks, G. D., and Malhotra, P. R. (1977). A device for separation of pupae from larvae of *Aedes aegypti* (Diptera: Culicidae). *J. Med. Entomol.* **14**, 241–243.

Anthony, D. W., Savage, K. E., and Wiedhaas, D. E. (1972). Nosematosis: Its effect on *Anopheles albimanus* Wiedemann, and a population model of its relation to malaria transmission. *Proc. Helminthol. Soc. Wash., Spec. Issue* **39**, 428–433.

Asahina, S. (1964). Food material and feeding procedures for mosquito larvae. *Bull. W. H. O.* **31**, 463–466.

Asman, M. M., Craig, G. B., Jr., and Rai, K. S. (1963). Heterosis in *Aedes aegypti*. *Bull. Entomol. Soc. Am.* **9**, 173.

Asman, S. M. (1975). Reduced temperature and embryonation delay in *Culex tarsalis*. *Mosq. News* **35**, 230–231.

Bailey, D. L., Dame, D. A., Munroe, W. L., and Thomas, J. A. (1978). Colony maintenance of *Anopheles albimanus* Wiedemann by feeding preserved blood through a natural membrane. *Mosq. News* **38**, 403–408.

Bailey, D. L., Thomas, J. A., Munroe, W. L., and Dame, D. A. (1979). Viability of eggs of *Anopheles albimanus* and *Anopheles quadrimaculatus* when dried and stored at various temperatures. *Mosq. News* **39**, 113–116.

Bano, L. (1958). Partial inhibitory effect of *Plistophora culicis* on the sporogonic cycle of *Plasmodium cynomolgi* in *Anopheles stephensi*. *Nature (London)* **181**, 430.

Barbosa, P., and Peters, T. M. (1969). A comparative study of egg hatching techniques for Aedes aegypti (L.). *Mosq. News* **29**, 548–551.

Barbosa, P., Peters, T. M., and Greenough, N. C. (1972). Overcrowding of mosquito populations: Response of larval *Aedes aegypti* to stress. *Environ. Entomol.* **1**, 89–93.

Bar-Zeev, M. (1957). The effect of density on the larvae of the mosquito and its influence on fecundity. *Bull. Res. Counc. Isr.* **66**, 220–228.

Bar-Zeev, M. (1958). The effect of temperature on the growth rate and survival of the immature stages of *Aedes aegypti* (L.). *Bull. Entomol. Res.* **49**, 157–163.

Bar-Zeev, M. (1962). A simple technique for obtaining standard numbers of newly hatched mosquito larvae. *Mosq. News* **22**, 171–175.

Bar-Zeev, M., and Galun, R. (1961). A magnetic method of separating mosquito pupae from larvae. *Mosq. News* **21**, 225–228.

Bates, M. (1949). "The Natural History of Mosquitoes." Macmillan, New York.

Belkin, J. N. (1962). "The Mosquitoes of the South Pacific (Diptera, Culicidae)" Vol. 1. Univ. of California Press, Los Angeles.

Bentley, M. D., Lee, H.-P., McDaniel, I. N., Stiehl, B., and Yatagai, M. (1974). A mosquito egg counter by simple modification of a colorimeter. *J. Econ. Entomol.* **67**, 790–791.

Bentley, M. D., McDaniel, I. N., Lee, H.-P., Stiehl, B., and Yatagai, M. (1976). Studies of *Aedes triseriatus* oviposition attractants produced by larvae of *Aedes triseriatus* and *Aedes atropalpus* (Diptera: Culicidae). *J. Med. Entomol.* **13**, 112–115.

Bertram, D. S. (1965). Double infection of mosquitoes with a virus and a malarial parasite. *Int. Congr. Entomol. 12th, 1964* pp. 766–767.

Bidlingmayer, W. L. (1971). Mosquito flight paths in relation to the environment. 1. Illumination levels, orientation, and resting areas. *Ann. Entomol. Soc. Am.* **64**, 1121–1131.

Bradley, G. H., Goodwin, M. H., Jr., and Stone, A. (1949). Entomologic techniques as applied to anophelines. *In* "Malariology. A Comprehensive Survey of All Aspects of this Group of Diseases from a Global Standpoint" (M. F. Boyd, ed.), pp. 331–378. Saunders, Philadelphia, Pennsylvania.

Bray, R. S. (1958). Studies on malaria in chimpanzees. V. The sporogonous cycle and mosquito transmission of *Plasmodium vivax schwetzi*. *J. Parasitol.* **44**, 46–51.

Bryan, J. H., and Southgate, B. A. (1978). Studies of forced mating techniques on anopheline mosquitoes. *Mosq. News* **38**, 338–342.

Burton, G. J. (1971). A simple inexpensive styrofoam chamber for long-term holding of adult mosquitoes. *Mosq. News* **31**, 220–221.

Canning, E. U., and Hulls, R. H. (1970). A microsporidian infection of *Anopheles gambiae* Giles, from Tanzania: Interpretation of its mode of transmission and notes on *Nosema* infections in mosquitoes. *J. Protozool.* **17**, 531–539.

Carroll, D. F., Jones, G. E., and Wills, W. (1976). A simple artificial feeding technique for mosquitoes: Further investigations. *Proc. 63rd Annu. Meet.—N. J. Mosq. Exterm. Assoc.* **63**, 182–185.

Chambers, D. L. (1977). Quality control in mass rearing. *Annu. Rev. Entomol.* **22**, 289–308.

Chapman, H. C. (1974). Biological control of mosquito larvae. *Ann. Rev. Entomol.* **19**, 33–59.

Chapman, H. C., and Barr, A. R. (1969). Techniques for successful colonization of many mosquito species. *Mosq. News* **29**, 532–535.

Chapman, H. C., Woodard, D. B., Kellen, W. R., and Clark, T. B. (1966). Host-parasite relationships of *Thelohania* associated with mosquitoes in Louisiana. *J. Invertebr. Pathol.* **8**, 452–456.

Christophers, S. R. (1960). *"Aedes aegypti* (L.) the Yellow Fever Mosquito. Its Life History, Bionomics and Structure.'' Cambridge Univ. Press, London and New York.

Clements, A. N. (1963). ''The Physiology of Mosquitoes.'' Pergamon, Oxford.

Craig, G. B., Jr. (1964). Applications of genetic technology to mosquito rearing. *Bull. W. H. O.* **31**, 469–473.

Craig, G. B., Jr., and Hickey, W. A. (1967). Genetics of *Aedes aegypti. In* ''Genetics of Insect Vectors of Disease'' (J. W. Wright and R. Pal, eds.), pp. 67–131. Am. Elsevier, New York.

Craig, G. B., Jr., VandeHey, R. C., and Hickey, W. A. (1961). Genetic variability in populations of *Aedes aegypti. Bull. W. H. O.* **24**, 527–539.

Crans, W. J., and Slaff, M. E. (1977). Growth and behavior of colonized *Toxorhynchites rutilus septentrionalis. Mosq. News* **37**, 207–211.

Dadd, R. H. (1973). Autophagostimulation by mosquito larvae. *Entomol. Exp. Appl.* **16**, 295–300.

Dadd, R. H., and Kleinjan, J. E. (1974). Autophagostimulant from *Culex pipiens* larvae: Distinction from other mosquito larval factors. *Environ. Entomol.* **3**, 12–28.

Dadd, R. H., and Kleinjan, J. E. (1976). Chemically defined dietary media for larvae of the mosquito *Culex pipiens* (Diptera: Culicidae): Effects of colloid texturizers. *J. Med. Entomol.* **13**, 285–291.

Dame, D. A., Haile, D. G., Lofgren, C. S., Bailey, D. L., and Munroe, W. L. (1978). Improved rearing techniques for larval *Anopheles albimanus:* Use of dried mosquito eggs and electric heating tapes. *Mosq. News* **38**, 68–74.

Davies, E. E., Howells, R. E., and Venters, D. (1971). Microbial infections associated with plasmodial development in *Anopheles stephensi. Ann. Trop. Med. Parasitol.* **65**, 403–408.

Davies, J. B. (1969). Field preservation and storage of mosquitoes for laboratory studies. *Mosq. News* **29**, 259.

De St. Jeor, S. C., and Nielsen, L. T. (1964). The use of antibiotics as an aid in rearing larvae of *Culex tarsalis* Coq. *Mosq. News* **24**, 133–137.

Edman, J. D., and Bidlingmayer, W. L. (1969). Flight capacity of blood-engorged mosquitoes. *Mosq. News* **29**, 386–392.

El-Gayar, F. H., Gawaad, A.A.A., and Watson, W. M. (1972). Development of a standardized technique for rearing larvae of *Anopheles pharoensis* Theo. (Dipt., Culicidae), and preparation of dosage-mortality curves for five larvicides. *Z. Angew. Entomol.* **70**, 316–322.

Focks, D. A., Hall, D. W., and Seawright, J. A. (1977). Laboratory colonization and biological observations of *Toxorhynchites rutilus rutilus. Mosq. News* **37**, 751–755.

Focks, D. A., Seawright, J. A., and Hall, D. W. (1978). Laboratory rearing of *Toxorhynchites rutilus rutilus* (Coquillett) on a non-living diet. *Mosq. News* **38**, 325–328.

Ford, H. R., and Green, E. (1972). Laboratory rearing of *Anopheles albimanus* Wiedemann. *Mosq. News* **32**, 509–513.

Ford, H. R., and Green, E. (1976). Methods for rearing *Aedes taeniorhynchus* (Wiedemann) in the laboratory. *U. S. Dep. Agric., Agric. Res. Serv.* **ARS-S-145**, 1–4.

Foster, W. A., and Lea, A. O. (1975). Sexual behavior maturation in male *Aedes triseriatus* (Diptera: Culicidae): A reexamination. *J. Med. Entomol.* **12**, 459–463.

Fowler, H. W., Jr. (1972). Rates of insemination by induced copulation of *Aedes vexans* (Diptera: Culicidae) treated with three anaesthetics. *Ann. Entomol. Soc. Am.* **65**, 293–296.

Fox, R. M., and Weiser, J. (1959). A microsporidian parasite of *Anopheles gambiae* in Liberia. *J. Parasitol.* **45**, 21–30.

French, F. E. (1970). Maintaining mosquito colonies of *Aedes atropalpus* and *Anopheles stephensi* with less than 5 hours labor per month. *Can. J. Zool.* **48**, 393–394.

Friend, W. G., and Smith, J.J.B. (1977). Factors affecting feeding in bloodsucking insects. *Ann. Rev. Entomol.* **22**, 309–331.

Furumizo, R. T., Cheong, W. H., and Rudnick, A. (1977). Laboratory studies of *Toxorhynchites splendens*. Part I. Colonization and laboratory maintenance. *Mosq. News* **37**, 664–667.

Garnham, P.C.C. (1956). Microsporidia in laboratory colonies of *Anopheles*. *Bull. W. H. O.* **15**, 845–847.

Gerberg, E. J. (1970). Manual for mosquito rearing and experimental techniques. *Am. Mosq. Control Assoc. Bull.* No. 5, pp. 1–109.

Gerberg, E. J., Gentry, J. W., and Diven, L. H. (1968). Mass rearing of *Anopheles stephensi* Liston. *Mosq. News* **28**, 342–346.

Gillett, J. D. (1967). Natural selection and feeding speed in a blood sucking insect. *Proc. R. Soc. London, Ser. B* **167**, 316–329.

Gillett, J. D. (1971). "The Mosquito: Its Life, Activities, and Impact on Human Affairs." Doubleday, New York.

Gillett, J. D. (1976). Apparatus for the routine production and collection of eggs of *Aedes aegypti*. *Trans. R. Soc. Trop. Med. Hyg.* **70**, 23.

Greenberg, G. (1970). Sterilizing procedures and agents, antibiotics and inhibitors in mass rearing of insects. *Bull. Entomol. Soc. Am.* **16**, 31–36.

Hagstrum, D. W., and Hagstrum, W. R. (1970). A simple device for producing fluctuating temperatures, with an evaluation of the ecological significance of fluctuating temperatures. *Ann. Entomol. Soc. Am.* **63**, 1385–1389.

Hamilton, D. R., and Bradley, R. E., Sr. (1977). An integrated system for the production of gnotobiotic *Anopheles quadrimaculatus*. *J. Inverteb. Pathol.* **30**, 318–324.

Hazard, E. I. (1967). Modification of the ice water method for harvesting *Anopheles* and *Culex* pupae. *Mosq. News* **27**, 115–116.

Hazard, E. I. (1970). Microsporidian diseases in mosquito colonies: *Nosema* in two *Anopheles* colonies. *Proc. Int. Colloq. Insect Pathol., 4th, 1970*, pp. 267–271.

Hazard, E. I., Turner, R. B., and Lofgren, C. S. (1967). Mosquito growth stimulating substances associated with infusions. *J. Med. Entomol.* **4**, 455–460.

Holzapfel, C. M., and Bradshaw, W. E. (1976). Rearing of *Toxorhynchites rutilus septentrionalis* (Diptera: Culicidae) from Florida and Pennsylvania with notes on their pre-diapause and pupal development. *Ann. Entomol. Soc. Am.* **69**, 1062–1064.

Horsfall, W. R. (1955). "Mosquitoes. Their Bionomics and Relation to Disease." Ronald Press, New York.

Horsfall, W. R., Fowler, H. W., Jr., Moretti, L. J., and Larsen, J. R. (1973). "Bionomics and Embryology of the Inland Floodwater mosquito *Aedes vexans*." Univ. of Illinois Press, Chicago.

Hudson, A., and McClintock, J. (1967). A chemical factor that stimulates oviposition by *Culex tarsalis* Coquillett (Diptera, Culicidae). *Anim. Behav.* **15**, 336–341.

Huffaker, C. B. (1944). The temperature relation of the immature stages of the malarial mosquito, *Anopheles quadrimaculatus* Say, with a comparison of the developmental power of constant and variable temperatures in insect metabolism. *Ann. Entomol. Soc. Am.* **37**, 1–27.

Ikeshoji, T., and Mulla, M. S. (1970a). Overcrowding factors of mosquito larvae. *J. Econ. Entomol.* **63**, 90–96.

Ikeshoji, T., and Mulla, M. S. (1970b). Overcrowding factors of mosquito larvae. 2. Growth retarding and bacteriostatic effects of the overcrowding factors of mosquito larvae. *J. Econ. Entomol.* **63**, 1737–1743.

Ikeshoji, T., and Mulla, M. S. (1974a). Overcrowding factors of mosquito larvae: Isolation and chemical identification. *Environ. Entomol.* **3**, 482–486.

Ikeshoji, T., and Mulla, M. S. (1974b). Overcrowding factors of mosquito larvae: Activity of branched fatty acids against mosquito larvae. *Environ. Entomol.* **3**, 487–491.

Ising, E. (1972). Provisorische Klimaraeume zur Laborzucht von Stechmuecken: 2. Ein klimatisierbares "Gebaeude" zur Verwendung im Freiland. *Z. Angew. Zool.* **59,** 141-151.

Jenkins, D. W. (1964). Pathogens, parasites and predators of medically important arthropods: Annotated list and bibliography. *Bull. W. H. O.* **30,** Suppl. 1-150.

Jupp, P. G., and Brown, R. G. (1967). The laboratory colonization of *Culex (Culex) univittatus* Theobald (Diptera: Culicidae) from material collected in the Highveld region of South Africa. *J. Entomol. Soc. South Afr.* **30,** 34-39.

Kalpage, K.S.P., and Brust, R. A. (1973). Oviposition attractants produced by immature *Aedes atropalpus. Environ. Entomol.* **2,** 729-730.

Kardatzke, J. T. (1976). Maintenance and transportation of female mosquitoes collected in the field. *Mosq. News* **36,** 527-529.

Kellen, W. R., Chapman, H. C., Clark, T. B., and Lindegren, J. E. (1965). Host-parasite relationships of some *Thelohania* from mosquitoes. *J. Invertebr. Pathol.* **7,** 161-166.

Killick-Kendrick, R. (1971). The collection of strains of murine malaria parasites in the field, and their maintenance in the laboratory by cyclical passage. *Symp. Br. Soc. Parasitol.* **9,** 39-64.

Klassen, W., and Gentz, G. (1971). Temperature-constant and temperature gradient-free insectary: Design and operation. *J. Econ. Entomol.* **64,** 1334-1336.

Knight, K. L. (1978). "Supplement to a Catalog of the Mosquitoes of the World," Thomas Say Found., Vol. VI, Suppl. Entomol. Soc. Am., Washington, D.C.

Knight, K. L., and Stone, A. (1977). "A Catalog of the Mosquitoes of the World," 2nd ed., Thomas Say Found., Vol. VI. Entomol. Soc. Am., Washington, D.C.

Kramer, J. P. (1964). Parasites in laboratory colonies of mosquitoes. *Bull. W. H. O.* **31,** 475-478.

Kuno, G., and Moore, C. G. (1975). Production of larval growth retardant in axenic cultures of *Aedes aegypti. Mosq. News* **35,** 199-201.

Laird, M. (1971). A bibliography on diseases and enemies of medically important arthropods 1963-67 with some earlier titles omitted from Jenkins' 1964 list. *In* "Microbial Control of Insects and Mites" (H. D. Burgess and N. W. Hussey, eds.), Appendix 7, pp. 751-789. Academic Press, New York.

Lang, C. A., Basch, K. J., and Storey, R. S. (1972). Growth, composition and longevity of the axenic mosquito (Dipt., Culicidae). *J. Nutr.* **102,** 1057-1066.

Lang, J. T., and Foster, W. A. (1976). Is there a female sex pheromone in the mosquito *Culiseta inornata? Environ. Entomol.* **5,** 1109-1115.

Laven, H. (1967). Formal genetics of *Culex pipiens. In* "Genetics of Insect Vectors of Disease" (J. W. Wright and R. Pal, eds.), pp. 17-65. Am. Elsevier, New York.

McClelland, G.A.H. (1967). Speciation and evolution in *Aedes. In* "Genetics of Insect Vectors of Disease" (J. W. Wright and R. Pal, eds.), pp. 277-311. Am. Elsevier, New York.

McCray, E. M., Jr. (1963). Escape-proof colony cage (*Aedes aegypti*). *Mosq. News* **23,** 309-311.

McCray, E. M., Jr., McCray, T. L., and Schoof, H. F. (1972). Effects of air currents upon the life span (longevity) of adult *Aedes aegypti* (L.) in the laboratory. *Mosq. News* **32,** 620-622.

McCuiston, L. J., and White, D. J. (1976). Laboratory colonization of *Aedes sollicitans* (Walker) with a review of the technique of induced copulation. *Proc. Annu. Meet.—N. J. Mosq. Exterm. Assoc.* **63,** 164-175.

Macdonald, W. W. (1962). The genetic basis of susceptibility to infection with semiperiodic *Brugia malayi* in *Aedes aegypti. Ann. Trop. Med. Parasitol.* **56,** 373-382.

Macdonald, W. W. (1967). The influence of genetic and other factors on vector susceptibility to parasites. *In* "Genetics of Insect Vectors of Disease" (J. W. Wright and R. Pal, eds.), pp. 567-584. Am. Elsevier, New York.

Macdonald, W. W. (1971). The maintenance of vectors of filariasis. *Symp. Br. Soc. Parasitol.* **9,** 123-149.

Mackauer, M. (1976). Genetic problems in the production of biological control agents. *Ann. Rev. Entomol.* **21**, 369–385.

Mattingly, P. F. (1967). Genetics of behaviour. *In* "Genetics of Insect Vectors of Disease" (J. W. Wright and R. Pal, eds.), pp. 553–566. Am. Elsevier, New York.

Mattingly, P. F. (1969). "The Biology of Mosquito-borne Disease." Allen & Unwin, London.

Meola, R. (1964). The influence of temperature and humidity on embryonic longevity in *Aedes aegypti. Ann. Entomol. Soc. Am.* **57**, 468–472.

Moody, D. S., Mastro, V. C., and Payne, T. L. (1973). Automatic light-dimming system to simulate twilight in environmental chambers. *J. Econ. Entomol.* **66**, 1334–1335.

Moore, C. G., and Whitacre, D. M. (1972). Competition in mosquitoes. 2. Production of *Aedes aegypti* larval growth retardant at various densities and nutrition levels. *Ann. Entomol. Soc. Am.* **65**, 915–918.

Morlan, H. B., Hayes, R. O., and Schoof, J. (1963). Methods for mass rearing of *Aedes aegypti* (L.). *Public Health Rep.* **78**, 711–719.

Mouchet, J. (1967). Quelques remarques sur le transport et l'expédition de *Culex pipiens fatigans. Bull. W. H. O.*. **37**, 329.

Nayar, J. K. (1972). Effects of constant and fluctuating temperatures on life span of *Aedes taeniorhynchus* adults. *J. Insect Physiol.* **18**, 1303–1313.

Nayar, J. K., and Sauerman, D. M., Jr. (1975). The effects of nutrition on survival and fecundity in Florida mosquitoes. Part 2. Utilization of a blood meal for survival. *J. Med. Entomol.* **12**, 99–103.

Nayar, J. K., and Sauerman, D. M., Jr. (1977). The effects of nutrition on survival and fecundity in Florida mosquitoes. Part 4. Effects of blood source on oocyte development. *J. Med. Entomol.* **14**, 167–174.

Nijhout, H. F., and Craig, G. B., Jr. (1971). Reproductive isolation in *Stegomyia* mosquitoes. III. Evidence for a sexual pheromone. *Entomol. Exp. Appl.* **14**, 399–412.

Novak, R. J., and Shroyer, D. A. (1978). Eggs of *Aedes triseriatus* and *Ae. hendersoni:* A method to stimulate optimal hatch. *Mosq. News.* **38**, 515–521.

Olson, J. K., and Horsfall, W. R. (1972). Thermal stress and anomalous development of mosquitoes (Diptera, Culicidae). VIII. Gonadal responses to fluctuating temperature. *Ann. Zool. Fenn.* **9**, 98–110.

Osgood, C. E. (1971a). Wet filter paper as an oviposition substrate for mosquitoes that lay egg rafts. *Mosq. News* **31**, 32–35.

Osgood, C. E. (1971b). An oviposition pheromone associated with the egg rafts of *Culex tarsalis. J. Econ. Entomol.* **64**, 1038–1041.

Pappas, L. G. (1973). Larval rearing technique for *Culiseta inornata* (Will.). *Mosq. News* **33**, 604–605.

Peters, T. M., and Barbosa, P. 1977). Influence of population density on size, fecundity, and developmental rate of insects in culture. *Ann. Rev. Entomol.* **22**, 431–450.

Peters, T. M., Chevone, B. I., Greenough, N. C., Callahan, R. A., and Barbosa, P. (1969). Intraspecific competition in *Aedes aegypti* (L.) larvae. I. Equipment, techniques and methodology. *Mosq. News* **29**, 667–674.

Polk, U. B. (1978). Use of sugar cubes as a carbohydrate source for adult *Culex quinquefasciatus* Say. *Mosq. News* **38**, 422.

Provost, N. W. (1957). The dispersal of *Aedes taeniorhynchus*. II. The second experiment. *Mosq. News* **17**, 233–247.

Reisen, W. K. (1975). Effects of selected antibiotics on the larval development of *Anopheles stephensi* Liston (Diptera: Culicidae). *Pak. J. Zool.* **7**, 113–115.

Reisen, W. K., and Emory, R. W. (1977). Intraspecific competition in *Anopheles stephensi* (Diptera:

Culicidae). II. The effects of more crowded densities and the addition of antibiotics. *Can. Entomol.* **109**, 1475-1480.

Reisen, W. K., and Siddiqui, T. F. (1978). The influence of conspecific immatures on the oviposition preferences of the mosquitoes *Anopheles stephensi* and *Culex tritaeniorhynchus*. *Pak. J. Zool.* **10**, 31-41.

Reynolds, D. G. (1971). Parasitism of *Culex fatigans* by *Nosema stegomyiae*. *J. Inverteb. Pathol.* **18**, 429.

Roberts, D. W., and Strand, M. A. (1977). Pathogens of medically important arthropods. *Bull. W. H. O.* **55**, Suppl., 1-419.

Rosales-Ronquillo, M. C., Simmons, R. W., and Silverman, P. H. (1973). Aseptic rearing of *Anopheles stephensi* (Diptera: Culicidae). *Ann. Entomol. Soc. Am.* **66**, 949-954.

Rozeboom, L. E., Rosen, L., and Ikeda, J. (1973). Observations on oviposition by *Aedes (S.) albopictus* Skuse and *A. (S.) polynesiensis* Marks in nature. *J. Med. Entomol.* **10**, 397-399.

Russell, P. F., West, L. S., Manwell, R. D., and MacDonald, G. (1963). "Practical Malariology." Oxford Univ. Press, London and New York.

Rutledge, L. C., Ward, R. A., and Gould, D. J. (1964). Studies on the feeding response of mosquitoes to nutritive solutions in a new membrane feeder. *Mosq. News* **24**, 407-419.

Rudledge, L. C., Sofield, R. K., and Piper, G. N. (1976). Rapid counting methods for mosquito larvae. *Mosq. News* **36**, 537-540.

Savage, K. E., Lowe, R. E., Hazard, E. I., and Lofgren, C. S. (1971). Studies of the transmission of *Plasmodium gallinaceum* by *Anopheles quadrimaculatus* infected with a *Nosema* sp. *Bull. W. H. O.* **45**, 845-847.

Schlosser, I. J., and Buffington, J. D. (1977). The energetics of r- vs. K-selection in two African strains of *Aedes aegypti*. *Ann. Entomol. Soc. Am.* **70**, 196-202.

Service, M. W. (1970). Insect mortality. *Nature (London)* **227**, 421.

Service, M. W. (1976). "Mosquito Ecology. Field Sampling Methods." Applied Science Publishers, London.

Sharma, V. P., Patterson, R. S., and Ford, H. R. (1972). A device for the rapid separation of male and female mosquito pupae. *Bull. W. H. O.* **47**, 429-432.

Sharma, V. P., Labreque, G. C., and Patterson, R. S. (9174). A device for the pupal separation of male from female mosquitoes in the field. *Mosq. News* **34**, 9-11.

Shelton, R. M. (1973). The effect of temperatures on development of eight mosquito species. *Mosq. News* **33**, 1-12.

Shroyer, D. A., and Sanders, D. P. (1977). The influence of carbohydrate-feeding and insemination on oviposition of an Indiana strain of *Aedes vexans* (Diptera: Culicidae). *J. Med. Entomol.* **14**, 121-127.

Smith, C. N. (1966). "Insect Colonization and Mass Production." Academic Press, New York.

Smittle, B. J., and Patterson, R. S. (1974). Container for irradiation and mass transport of adult mosquitoes. *Mosq. News* **34**, 406-408.

Sneller, V. P., and Dadd, R. H. (1977). Requirement for sugar in a chemically defined diet for larval *Aedes aegypti* (Diptera: Culicidae). *J. Med. Entomol.* **14**, 387-392.

Sollers-Riedel, H. (1963-present). Literature references to mosquitoes and mosquito-borne diseases. *Mosq. News* **23**,-present (various pp.) (See also Sollers, H., Stage, H. H. and Sollers, H., and Stage, H. H. in earlier volumes.)

Soman, R. S., and Reuben, R. (1970). Studies on the preference shown by ovipositing females of *Aedes aegypti* for water containing immature stages of the same species. *J. Med. Entomol.* **7**, 485-489.

Spielman, A., and Kitzmiller, J. B. (1967). Genetics of populations of medically important arthropods. *In* "Genetics of Insect Vectors of Disease" (J. W. Wright and R. Pal, eds.), pp. 459-485. Am. Elsevier, New York.

Starratt, A. N., and Osgood, C. E. (1972). An oviposition pheromone of the mosquito *Culex tarsalis:* Diglyceride composition of the active fraction. *Biochim. Biophys. Acta* **280**, 187–193.

Trembley, H. L. (1955). Mosquito culture techniques and experimental procedures. *Am. Mosq. Control Assoc. Bull.* No. 3, pp. 1–73.

Trimble, R. M., and Corbet, P. S. (1975). Laboratory colonization of *Toxorhynchites rutilus septentrionalis* (Diptera: Culicidae). *Ann. Entomol. Soc. Am.* **68**, 217–219.

Trpis, M., and Gerberg, E. J. (1973). Laboratory colonization of *Toxorhynchites brevipalpis. Bull. W. H. O.* **48**, 637–638.

Tubergen, T. A., Breaud, T. P., and McConnell, E. (1978). A technique for drying eggs of *Anopheles stephensi* and its effect on their viability after storage at 4°C. *Mosq. News* **38**, 583–585.

Undeen, A. H., and Alger, N. E. (1975). The effect of the microsporidian, *Nosema algerae,* on *Anopheles stephensi. J. Inverterbr. Pathol.* **25**, 19–24.

VandeHey, R. C. (1964). Genetic variability in *Aedes aegypti* (Diptera: Culicidae). III. Plasticity in laboratory populations. *Ann. Entomol. Soc. Am.* **57**, 488–496.

Vavra, J., and Undeen, A. H. (1970). *Nosema algerae* n.sp. (Cnidospora, Microsporida), a pathogen in a laboratory colony of *Anopheles stephensi* Liston (Diptera, Culicidae). *J. Protozool.* **17**, 240–244.

Wade, J. O. (1975). An improved method for the membrane feeding of mosquitoes. *Trans. R. Soc. Trop. Med. Hyg.* **69**, 19.

Wade, J. O. (1976). A new design of membrane feeder incorporating an electrical blood stirring device. *Ann. Trop. Med. Parasitol.* **70**, 113–120.

Walker, P. J., and Rogers, A. (1971). A simple method for obtaining a circadian temperature cycle from an air conditioner in an insectarium. *J. Med. Entomol.* **8**, 613–614.

Wallis, R. C., and Lite, S. W. (1970). Axenic rearing of *Culex salinarius. Mosq. News* **30**, 427–429.

Ward, R. A. (1963). Genetic aspects of the susceptibility of mosquitoes to malarial infection. *Exp. Parasitol.* **13**, 328–341.

Ward, R. A., and Savage, K. E. (1972). Effects of microsporidian parasites upon anopheline mosquitoes and malarial infection. *Proc. Helminthol. Soc. Wash., Spec. Issue* **39**, 434–438.

Weathersby, A. B. (1963). Harvesting mosquito pupae with cold water. *Mosq. News* **23**, 249–251.

Whitten, M. J., and Foster, G. G. (1975). Genetical methods of pest control. *Ann. Rev. Entomol.* **20**, 461–476.

Williams, R. W. (1953). The growth stimulating effect of APF, terramycin hydrochloride, vitamin B_{12} and an undetermined factor "X" upon *Aedes aegypti* (L.) (Diptera: Culicidae). *Am. J. Trop. Med. Hyg.* **2**, 109–114.

Williams, R. E. (1962). Effect of coloring oviposition media with regard to the mosquito *Aedes triseriatus* (Say). *J. Parasitol.* **48**, 919–925.

Wills, W., Carroll, D. F., and Jones, G. E. (1974). A simple method for artificially feeding mosquitoes. *Mosq. News* **34**, 119–121.

Wilton, D. P. (1968). Oviposition site selection by the tree-hole mosquito, *Aedes triseriatus* (Say). *J. Med. Entomol.* **5**, 189–194.

World Health Organization (1967). Genetics of vectors and insecticide resistance. *In* "Genetics of Insect Vectors of Disease" (J. W. Wright and R. Pal, eds.), Appendix A and B, pp. 735–758. Am. Elsevier, New York.

World Health Organization (1975). "Manual on Practical Entomology in Malaria. Part II. Methods and Techniques" W.H.O. Offset Publ. No. 13, W.H.O., Geneva.

Yen, J. H., and Barr, A. R. (1973). The etiological agent of cytoplasmic incompatability in *Culex pipiens* L. *J. Invertebr. Pathol.* **22**, 242–250.

Yoeli, M., and Boné, G. (1967). Studies on *Anopheles dureni* Edwards. *Riv. Malariol.* **46**, 3–13.

The Transmission by Mosquitoes of Plasmodia in the Laboratory

Jerome P. Vanderberg and Robert W. Gwadz

I. INTRODUCTION

Malarial infections are normally initiated when an infected mosquito, in the act of feeding, injects sporozoites into a susceptible host. However, the majority of experimental studies start with infections initiated by the injection of infected blood. Indeed, a stranger surveying the literature on the subject might easily come to the conclusion that malaria is a blood disease transmitted by the bite of a hypodermic needle. Because of the relative ease of working with blood-induced infections, and the difficulty in working with mosquitoes, research requiring mosquito passage of the parasite has been rather neglected. Nevertheless, there are a number of problems that can be approached only through the use of laboratory infections induced with the mosquito stages of the parasite.

The course of sporozoite-induced malaria infections may differ significantly from that of blood-induced infections. In *Plasmodium vivax* malaria in humans, characteristics of the infection such as length of the prepatent period, duration and severity of clinical attacks, tendency to relapse, and the latent period between relapses are determined by the number of sporozoites injected to initiate infection. Indeed, relapses of mammalian malarias can only occur in sporozoite-induced infections (James, 1931; Boyd and Stratman-Thomas, 1933b; James *et al.*, 1936; Craige *et al.*, 1947; Shute and Maryon, 1968; Shute *et al.*, 1976). Because sporozoites are involved in the natural transmission of malaria, it follows that sporozoite-induced laboratory infections more closely mimic what actually occurs in nature.

There is considerable interest in developing effective means of prophylaxis against mosquito-transmitted sporozoites, either by drugs which prevent infection (see Chapter 3, Vol. 1) or by immunization with sporozoites (see Chapter 4, Vol. 3). Research in these areas requires routine production of sporozoites, and studies on mosquito transmission should be considered a necessary prerequisite for these pharmacological or immunological studies.

A number of areas of malaria research require the regular use of mosquitoes. Sexual development of the parasite takes place in the mosquito gut, and studies on the genetics of the parasite require the establishment of a system of mosquito transmission in order to understand the mechanisms involved. An overall understanding of the differentiation of the malaria parasite requires a study of the mosquito stages which occupy important transitional phases between the vertebrate and the invertebrate host. The gametocytes taken up by the feeding mosquito bridge the gap between the vertebrate host and its mosquito vector, while the sporozoites injected by the mosquito link the insect with the host on which it feeds and subsequently infects. The adaptive changes which occur within the parasite during its differentiation in the mosquito are interesting and instructive biological phenomena, e.g., the shifts in energy metabolism that the parasite undergoes as it moves between its mammalian and mosquito hosts (Mack and Vanderberg, 1978).

One of the more active areas of malaria research concerns the problem of host cell penetration by the parasite. Yet, nearly 100 years after the discovery of the malarial parasite, we still do not understand how the initial infective stage, the sporozoite, invades the liver of its mammalian host, or even which cells are initially invaded. Solution of this basic question requires laboratory-produced sporozoites.

One of the aims of this chapter is to point out some of the unsolved problems relating to sporozoite-induced malaria infections and to review the laboratory procedures and technology available. The first portion of this chapter considers the general principles and procedures involved in the transmission of malaria by mosquitoes. It covers such aspects as the susceptibility of mosquitoes to the parasite, the raising of infectious gametocytes in the vertebrate host, the infective blood meal taken by the mosquito, the laboratory maintenance of infected mosquitoes, the harvesting of sporozoites and assessment of their infectivity, and finally the challenge of the vertebrate host with sporozoites. In addition to general principles that apply to all species of malaria, there are certain specialized procedures that are unique to the malarias of birds, rodents, simians, and humans. Consequently, the final portion of the chapter deals specifically with each of these model systems.

II. SUSCEPTIBILITY OF MOSQUITOES TO *PLASMODIUM*

A. Introduction

Ronald Ross, in his original studies on mosquito transmission of malaria, recognized that different types of malaria were transmitted by different species of mosquitoes. He found that human malaria could infect ''dapple-winged mosquitoes'' (probably *Anopheles stephensi* and *A. culicifacies*), while avian malaria infected "grey or barred back mosquitoes" (probably *Culex quinquefasciatus*) and "brindled mosquitoes" (probably *Aedes* spp.) (Ross, 1923). This basic difference, i.e., avian malarias are transmitted by culicine mosquitoes while mammalian malarias are transmitted by anophelines, has generally held true, though the divisions have now always been clear-cut. Anophelines have been shown on numerous occasions to be capable of transmitting avian malaria parasites (review by Huff, 1965).

Studies conducted by many workers have shown that there is often a high degree of specificity in the relationship between the mosquito and the parasite (MacDonald, 1967). Spielman and Kitzmiller (1967) have pointed out that "many important vector species are polymorphic. In some cases sharply contrasting forms are found in different geographical areas or in differing ecological circumstances. . . . In some cases, one population may be of much greater importance as a disease vector than its subtly differing neighbor." Well-known examples of this are the *A. maculipennis* complex in Europe, the *A. stephensi* complex in Asia, the *A. gambiae* complex in Africa, and the *A. leucosphyrus* group in Southeast Asia.

Thus, in developing a laboratory system for mosquito transmission of malaria, one must carefully choose a parasite–vector combination which will allow for consistent, efficient mosquito infection, parasite maturation, and mosquito infectivity. Even with an established and efficient laboratory transmission system, however, there may be genetic drift in the susceptibility of the mosquito population or the infectivity of the parasite. Rutledge *et al.* (1970) measured the susceptibility of laboratory colonies of *A. quadrimaculatus* and *A. stephensi* to a strain of *P. cynomolgi* over the course of a year and found marked fluctuations in relative susceptibility. This problem may be due to the fact that laboratories often maintain continuous breeding colonies of vector mosquitoes and regularly remove mosquitoes from these colonies for infective feedings. The infected mosquitoes are ordinarily not used for breeding purposes. Thus, there is an unconscious artificial selection for mosquito fecundity and survival under the peculiar environmental maintenance conditions of the breeding colony. Generally, no special attempts are made to select for vector potential. A number of workers, however, have had considerable success in selecting mosquitoes for increased susceptibility to the parasite.

B. Selection of Mosquitoes for Increased Susceptibility to Malaria

The fact that certain individual mosquitoes within a population are more susceptible to malaria infection than others has long been known (review in Boyd, 1949). Huff (1927) showed that the disparate susceptibility of different members of a population of *C. pipiens* feeding on a *P. cathemerium*-infected host could not be explained as being due to the ingestion of larger or smaller numbers of gametocytes. He introduced the concept of individual mosquito immunity which he defined as "that characteristic of certain individuals belonging to a species susceptible to a given infection of being able to resist entirely that infection when given even very high inoculations of the parasite." By giving individual mosquitoes repeated meals of infected blood, Huff (1930) was able to show that the susceptibility or refractoriness of individual mosquitoes was a relatively fixed condition. Thus, it has been subsequently possible for several workers to select artificially for strains of mosquitoes with increased or decreased susceptibility to malarial infection [Huff (1929) for increased or decreased susceptibility of *C. pipiens* to *P. gallinaceum;* Huff (1931) for increased or decreased susceptibility of *C. quinquefasciatus* to *P. cathemerium;* Trager (1942) for increased susceptibility of *Aedes aegypti* to *P. lophurae;* Micks (1949) for increased susceptibility of *C. pipiens* to *P. elongatum;* Ward (1963) for increased or decreased susceptibility of *A. aegypti* to *P. gallinaceum*]. One of the chief difficulties associated with many of these studies was that the highly inbred lines of selected mosquitoes rapidly lost their fertility and could no longer be maintained as breeding colonies in the laboratory. This problem was somewhat resolved by Kilama and Craig (1969) who initiated their selection studies with two geographically distinct populations of *A. aegypti,* one of which was already highly susceptible to and the other almost entirely refractory to *P. gallinaceum.* By cross-breeding experiments, these workers found that refractoriness in this case was controlled by a single recessive mendelian factor.

Artificial selection of strains of *Anopheles* mosquitoes with increased susceptibility to human malaria has been less successful. Workers at the Rockefeller Foundation (1948, 1950) selected *A. quadrimaculatus* for increased or decreased susceptibility to *P. gallinaceum,* but Boyd and Russell (1943) were unable to change the susceptibility of *A. quadrimaculatus* to *P. vivax* by six generations of selective breeding. As previously indicated, it is well known that populations of anophelines from different geographic areas may have different susceptibilities to a parasite [e.g., Rutledge *et al.* (1970) who demonstrated different susceptibilities of various geographic strains of *A. stephensi* to *P. cynomolgi*]. More recently, Warren *et al.* (1977) described three morphologically different, true-breeding phenotypes within a single geographic strain of *A. albimanus* from El Salvador. These variants differed significantly in their susceptibility to a geographically coindigenous strain of *P. vivax.* Differences in their susceptibility to *P. falciparum,* however, were considerably less marked. The failure of Boyd and Russell (1943) to select successfully for increased susceptibility of *A. quadrimaculatus* to *P. vivax* may have been due to the detrimental effects of mosquito inbreeding induced by repeated brother–sister matings (as suggested by Huff, in Boyd and Russell, 1943). Recent reports have described selection for lines of *A. gambiae* (Mashadeni-Al and Davidson, 1978) and *A. atroparvus* (Van der Kaay *et al.,* 1978) susceptible and refractory to *P. berghei.*

Laboratory workers planning further studies on artificial selection of more-or-less susceptible strains of vector mosquitoes might do well to follow the lead of Kilama and Craig (1969) in starting selection with geographic strains of mosquitoes that have already attained a high degree of susceptibility or nonsusceptibility under natural conditions. Aside from the fact that fewer generations would be required to reach homozygosity, there would be less chance of the loss of colony fertility due to extreme inbreeding. Many genetically well-defined lines of vector mosquito species are now being described, and further work on their relative susceptibility to malaria is in order.

C. Factors Governing Choice of Vector for Laboratory Transmission

In the studies noted above, selection for susceptibility has been based on a common criterion, the development of oocysts on the gut of the subject mosquito. However, ''susceptibility'' is a relative term and can be expressed in different ways in various mosquito hosts. Parasite development can be aborted prior to fertilization, ookinete formation, or early oocyst development. In some mosquitoes, oocysts develop but fail to rupture, in others oocysts rupture but sporozoites are destroyed in the mosquito hemocoel. In other mosquitoes, sporozoites reach the salivary glands but are not infectious. A mosquito species can be refractory to one species of malaria, support partial development of a second, and support full maturation of yet a third closely related parasite. As a result, several mosquito species may be available for a particular study, and such factors as longevity and ease of mass rearing become important considerations. An illustration of this choice can be seen in studies measuring gamete infectivity and completion of the sexual cycle in various primate malarias. Oocyst development is used as a measure of the effective conversion of gametocytes to gametes to ookinetes in the mosquito gut. *Anopheles balabacensis* is a difficult species to rear; female mosquitoes must be individually force-mated, and larvae must be carefully tended. However, it is the only species in laboratory colonization which can develop heavy salivary gland infections with the monkey malaria *P. knowlesi*. *Anopheles freeborni* is an easily reared species which supports *P. knowlesi* development only to oocyst maturation; sporozoites are seldom seen in the salivary glands of this species. For studies on gamete infectivity *A. freeborni* is a logical choice, since only oocyst development is needed for monitoring infectivity. For studies requiring mature sporozoites, only *A. balabacensis* is acceptable.

III. GAMETOCYTES IN THE VERTEBRATE HOST

Mosquitoes become infected with malaria when they ingest gametocytes in a blood meal taken from an infectious vertebrate host. Efficient laboratory transmission of malaria by mosquitoes thus requires an understanding of the factors that influence the formation, maturation, and survival of gametocytes within the vertebrate.

A. The Origin of Gametocytes

Early in the history of malaria research, workers began to recognize that gametocytes were formed by the differentiation of asexual parasites within the red blood cell. Thus, Marchiafava and Bignami (1900) in writing about the development of the gametocyte (''semilunar'' or ''crescent'' stage) of *P. falciparum* (estivoautumnal malaria) were already able to state:

> The researches carried on in Rome have for a long time shown that the bodies of the semi-lunar stage are developed from the estivoautumnal parasites, of which they represent a constant life phase.
>
> The young parasitic forms from which the crescents originate are distinguishable from other forms of this species of parasite, even when they are less than a quarter of the size of a red blood cell. They occur as small, round, ovoid, or spindle-shaped bodies, which when seen in a fresh specimen appear to be quite homogenous and to contain a greater amount of black pigment than do the bodies of equal size of the preceding cycle; the pigment, moreover, is in the form of little rods or of somewhat large granules, and is either irregularly disseminated in the body of the parasite, or collected chiefly towards the periphery. These forms are not motile, they always occupy the lateral portion of the red corpuscle, and in their development always tend to adapt their convex surface to the edge of the corpuscle itself.
>
> As the development proceeds, even the bodies which were originally round tend to take on a long ovoid or rather spindle form, so long as the distance between the poles of the ovoid or the spindle does not exceed the diameter of the red corpuscle; when it does, the body either keeps the same shape or it becomes curved and forms the true crescent.

This accurate description of *P. falciparum* gametocyte development, as well as the descriptions of other early workers, were arrived at by conjecture. Microscope slides showing an apparently graded series of developmental stages ranging from asexual parasites to mature gametocytes were fitted together to form a logical series of developmental steps. However, absolute proof that gametocytes must arise from asexual parasites awaited the cloning studies of Walliker *et al.* (1973) who showed that rodent infections initiated with individual asexual parasites of *P. berghei* gave rise to parasitemias consisting of both asexual parasites and gametocytes. Gametocytes have also been shown to arise from exoerythrocytic (EE) merozoites, both in avian malaria (Adler and Tchernomoretz, 1941) and in mammalian malaria (James *et al.*, 1936; Killick-Kendrick and Warren, 1968).

B. Gametocyte Induction

1. Parasite Factors

The specific factors that induce the formation of gametocytes from asexual parasites (gametocytogenesis) are still not understood. The ability to produce greater or lesser numbers of gametocytes seems to be an inherent characteristic of a given parasite strain. For instance, some strains of *P. falciparum* produce many gametocytes, while others produce few (Marchoux, 1922). Similarly, differences in the degree of gametocyte production by different strains of *P. vivax* was observed by Korteweg (1930). There are numerous further examples of "good" versus "poor" gametocyte-producing strains of both avian and mammalian malaria species (reviews in Coatney *et al.*, 1971; Garnham, 1966).

In some strains, the inherent ability to produce gametocytes may become reduced or even entirely lost. This has been noted especially after repeated blood passage of the parasite by syringe, without occasional interposition of sexual reproduction through the mosquito. Huff and Gambrell (1934) and Gambrell (1937) observed that, when *P. cathemerium* was passed from canary to canary over a long period, by inoculation of blood from acutely infected birds, the number of gametocytes produced in each infection gradually decreased, and in two strains gametocyte production ceased completely. An even more striking example is that of *P. lophurae*, an avian malaria parasite that has been one of the most important experimental models for biochemical, physiological, and *in vitro* culture studies on malaria. The only existing strain of this parasite, originally isolated at the New York Zoological Park from pheasants imported from Borneo (Coggeshall, 1938), has essentially lost its ability to produce gametocytes (Garnham, 1966). Rodent malaria parasites seem to be especially prone toward losing the ability to produce infective gametocytes. Different strains vary, however, in the number of syringe passages tolerated before gametocyte viability deteriorates. Some commonly used strains, such as the NYU-2 strain of *P. berghei,* have completely lost gametocyte-producing potential. If a high degree of continued gametocyte infectivity is desired with rodent malaria, it is wise as a general rule not to permit more than three to five blood-to-blood passages before interposition of a mosquito passage. Similar findings have been made with human malaria. Not long after the introduction of malaria therapy for the treatment of general paralysis of the insane, it was found that some strains of *P. vivax* maintained by blood passage lost their ability to produce gametocytes (Barzilai-Vivaldi and Kauders, 1924; Schulze, 1925; Cuboni, 1926).

Loss of gametocyte-producing ability does not, however, invariably accompany continued passage of a parasite strain by syringe. *Plasmodium gallinaceum, P. knowlesi,* and *P. cynomolgi* may be syringe-passaged repeatedly over a period of years without any apparent diminution of gametocyte production. Strains of *P. vivax* passaged by blood between patients over a 5-year period continued to produce gametocytes during this time (Mühlens and Kirschbaum, 1924). It should especially be noted that the first demonstration of *P. falciparum* EE forms was with sporozoites obtained by feeding mosquitoes with a parasite strain that had just previously undergone 15 serial blood passages by syringe (Shortt *et al.,* 1949).

The loss of gametocytes due to repeated blood passage has often been referred to as "senescence of the strain." This rather imprecise phrase does not, however, tell us anything about the biological mechanisms involved. The actual mechanism responsible for this loss may result from selection for parasites that multiply rapidly in the blood, with no selective pressure in favor of gametocyte production. In some cases, the component of the genome controlling gametocyte formation may be entirely lost. In other cases it may be merely repressed, as evidenced by the ability of some strains to again produce gametocytes after appropriate manipulations.

A number of methods have been reported to reinduce gametocyte production in *Plasmodium* strains that have lost this ability, or to increase production in low-level producers. Several antimalarial drugs given in low doses have been found to induce increased numbers of *P. falciparum* gametocytes in human infections. though these gametocytes have not always been shown to be infective (Findlay *et al.*, 1946; Ramakrishnan *et al.*, 1952; Shute and Maryon, 1951). Chloroquine, which has been shown to enhance the infectivity of gametocytes of chloroquine-resistant strains of rodent malaria (Ramkaran and Peters, 1969; Wilkinson *et al.*, 1976), also appears to be able to induce new gametocyte formation in strains that have lost this ability. Peters *et al.* (1978) reported that this drug appeared to trigger the formation of normal gametocytes in an agametocytic strain of *P. yoelii* spp. that had been carried through about 20 years and countless passages in the laboratory by blood transfer. Other treatments shown to restore gametocytes to agametocytic strains of rodent malaria have been cryopreservation, with subsequent thawing (Bafort *et al.*, 1965; Vincke *et al.*, 1965), and passage through more susceptible rodent hosts (Jadin *et al.*, 1959). Increased formation of gametocytes has also been associated with the acquisition of drug resistance. Lines of *P. gallinaceum* selected for resistance to sulfadiazine showed marked increases in gametocyte production (Bishop, 1955).

Attempts to reinstitute gametocyte production in an agametocytic strain have not been uniformly successful, however. Hawking (1972) unsuccessfully attempted to initiate gametocyte production in two strains of *P. berghei* that had lost this ability. The procedures he tried included induction of resistance to chloroquine, sulfadiazine, and pyrimethamine, repeated treatment with subeffective doses of acriflavin, ethidium, colchicine, testosterone, and dexamethasone, and exposure to gamma irradiation or cryopreservation.

2. Environmental Factors

In addition to the inherent genetic ability of malaria parasites to develop into gametocytes, it seems clear that the developmental process itself must be initiated by external stimuli. The gametocyte productivity of a given plasmodial strain may be enhanced under one set of conditions and reduced under another. Thompson and Huff (1944) found that *P. mexicanum*, a parasite normally found in the lizard *Sceloporus ferrariperezi,* lost its gametocytes when transferred to another lizard, *S. collaris.* However, gametocyte production was again initiated when the parasite was transferred to a third host species, *S. olivaceous.* Similarly, the experimental adaptation of the avian malaria parasite *P. lophurae* to mice by McGee (1951) was accompanied by the loss of gametocyte production, though this capacity was regained when the adapted strain was returned to chick embryos. Likewise, in the case of rodent malaria, a strain of *P. berghei* that had lost its ability to produce gametocytes during serial passages in mice was induced to begin producing gametocytes again by repeated passage through young hamsters or the natural host, *Thamnomys* (Jadin *et al.,* 1959).

The physiological status of the host species may also affect the parasite. Gametocyte production of avian malarias as well as of other hemosporidian parasites of birds has been shown to vary seasonally with the endocrine cycle of the bird (review in Bishop, 1955). Many free-living protozoa have been shown to begin producing sexual stages as a response to nutritional stresses (review in Crandall, 1977).

Early malariologists subscribed to the view of Koch (1898) that the production of gametocytes in falciparum malaria was a response to the development of immunity by the human host. Thus, Stephens and Christophers (1908), as well as Thomson (1911), proposed that the sexual cycle was initiated when conditions became unfavorable for the asexual trophozoites, and that the gametocytes actually developed as a response to the ensuing immunity. However, field studies by Schüffner (1919) in Sumatra suggested quite the contrary. Schüffner pointed out that, if Koch's theory were accurate, there ought to be increasing gametocytemia with increasing host immunity. The epidemiological data, however, indicated otherwise. In children up to 2 years of age, 51% of those infected with *P. falciparum* had gametocytes in their circulation, while only 8% of the adults surveyed were found to have gametocytes. Similar findings have since been made by many other workers (reviews in Bishop, 1955; Covell, 1960). There has been some controversy as to whether the dissimilar *P. falciparum* gametocytemias found in children versus adults in endemic areas merely reflect the higher overall degree of parasitemia found in children, or whether these differences actually result from a higher gametocyte/asexual parasite ratio in children. The latter suggests an environmental enhancing effect on gametocyte production in children. Christophers (1924) and Sinton *et al.* (1926) found that the number of gametocytes produced was proportional to the overall parasitemia, whereas Garnham (1931) found no such correlation.

The erroneous assumption that gametocyte production in *P. falciparum* is a response to the development of host immunity may have come about because of the extended period of development required for the gametocytes of this species. These gametocytes are known to develop in the internal organs (chiefly the spleen and bone marrow) for a period of about 10 days, after which time they are released into the general circulation. This release often occurs at about the same time there is a reduction in asexual parasitemia. Early workers may have considered these two distinct processes, i.e., the appearance of gametocytes and the reduction in asexual parasitemia, to be causally related. The recent demonstration that *P. falciparum* gametocyte production can take place in an *in vitro* culture system obviously establishes the irrelevancy of immunity as a requirement for this developmental process. The specific environmental factors responsibel for the induction of gametocyte formation have still not been identified, though the *in vitro* studies of Carter and Miller (1980) with *P. falciparum* clearly show that such environmental factors are definitely involved.

C. Gametocyte Morphology

Gametocytes can be readily identified in blood smears conventionally stained with Giemsa stain, as described in Chapter 4, Vol. 1. In most instances, gametocytes are easily distinguishable morphologically from asexual trophozoites. Gametocytes typically take longer to develop than trophozoites and tend to be somewhat larger at maturity. Even when young, they can often be distinguished on the basis of their denser, more compact appearance and their lack of a vacuole. At all stages of their development, gametocytes tend to be characterized by a general distribution of pigment granules throughout their cytoplasm, compared with the clumping of granules commonly observed in trophozoites. There are some exceptions in the ease with which gametocytes can be identified. Macrogametocytes of *P. malariae,* for instance, are extremely difficult to distinguish from the large uninucleate trophozoites they often resemble. Most gametocytes are compact and rounded in appearance, as observed in a stained smear. Some species, however, have gametocytes with a conspicuously elongate shape. These include *P. falciparum* in mammalian malaria, and three of the four known subgenera of avian malaria (including the important species *P. fallax* and *P. lophurae*).

Macrogametocytes can generally be distinguished from microgametocytes with ease. The former tend to be larger, often taking up virtually all the cytoplasm of the host red blood cell. The nucleus of the macrogametocyte is generally compact in size and eccentric in location. The cytoplasm is usually quite basophilic and stains blue with Giemsa, reflecting the greater concentration of ribosomes in macrogametocytes, as observed by electron microscopy. Fine-structural studies also indicate that macrogametocytes have a greater concentration of electron-dense, osmiophilic bodies similar to micronemes (Sinden *et al.*, 1976).

Microgametocytes, on the other hand, tend to be somewhat smaller, usually not filling the entire red blood cell cytoplasm. The nucleus is considerably larger than that of the macrogametocyte, sometimes occupying as much as one-half of the entire parasite. This presumably reflects the polyploid nature of the microgametocyte nucleus prior to the formation of microgametes. The microgametocyte cytoplasm is less basophilic than that of the macrogametocyte, tending to be more gray than blue.

For accurate identification of gametocytes of a given species of malaria, the laboratory worker should consult color plates in standard monographs, such as Garnham (1966) and Coatney et al. (1971).

D. Kinetics of Gametocytes and Gametocyte Infectivity in the Blood

1. First Appearance in the Blood

Gametocytes may be seen quite early in an infection, often with the first asexual parasites, or their appearance may be delayed until much later. They have been observed to appear together with the first asexual trophozoites in experimentally induced infections of different species of avian malaria (Shah, 1934; Lumsden and Bertram, 1940; Bishop, 1943; Eyles, 1951), rodent malaria (Killick-Kendrick and Warren, 1968), and human (vivax) malaria (Boyd et al., 1936b). In *P. falciparum,* where gametocyte development is prolonged in the internal organs, there is generally at least a 10-day period between the appearance of the first asexual parasites in a primary attack and the appearance of gametocytes in the peripheral circulation (Jeffery, 1960; Kitchen and Putnam, 1942). However, *P. falciparum* gametocytes may not be observed in a primary attack for over 3 weeks (Shute and Maryon, 1951). It had been observed by Bignami and Bastianelli (1890) that "after the formation of the young crescent-shaped forms has thus commenced . . . their production continues with each successive paroxysm, so that after a series of attacks the blood contains an accumulation of crescent-shaped forms." Gametocytes of human and simian malarias do not seem to appear gradually and in steady numbers. Rather they have been described as appearing in "showers" in vivax malaria (Boyd et al., 1936b), while Garnham (1931) has described the appearance of gametocytes in falciparum malaria as a sudden flooding of the blood with them. Hawking (1975) has reported "bursts" of exflagellating gametocytes in rhesus monkeys infected with *P. cynomolgi.* The pattern of appearance of the gametocytes in falciparum malaria has been noted by Brumpt (1949) as follows:

> They increase rapidly in number on successive days for about a week; often there is a marked coincident decline in the trophozoites, which may almost disappear. Thus, the appearance of the "gametocyte wave" often coincides with a remission. At about the crest of the gametocyte wave trophozoites again increase and may regain pyrogenic levels in a few days, to be followed by another gametocyte wave. *Falciparum* infections invariably exhibit these successive and consecutive waves of trophozoites and gametocytes.

2. Parameters of Gametocyte Infectivity

The appearance of gametocytes in the blood is no guarantee of their infectivity. They must often undergo a further period of development to reach functional maturity. This functional maturity is generally measured either by the ability of the microgametocytes to exflagellate or infectivity of the gametocytes to mosquitoes.

a. Demonstration of Exflagellation. A consideration of the factors involved in the induction of exflagellation has been presented elsewhere in this volume. Exflagellation is commonly demonstrated and quantified in one of two ways: (1) by allowing it to proceed within a drop of blood on a microscope slide, after which the preparation is stained for microscopic observation, or (2) by preparing a wet mount slide and observing exflagellation directly as it occurs.

The stained slide method is generally known as the Shute technique, and has been described by James (1934) and in Shute and Maryon (1966). Moist petri dish chambers are prepared by inserting a piece of filter paper cut to fit in the lid and in the bottom of each dish. As much water as the paper can absorb is added, and the dishes are closed. Tubing or glass rods are placed in each dish to support the microscope slides above the saturated filter paper. Blood taken directly from patients or from experimental animals is applied to the slide as a film slightly thicker than an ordinary thin film and is generally breathed upon lightly before being placed in the chamber. *In vitro* preparations with hematocrits lower than that of whole blood should of course have correspondingly more material applied to the slide. The slides are then incubated at an appropriate temperature (generally at about 23°–25°C), and individual slides may be removed at intervals to determine the optimal time for exflagellation under the prevailing conditions. At 25°C exflagellation is complete in 15 minutes for *P. vivax* and *P. ovale* and in 15–30 minutes for *P. falciparum* (Shute and Maryon, 1966). Slides found to be already dry upon removal are discarded; others are allowed to air-dry or may be rapidly dried by passing them over a flame. The slides may then be fixed with methanol and stained with Giemsa stain, as for ordinary cytological staining of blood films. For special cytological studies, slides removed from the humid petri dish chamber may be allowed to dry in an atmosphere of osmium tetroxide vapor.

Direct observation of exflagellation while it is occurring is easier because of the agitation and movement of adjacent red blood cells. This can often be seen by scanning slides at relatively low magnifications. Observations are best made with phase-contrast illumination at magnifications approximating 400×. The cells should be diluted so that exflagellation can be readily seen and not obscured by overlying erythrocytes. Sinden and Croll (1975) made observations by diluting whole blood collected from mice 10-fold with various types of media. Carter and Nijhout (1977) diluted blood collected from chickens to a 0.3% hematocrit so that the erythrocytes settled out in a monolayer in their observation chamber. Determination of the proper drop size and hematocrit to use will obviously vary with the size of the coverslip placed on top. To prevent drying around the edges, the coverslip may be sealed with Vaseline or nail polish.

The presence of exflagellating microgametocytes in a preparation is a useful indicator of gametocyte infectivity but is not necessarily an absolute indication. James (1931), for instance, found the presence of exflagellation to be a dependable guide to the infectiousness of vivax patients, but not so in the case of falciparum infections, while Boyd (1942) reported several instances of poor infectivity when mosquitoes were fed upon vivax patients with high gametocytemias and abundant exflagellations. One should also recognize that the inability to demonstrate exflagellation may not mean that the gametocytes are incapable, but that the method being used is not working properly.

b. Infectivity to Mosquitoes. The ultimate way to measure the infectivity of gametocytes is to test their ability to develop further within susceptible mosquitoes. After giving the mosquitoes the test blood meal, they can be examined the following day for the presence of ookinetes in the lumen of the midgut, or several days later for the presence of oocysts on the midgut wall. During the first several days after their initial appearance in the blood, *P. falciparum* gametocytes are often found to be immature, as evidenced by their lack of infectivity to mosquitoes (Basu, 1939; Collins, 1962; McCarthy and Clyde, 1973). That this is actually due to gametocyte immaturity rather than a lack of gametocyte numbers early in the infection was demonstrated by Jeffery and Eyles (1955). In general, the higher the gametocyte level present in a host, the greater the percentage of mosquitoes that can be infected and the heavier the ensuing mosquito infection (as measured in oocysts or sporozoites per mosquito). When gametocytes are highly infective, relatively small numbers will infect mosquitoes. In the case of falciparum malaria, a gametocyte density of less than $100/mm^3$ of blood in generally sufficient for minimal infection of susceptible mosquitoes (Boyd and Kitchen, 1937; Collins, 1962; James, 1931). A number of workers have been able to infect mosquitoes by feedings on humans with gametocytemias of less than $1/mm^3$, or even with gametocyte levels so low as to be nondetectable by ordinary microscopic techniques (Muirhead-Thomson and Mercier, 1952; Robertson, 1945; Young et al., 1948).

3. Duration of Time That a Gametocyte is Infective

Once a given gametocyte in the peripheral circulation has attained complete infectivity, there is some question as to how long this infectivity may be retained. This has proved to be a difficult problem to resolve experimentally. Under ordinary circumstances new gametocytes are continually being recruited into the population of existing gametocytes, and one cannot distinguish the infectivity of these new gametocytes from that of the older ones. An experimental approach used has been to stop recruitment of new gametocytes with antimalarial drugs that inhibit this process.

It was recognized early that antimalarial drugs which act against asexual parasites may have no detectable activity against gametocytes that have already been formed. Indeed, the process of microgametocyte exflagellation was discovered by Laveran (1880) in blood from a patient being treated with quinine. Bastianelli and Bignami (1900) found that gametocytes of *P. falciparum* could be observed in the circulation for only up to 1–2 weeks after quinine treatment, thus suggesting that new gametocyte formation had been stopped. Similar findings have been made with chloroquine. Jeffery *et al.* (1956) and Smalley and Sinden (1977) used chloroquine to eradicate *P. falciparum* asexual parasites from patients that exhibited gametocytes. Both groups of workers found that gametocytes persisted for a period of about 20 days after chloroquine treatment, though the formation of new gametocytes appeared to have stopped. Exflagellation and mosquito infectivity were demonstrated, thus establishing that at least some of the residual gametocytes had retained their infectivity. These studies showed that *P. falciparum* gametocytes appeared to be able to circulate in an infective state for at least several days after they attained their infectivity in the peripheral circulation.

This conclusion is at variance with the suggestion of Hawking (1975) that ''the mature male gametocyte is quite a short-lived organism,'' that ''it seems to be in an unstable state which cannot be maintained for more than 6–12 hours,'' and that, ''if the gametocyte cannot be taken up by a mosquito within this period, then it breaks down and has to be replaced by another.'' Nocturnal periodicity of morphologically mature gametocytes was first reported by Shah (1934) for *P. cathemerium* gametocytes in canaries. When susceptible mosquitoes were fed on these birds, a significantly higher percentage of those feeding at night (when mature gametocytes were more prevalent) became infected, compared with those that fed during the day (Shah *et al.*, 1934). Similar morphological observations were made by Gambrell (1937) who showed that the periodicity of gametocyte production and maturation was correlated with the periodicity of the asexual parasites. When this periodicity was shifted in time by changing the light–dark cycle the birds were exposed to, the periodicity of the gametocytes was correspondingly shifted. Furthermore, a strain of *P. cathemerium* that lacked pronounced asexual synchronism was shown not to produce any gametocytes. More recently, periodicity of gametocyte maturation within the blood has been reported for *P. knowlesi, P. cynomolgi, P. coatneyi, P. inui, P. berghei,* and *P. cathemerium* (review in Hawking, 1975).

On the basis of exflagellation studies, Hawking *et al.* (1971) also suggested a

48-hour synchronicity for maturation of *P. falciparum* microgametocytes, but their evidence for this seems weak. By feeding mosquitoes on infected humans at various times during the day and night, neither McCarthy and Clyde (1973) nor Bray *et al.* (1976) could find evidence for a circadian rhythm in the ability of the *P. falciparum* gametocytes to infect mosquitoes. Finally, as previously discussed, Smalley and Sinden (1977) have shown that *P. falciparum* gametocytes are not short-lived, but that they may persist in a mature condition in the circulation for at least several days.

In summary, the evidence is quite strong that several different species of malaria have a nocturnal periodicity of mature gametocytes. This is especially true in simian malarias, where several different investigators have confirmed that better infections of mosquitoes may be obtained by feeding the mosquitoes on monkeys at night. For maximal production of sporozoites in the laboratory it may be necessary to correlate mosquito feedings with these peaks in gametocytemia. It should be pointed out, however, that this is not an absolute necessity for adequate production of sporozoites. Satisfactory if not ideal results have been obtained for years by investigators who have fed their mosquitoes on infected monkeys during normal laboratory daylight hours. An alternative laboratory approach may be to reverse the light–dark cycle the monkeys are exposed to in order to shift the peak of infective gametocytes to a more convenient (for the investigator) daylight hour. The evidence for synchronous maturation of gametocytes in other species of malaria, such as *P. falciparum,* and rodent malarias is not so convincing, and "ideal" feeding times have yet to be established in these cases.

4. Loss of Gametocyte Infectivity during the Course of an Infection

Many workers have observed that gametocyte infectivity may be relatively high early in an infection with malaria but may decrease dramatically later when the parasitemia reaches a peak. Surprisingly, this reduction in gametocyte infectivity often occurs in the face of rising numbers of gametocytes in the blood. This phenomenon has been reported for avian malaria (Lumsden and Bertram, 1940; Cantrell and Jordan, 1946; Eyles, 1951, 1952a,b; Huff and Marchbank, 1955), for rodent malaria (Vanderberg *et al.,* 1968), and for simian malaria (Gwadz and Green, 1978).

Eyles (1951) described this loss of gametocyte infectivity in chickens that had received blood-induced infections of *P. gallinaceum.* However, he observed no such falloff in gametocyte infectivity when the infections were induced with sporozoites, which normally produce milder parasitemias. Three possible reasons were proposed to account for the loss of gametocyte viability in severe infections: (1) immune factors that act against the gametocytes, (2) depletion of necessary growth factors by the parasite, and (3) production of toxic factors active against the gametocyte. To test these possibilities, Eyles (1952a,b) conducted a series of ingenious mosquito infection experiments. Gametocyte-containing blood was removed from infected chickens, after which the cellular components were washed and resuspended in various media. This was then fed to susceptible mosquitoes through a membrane. The results showed that gametocytes which had lost their infectivity within the infected chicken could regain a significant portion of this infectivity if they were resuspended in normal serum or mixed with normal erythrocytes from noninfected chickens. Resuspension of the gametocytes in serum taken from chickens at the peak of their infection caused a decrease in gametocyte infectivity.

Other workers have used *in vivo* studies, instead, to investigate the loss of gametocyte infectivity during a malaria infection. Cantrell and Jordan (1946) transfused infected chickens with blood collected from healthy uninfected ones and found that in two of three experiments there was an increase in gametocyte infectivity to mosquitoes fed after the transfusion. They attributed these results to the restoration, by means of transfusion, of essential growth factors that had become depleted in the blood of infected chickens. Even more extensive types of supplementation experiments were conducted by Huff *et al.* (1958). Chickens infected with *P. gallinaceum* were given supplements of various substances such as whole blood, CoA, ferrous sulfate, glutathione, pantothenate, and sucrose. None of these substances had any enhancing effect on the course of gametocyte infectivity during the infection. Attempts were also made to exaggerate the loss of gametocyte infectivity by nutrient depletion procedures. Repeated bleedings of birds during the infections, however, had no notable effect on gametocyte infectivity. These authors concluded that the decreasing infectivity of gametocytes during an infection could better be explained on the basis of the development of an active immunity, rather than by a depletion effect within the infected host. It should be pointed out that, if the loss of gametocyte infectivity is related to the effects of an immune response, the immunity does not act directly upon the circulating gametocyte. Evidence for this comes from the studies of Eyles (1952b) and Gwadz (1976) showing that a loss of gametocyte infectivity is reversible when the gametocytes are resuspended in another medium. Immunity, however, may exercise its control by acting against newly formed gametes within the mosquito midgut, as discussed in the next section of this chapter.

In summary, the loss of gametocyte infectivity during an infection may be caused by all three of the postulates mentioned previously: immune factors, depletion effects, and toxic factors. All three occur during a malaria infection, and all or any of the three may act against gametocyte infectivity to various degrees depending upon the circumstances. Investigators involved in the experimental transmission of malaria must be aware of this phenomenon and take steps to guard against it. This generally involves use of the gametocytes relatively early in the infection, at a time when gametocyte density in the blood is at an acceptably high level but when a significant loss of gametocyte infectivity has not yet occurred. Because this may vary for each host–parasite relationship, it will be discussed later in this chapter in more specific detail for each of the various types of experimental malaria.

E. Antibodies against Gametocytes and Gametes

As noted in the preceding section, infectivity of the sexual stages of various malaria species to mosquitoes is often reduced at times of peak asexual parasitemia. This reduction occurs in spite of the fact that peak asexual parasitemias are usually accompanied by or just precede peak numbers of gametocytes. In discussing this phenomenon, Carter and Gwadz (see Chapter 7, Vol. 3) concluded that reduced infectiousness of gametocytes was mediated in large part by detrimental conditions in the plasma associated with high asexual parasitemias. These factors may cause reduced infectivity of the gametocytes after ingestion by a mosquito or may irreversibly damage gametocytes in the circulation. Conditions of this type are characteristic of blood-induced infections with such parasites as *P. gallinaceum, P. berghei,* and *P. knowlesi.* However, these antigametocyte environmental factors are not always associated with antibodies specific against sexual parasites.

As a practical consideration, antigametocyte or antigamete antibodies need not hinder laboratory studies requiring the infection of mosquitoes. Chickens infected with *P. gallinaceum* first begin producing antigamete antibodies after the peak of parasitemia and subsequent to the time when mosquitoes are generally fed on them (Carter *et al.,* 1979b). By the time the antibodies appear, few if any parasites are demonstrable in the circulation. Because once-infected chickens enjoy lifelong premunition, they will not support a recrudescence or reinfection and cannot be used further for infecting mosquitoes. Similarly, rodents with high asexual parasitemias of *P. yoelii* show reduced infectiousness to mosquitoes (Mendis and Targett, 1979), but satisfactory mosquito infections may be obtained early during the rodent infection. With *P. chabaudi,* gametocyte infectivity to mosquitoes follows the peak of asexual parasitemia and shows no evidence of being antibody-suppressed (Wéry, 1968). Indeed, high mosquito infectivity may be obtained quite late in the infection with this species of rodent malaria.

Rhesus monkeys repeatedly infected with *P. knowlesi* develop immunity against the asexual stages of the parasite, control their asexual parasitemias, produce fewer gametocytes, and therefore are less infectious to mosquitoes. However, if these monkeys are splenectomized and reinfected, asexual parasitemias rise rapidly, gametocytes are produced, and mosquitoes are uniformly infected. There is no evidence of antigamete or gametocyte antibodies produced (Gwadz and Green, 1978). Moreover, antigamete or gametocyte antibodies cannot be demonstrated from these repeatedly infected monkeys by the immunofluorescent antibody test (R. Carter, personal communication, 1979).

Antigamete antibodies which effectively block mosquito infection can be produced in chickens (Gwadz, 1976; Carter and Chen, 1976), in mice (Mendis and Targett, 1979), and in monkeys (Gwadz and Green, 1978). Details of these artificial immunization schemes have been reviewed by Carter and Gwadz (see Chapter 7, Vol. 3).

Numerous reports beginning with Ross (1896) and Darling (1910), and extending through Sinden and Smalley (1976), have noted the *in vitro* phagocytosis of extracellular gametocytes and exflagellating microgametes. However, Sinden and Smalley (1976) concluded that phagocytosis was significantly inhibited within the mosquito gut and was unlikely to affect successful transmission. Antigamete phagocytic activity probably has little effect on the sexual development of the malaria parasite within the mosquito gut and consequently little influence on laboratory transmission studies.

F. Experimental Manipulations of the Vertebrate Host for Increasing Infectiousness to Mosquitoes

The vertebrate hosts of avian and rodent malarias usually require no pretreatment to ensure that subsequent infections are consistently infectious to mosquitoes. Factors involved in choosing appropriate malaria–host combinations, host or malaria strains, or environmental conditions will be discussed below. However, a number of experimental protocols have evolved which can improve the infectiousness of primate malarias to mosquitoes.

Surgical removal of the spleen is a routine procedure for improving the general susceptibility of primates to malaria infection and is often a means of increasing infectiousness to mosquitoes. Collins and his co-workers (Coatney *et al.*, 1971; Sodeman *et al.*, 1970; Collins and Aikawa, 1977) have noted that infectivity of many primate malarias to mosquitoes is improved if the monkey hosts are splenectomized prior to or, in some cases, after infection. These procedures have been used to improve the infectiousness of *P. falciparum*, *P. vivax*, and *P. malariae* in *Aotus* monkeys. Similarly, rhesus monkeys repeatedly infected with *P. knowlesi* or *P. cynomolgi* and showing little or no infectivity to mosquitoes will, after splenectomy, produce infections highly infective to mosquitoes.

A second procedure which appears to alter the general infectiousness of a monkey host involves preinfection of the animal with a heterologous species of malaria. Collins *et al.* (1979) found that *Aotus trivirgatus griseimembra* monkeys previously infected with *P. vivax* or *P. fragile* sustained *P. falciparum* infections which were more likely to infect mosquitoes than were infections in monkeys without previous malaria experience. De Arruda-Mayr *et al.* (1979) noted a similar finding in the increased infectiousness of *P. cynomolgi* in rhesus monkeys previously infected with *P. knowlesi.*

Immunosuppressant drugs have been shown to influence gametocyte maturation and subsequent infectivity to mosquitoes with one strain of *P. falciparum* in *Aotus* monkeys, but the results were not consistent (Ward *et al.*, 1972).

IV. THE INFECTIVE BLOOD MEAL

The early studies of Ronald Ross, and soon thereafter those of Grassi, Bignami, and Bastianelli, demonstrated that mosquitoes could be infected by feeding on malarious hosts. Experimental protocols for infecting mosquitoes quickly became a feature of malaria research. Indeed, Ross (1898) first demonstrated the cyclic transmission of malaria through mosquitoes, using an animal model, a bird malaria (probably *P. relictum*) in sparrows.

Two methods for infecting mosquitoes have been used since those early experiments. The most common method consists of applying caged female mosquitoes to the exposed skin of a malarious host and allowing them to feed through the cage netting. A second method allows mosquitoes to feed directly on blood, usually through a membrane after the infected blood had been removed from a host and suspended within a feeding device.

The process by which the female mosquito feeds on blood has been described in detail by a number of authors (e.g., Gordon and Lumsden, 1939; Griffiths and Gordon, 1952; Clements, 1963). Before attempting to induce mosquitoes to take an infectious blood meal, several factors must be considered. As previously noted (Section II,A), mosquito–malaria relationships can be quite precise, and only certain mosquito species or even certain selected strains may support development of a particular malaria species. Mosquitoes also exhibit host preferences and may not feed on all animals. However, after an appropriate vector-parasite combination has been selected, some general guidelines should be followed.

1. Mosquitoes should be well reared, of uniform size, and usually 3-6 days old (postemergence). Younger mosquitoes are usually reluctant to feed, while older mosquitoes may not survive long enough to allow sporozoite maturation. Mosquitoes reared under crowded conditions often feed poorly or die before the parasite can develop fully.

2. Male mosquitoes are best removed from a cage prior to feeding. Excess males crowd the cage and may tend to disturb females trying to feed. Alternatively, males and females may be separated as pupae (see this volume, Chapter 3), since female pupae are distinctively larger. Some investigators, however, ignore the presence of males.

3. Female mosquitoes should be starved 12–24 hours before feeding. Starving consists of removing external sugar and water sources from a cage of mosquitoes. A sugar source should be offered after the infectious blood meal, and the infected mosquitoes maintained on a sugar solution until they are used. Particular care must be taken to ensure proper humidity during the starvation period to prevent excessive desiccation.

4. Some mosquito species feed best in the dark, and a few will feed only at night. At the same time, some malaria species are highly synchronous and give maximal mosquito infections at night, e.g., *P. knowlesi* (Hawking *et al.*, 1968) and *P. coatneyi* (Coatney *et al.*, 1971), and night feedings in these cases are necessary (see Section III,D,3).

5. The malarious host should be restrained to allow undisturbed mosquito feeding. Rodents usually require an anesthetic such as sodium pentobarbital injected intraperitoneally to induce a state of unconsciousness. Once anesthetized, they can be placed directly on a cage of mosquitoes. Birds (e.g., chickens or canaries) are seldom given anesthetics but must be physically restrained to permit feedings. Gerberg *et al.* (1966) described a device for holding chickens during mosquito feedings. A simpler method involves strapping chickens or pigeons to a light board with twine. Canaries can be restrained by wrapping snuggly in cheesecloth; the restrained bird can then be placed directly in a cage of mosquitoes. Alternatively, a canary may be placed in a small cage and the cage placed directly in a cage of mosquitoes. Left overnight in the dark, the canary will remain quiescent and the mosquitoes will feed *ad lib*.

Larger primates must be anesthetized before feeding is attempted. After injection with a fast-acting compound such as ketamine hydrochloride, an unconscious monkey can be strapped to a board, and caged mosquitoes applied to shaved areas of skin. Smaller monkeys such as *Aotus* and *Saimiri* can be restrained without anesthetic for mosquito feedings.

The status of the infection in the malarious host is a major consideration in determining when to attempt to infect mosquitoes. As noted earlier, gametocytes must be present, although not necessarily in high numbers, and must be infectious. As a general rule, feedings for most rodent, avian, and primate malarias are most successful during the initial phase of rising asexual parasitemia up to, but not including, the day of peak asexual parasitemia. Characteristics of individual malarias will be discussed in Section X.

Membrane-covered devices for the artificial feeding of hematophagous insects have been used since 1912 when Rodhain *et al.* developed a method for feeding tsetse flies on blood through rat skin. Most of the devices used today are patterned on the units described by Bishop and Gilchrist (1946), Rutledge *et al.* (1964), and Ward *et al.* (1978), among others. A typical membrane feeding system consists of an external unit for heating and circulating water and a water-jacketed feeding chamber covered at one end with a membrane. Blood in the chamber is warmed by water circulating through the water jacket to about 37°C, and mosquitoes feed through the cage netting, through the membrane, and on the blood. Baudruche membranes (Long and Long Company, Belleville, New Jersey) derived from bovine intestine are particularly effective, but chick or rat skin or washed condoms have been used.

Blood from a malarious host can be drawn into a syringe containing heparin (10 units/ml blood). Heparin should be preservative-free and is best prepared from powdered sodium heparin in sterile saline. Preservatives used in commercially prepared heparin solutions often have a gametocidal effect and may preclude infections through membranes. Blood may be put directly into the feeder, or washed and resuspended in serum or plasma to remove any antigamete factors inhibiting infection (Eyles, 1952b; Gwadz, 1976). Membrane feeding is particularly effective with some avian and primate malarias. Infections in mosquitoes fed through membranes usually equal or exceed infections in mosquitoes fed directly on the animal from which the blood has been drawn. Attempts to infect mosquitoes with various rodent malarias have met with less success.

Adenosine triphosphate (ATP) acts as a potent phagostimulant to most species of mosquitoes (Galun *et al.*, 1963) and can be used in membrane feeders to encourage mosquito engorgement on a variety of fluids with or without blood. However, under most conditions, mosquitoes will engorge on fresh or washed blood cells in plasma or serum without need of added stimulants.

V. MAINTENANCE OF INFECTED MOSQUITOES

A. General Procedures

In general, infected mosquitoes should be maintained under the same conditions of temperature and humidity, and receive the same treatment with regard to food and water, as uninfected mosquitoes of the same species. One notable exception is for mosquitoes infected with the commonly used rodent malaria *P. berghei*. Details of the temperature requirements of this species and others will be discussed in Section X, but in general infected mosquitoes infected with *P. berghei* must be maintained at about 21°C for sporozoites to develop (Vanderberg and Yoeli, 1966). Most other malaria species will complete development at normal insectary temperatures (24°–27°C) and humidities (55–75% RH).

Other required insectary conditions and procedures such as isolation of mosquitoes from toxic fumes, insecticides, and pathogens apply equally to infected and noninfected mosquitoes. Certain insect pathogens can affect both infected and noninfected mosquitoes and have on occasion destroyed whole laboratory colonies. In some instances, even though mosquitoes may not be killed outright, low-level concomitant infection with certain microsporidia can render them less susceptible to malaria infection by interfering with oocyst development (Garnham, 1956; Bano, 1958; Hulls, 1971; Ward and Savage, 1972). Cryptic microsporidian infections can readily alter the susceptibility of a laboratory colony to an otherwise compatible infection.

B. Safety Procedures for Handling Infected Mosquitoes

As a general rule, an insectary operation should tolerate no loose mosquitoes and operate on the principle that any loose mosquito may be infected. Avian and rodent malarias are not known to infect humans, and mosquitoes infected with these parasites present no known health hazard. The chicken malaria *P. gallinaceum* must be held under strict quarantine conditions because of its potential for infecting local chicken flocks.

Simian and human malarias, and particularly mosquitoes infected with these parasites, present a clear hazard for accidental infection of laboratory workers and casual visitors. Individuals at risk to infection should be aware of the symptoms associated with malaria infections and be prepared to alert a physician to the possibility of having been infected. A number of laboratory infections have been traced to workers being bitten by infected mosquitoes (e.g., Eyles *et al.*, 1960; Coatney *et al.*, 1971). The following is a list of safety procedures. All should be adjusted and modified to fit individual laboratory situations. However, common sense and attentive mosquito-handling procedures remain the best defense against accidental escape and infection.

1. Infected mosquitoes should be held in secure cages with the netting unbroken and firmly attached. The ''cage-within-a-cage'' procedure is not an unreasonable method for use with potential human pathogens.

2. Infected mosquitoes should be held in a secure, lockable insectary, away from noninfected mosquitoes or rearing facilities. In an isolated insectary reserved for infected mosquitoes, a loose mosquito would thus indicate a breakdown in safety precautions.

3. Handling of infected mosquitoes, transfers from cage to cage, dissection, etc., should *not* be done in the holding room. Rather, a special ''transfer room'' should be used for all manipulations of infected mosquitoes. A typical transfer room is a well-lit, closetlike unit with bare, light-colored walls, a low ceiling, and a mosquito-proof door. In such a room, escaped mosquitoes can be readily observed and recaptured.

4. Only small numbers of mosquitoes should be handled at any time. Aspirators and cages should be constantly checked for mosquitoes left behind in tubes or on the aspirator netting. Aspirators should be constructed of shatterproof plastic rather than glass, and entirely of transparent materials.

Any number of safety precautions can be instituted; however, the primary deterrent to accidental release of infected mosquitoes is careful attention to detail and established procedure.

VI. SAMPLING PROCEDURES FOR DETERMINING THE DEGREE OF MOSQUITO INFECTION

After its ingestion by a susceptible mosquito, the parasite passes through a series of developmental stages, namely, the ookinete within the lumen of the midgut, the oocyst on the midgut wall, and the sporozoite that travels from the oocyst through the hemocoel to its final localization within the salivary gland. Thus, a satisfactory assessment of mosquito infection requires an examination of the appropriate organ of the mosquito at a suitable time in parasite development. In general, three procedures have been used to assay mosquito infections: (1) ookinete determination by examining the partially digested blood meal recovered from the lumen of the midgut about 1 day after the infective blood meal, (2) oocyst determinations from counts made on the dissected midguts several days later, (3) sporozoite determinations made by examining the salivary glands subsequent to parasite maturation.

Finding any of the early stages of sporogonic development within a mosquito does not necessarily establish its vectorial capacity. In an unfavorable vector–parasite combination, parasite development may proceed quite normally at first and then be blocked at almost any point. Thus, ookinetes can be formed but may not develop further into oocysts; oocysts can be produced but may not form sporozoites within them; or sporozoites can be formed but may not have the capacity to invade the salivary glands (Bennett *et al.*, 1966; Yoeli, 1973). However, in an established laboratory system of malaria, where mosquitoes are known to produce infective salivary gland sporozoites within a given period under carefully controlled conditions, a quantitative assessment of the younger parasite stages (ookinetes and oocysts) may be used to assay the level of infection in a given batch of mosquitoes. Mosquitoes to be dissected for parasite stages are usually anesthetized with ether, chloroform, or cold and immediately examined. However, when examination must be delayed for any reason, intact mosquitoes

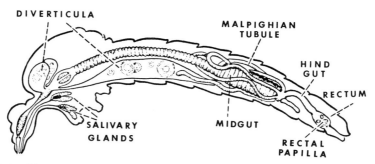

FIG. 1. Diagrammatic lateral view of a mosquito showing internal organs with ovaries omitted (modified from Hunter *et al.*, 1946).

may be stored indefinitely at $-20°C$ prior to dissection (Ward, 1962). The location of the midgut and salivary glands within the mosquito is seen in Fig. 1. A more detailed consideration of mosquito anatomy may be found in Christophers (1960) and Clements (1963).

A. Dissections for Ookinetes

Mosquitoes are usually examined for ookinetes the day following the infective blood meal. Ookinetes, if present, will be found in the semidigested blood clot after it is removed from the midgut, although some of them may have already disappeared into the midgut wall by the time the lumen contents are examined.

Mosquitoes are best anesthetized by exposure to ether vapors. For special precautions to be taken when mosquitoes have been infected with human pathogens, see Section V,B. The anesthetized mosquito should be transferred to a microscope slide and covered with a small drop of either a saline solution or of the media used for harvesting and maintaining sporozoites (Section VII,E). Dissecting the midgut is most readily done with the aid of a binocular dissecting microscope. Various instruments have been used by different investigators. Shute and Maryon (1966) have advocated the use of a bayonet-shaped needle with a sharp cutting edge (the Shute dissecting needle, manufactured by Baird and Tatlock, Ltd., England). Others prefer fine jewelers forceps made of stainless steel (either no. 5 straight or no. 7 curved). An especially useful and easily prepared dissecting instrument is the outer barrel of a 1-ml glass injection syringe to which has been fitted an injection needle. Depending upon how it is manipulated, the needle may serve as a blunt instrument for pressing and holding a specimen, a pointed piercing device, a scalpel with a sharp cutting edge, or a scoop for picking up dissected material (needle sizes between no. 20 and no. 25 are satisfactory, and different sizes may serve for different types of dissections).

Detailed instructions for removing midguts and salivary glands from infected mosquitoes have been given by several authors (Blacklock and Wilson, 1942; Hunter *et al.*, 1946; Boyd *et al.*, 1949; Garnham, 1966; Shute and Maryon, 1966). Most suggest removing the legs and wings from the anesthetized mosquito prior to the dissection, but this serves no useful purpose and seems unnecessary. To remove the midgut, the thorax is held firmly with a forceps or blund instrument, while the posterior two segments of the abdomen are gently and slowly pulled away from the anterior portion of the abdomen (Fig. 2). Some workers prefer to nick the abdominal wall on both sides of the pulling site prior to applying traction. In a successful dissection, the blood-filled midgut will be pulled into the drop of dissecting fluid, and the portions of the digestive tract anterior and posterior to the midgut may be cut off and removed. Blood-filled midguts are so fragile that they often rupture during dissection. Thus, considerable practice may be necessary before one learns to do these dissections on a

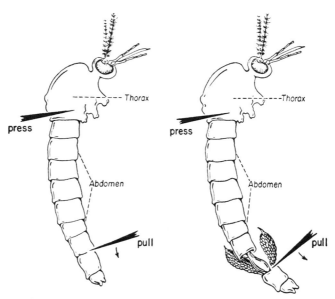

FIG. 2.   Method of pulling the posterior segments of a mosquito abdomen to remove the midgut (from Hunter *et al.*, 1946).

regular basis to obtain intact midguts. The isolated midgut is next transferred to a tiny drop of dissecting fluid on a clean slide. This too requires practice to avoid rupturing the fragile midgut. The midgut is then teased apart, and the blood meal mass is mixed together with the dissecting fluid as thoroughly as possible. The drop may then be used to make thick or thin smears which are stained with Giemsa stain. Ookinetes are readily observed with a high-power oil immersion lens. Ookinetes obtained in this manner have also been used for *in vitro* studies on their locomotion and behavior (Freyvogel, 1966).

It is difficult to quantify ookinete formation within a batch of mosquitos, because many ookinetes may be lost in the clotted blood meal mass and in the midgut wall. The main advantage gained from examinations for ookinetes lies in the early determination of whether mosquitoes fed on a gametocyte carrier have become infected. The presence of ookinetes does not necessarily establish that oocyst and sporozoite formation will follow, but the absence of ookinetes indicates that sporogony is not progressing.

Another procedure for obtaining ookinetes from mosquitoes has been described by Weiss and Vanderberg (1976). Free midguts are homogenized and then treated with collagenase and hyaluronidase to release the ookinetes. These are then concentrated by centrifugation on a density gradient. A method for quantifying the numbers of ookinetes recovered has also been described by these authors, but it is too time-consuming for routine assessment of ookinete formation. Its value lies in its ability to yield large numbers of *in vivo-* formed ookinetes for further experimental study.

B. Dissections for Oocysts

Counting of oocysts growing on mosquito midguts is the most common procedure used to determine the degree of mosquito infection. It is much easier to remove midguts than salivary glands, and infected midguts yield absolute oocyst counts, whereas sporozoite numbers in salivary glands can only be estimated. The timing of the midgut dissection may be important. If done too early after the infective meal, the oocysts may be too small to be readily observed; if done too late, some of the oocysts may have already ruptured and disappeared. Most workers find a period of 4–10 days after the infective blood meal to be satisfactory for oocyst determinations.

Removing midguts for oocyst counts is done as previously described for ookinete determinations, except that the midgut in this case is less fragile than the blood-filled one, and the dissection is generally more easily accomplished. Some workers prefer to put a drop of 2% Mercurochrome on top of the isolated midgut prior to covering it with a cover glass. Oocysts tend to stain more darkly than the midgut. Wet mount preparations of pressed oocysts are best observed under phase-contrast microscopy. If such a microscope is not readily available, satisfactory observations can be made with a normal compound microscope by partially closing down the iris diaphragm. Careful morphological observation is often necessary to distinguish oocysts from mosquito midgut tissues such as adipose cells, hemocytes, and cellular outpocketings of the midgut epithelium, all of which may superficially resemble oocysts. However, with experience the oocysts are readily identifiable. Young oocysts are easily distinguished by their characteristic patterns of pigment granules (Shute and Maryon, 1966); older oocysts may show prominent cleavage of the internal sporoblastoid material and the subsequent formation of sporozoites.

Midgut infections with oocysts are generally quantified in any of three ways: percentage of positive mosquitos with oocysts, mean number of oocysts per positive mosquito, as in Burgess (1960), and mean number of oocysts per total number of mosquitoes dissected, as in Collins (1962) and Collins *et al.* (1977). The latter authors multiply this mean number by 100 to obtain the *gut infection index* (GII). Different species or strains of vectors can then be compared with one another for vector efficiency on the basis of their GII determinations (Collins *et al.*, 1977). Another modification used is that, instead of actual oocyst counts, the degree of oocyst load is given in terms of a defined range of classes, e.g., 0 oocysts, >10 oocysts, >30 oocysts, and >50 oocysts (Collins *et al.*, 1977).

A parameter of infection sometimes used to assess the rate at which an infection is progressing is mean diameter of oocysts on a given day of development.

One must be cautious about this, however, because the apparent diameter of the oocysts may increase under pressure from the coverslip. This obviously varies with the amount of fluid under the coverslip.

C. Dissections for Salivary Gland Sporozoites

The ultimate indicator of the vectorial capacity of mosquitoes is the presence of mature sporozoites in their salivary glands. As with oocysts, the time of dissection is crucial. If the mosquitoes are dissected too early, the sporozoites may not yet have reached the glands. If they are dissected too late, some of the sporozoites may have been lost as a result of degeneration (Porter *et al.*, 1954). Also, an extremely high infection rate may induce excessive mosquito mortality. Dissection of the survivors (with relatively lower infections) would thus give an erroneous impression of the overall infection rate. It is therefore helpful to standardize quantitation by choosing standard days of dissection for each vector–parasite combination under given environmental conditions. This especially may be a problem when one is comparing two different growth rates for the parasites, as for instance when one is comparing growth at two different temperatures or in two different vector species. In this case, dissections have to be done over a period of several days to determine the peak infection day for parasites developing under each set of conditions.

Many different techniques have been described for removing salivary glands from mosquitoes (review in Blacklock and Wilson, 1942). It should be noted that the salivary glands, though attached to the head via the salivary duct, actually lie entirely within the thorax (Fig. 1). Either of two different procedures is generally followed to remove them: (1) Gentle pressure is applied to the thorax until the neck bulges slightly. At the same time, a probe or needle is placed on the neck just behind the head, and the head is pulled gently away from the thorax (Fig. 3). If this procedure is successful, the salivary glands will be pulled out trailing behind the head, and they can be severed and transferred to another slide. (2) The head is removed with a sharp cut, after which the thorax is firmly pressed to make the glands protrude. While the pressure is maintained, the glands (as well as

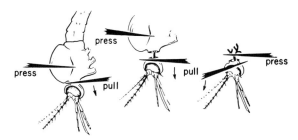

FIG. 3.   Steps in removing salivary glands from a mosquito (from Hunter *et al.*, 1946).

other tissue emerging from the anterior end of the thorax) are cut off and transferred to a small drop of fluid on another slide (see Fig. 3 in Shute and Maryon, 1966; or Fig. 24 in Garnham, 1966).

Salivary glands can be dissected into a fluid colored with either 0.5% brilliant cresyl blue or 0.1% methylene blue to stain the glands vitally and make them more readily visible. With experience, one can adjust the light to make the glands more visible without staining. The angle of the reflecting mirror under the stage of the dissecting microscope can be varied until the glands are revealed as refractile structures easily distinguished from other mosquito tissues. With practice, any of the instruments or techniques described can be used to make satisfactory midgut or salivary gland dissections. Each worker should experiment to find the most suitable procedure.

If the coverslip on top of the isolated salivary glands is tapped or pressed gently, the glands will be slightly crushed, and sporozoites released into the immediate vicinity. The sporozoites can be seen more readily by reducing the light intensity with the iris diaphragm of the microscope. The simplest way of assessing salivary gland infections is by determining the percentage of mosquitoes with salivary gland infections. This percentage has often been referred to as the *sporozoite rate* (Pringle, 1966). Quantitation of the degree of these infections is somewhat more difficult. Because of the problem of making accurate sporozoite counts, estimates are usually resorted to. A commonly used scheme, the *gland index*, divides the estimated degree of infection into 5 classes: 0 (no sporozoites), 1+ (1–10 sporozoites), 2+ (11–100 sporozoites), 3+ (101–1000 sporozoites), 4+ (more than 1000 sporozoites). By determining the average gland rating of the positive mosquitoes that have been dissected, one can obtain the *positive gland index* (Collins *et al.*, 1977).

More accurate assessments of the actual numbers of sporozoites in the glands are considerably more time-consuming. A laborious but sometimes useful technique for estimating the numbers of sporozoites in the salivary glands of individual mosquitoes has been described by Shute *et al.* (1965) and modified by Pringle (1966). Salivary glands from individual mosquitoes are removed, macerated, and spread over a defined platform area on a slide. After staining with Giemsa, sporozoite counts are made over defined sampling areas. A more easily done procedure, suitable for determining the mean number of sporozoites per gland in a batch of glands, involves maceration of the glands and counts of sporozoites using one of the counting procedures described in Section VII,G. In this way, Vanderberg (1977) was able to compare the relative intensity of infections with salivary gland sporozoites in different batches of mosquitoes.

D. Histological Procedures

It is sometimes desirable to make stained whole-mount preparations of infected midguts or salivary glands or to prepare histological sections for more careful study. Various procedures have been described for making fixed and stained whole-mount preparations of midguts (Boyd *et al.*, 1949; Garnham, 1966; Shute and Maryon, 1966). Another and much simpler way is to place the slide preparation on a piece of dry ice and allow the fluid under the coverslip to freeze. The slide is then removed from the dry ice, and the coverslip is quickly flipped off by inserting a razor blade under a corner of the still frozen-on coverslip. With practice, one finds that the flattened midgut tends to remain firmly attached to the slide. This attachment can be enhanced by prior coating of the slide with a small drop of albumin smeared along its surface. Once the coverslip is removed, the slide is plunged into Carnoy's solution (6 parts absolute ethanol, 3 parts chloroform, and 1 part glacial acetic acid) for 5–15 minutes of fixation. After washing for a few minutes in absolute ethanol, the preparation can be hydrated via a graded series of ethanol concentrations and then stained with any histological stain desired. A color plate showing oocysts so prepared is presented in Vanderberg *et al.* (1967). A similar procedure may be used for making whole mounts of infected salivary glands.

To prepare histological sections of infected midguts, or salivary glands, one may embed either the dissected-out organs themselves, or the entire mosquito. Any standard fixation and paraffin-embedding procedure may be used for the isolated midguts and salivary glands. Because of their small size, great care must be used in carrying these organs through the various histological solutions. Many workers thus prefer working with the entire mosquito for histological purposes. This poses its own problems because insect cuticle is somewhat impervious to penetration by histological reagents and because it tends to become quite hard and brittle during embedding, so that shattering often occurs during the sectioning procedure.

For better penetration through the cuticle, fixatives containing a lipid solvent are much more satisfactory than aqueous fixatives. Carnoy's (6:3:1) fixative for 30 minutes to 2 hours gives satisfactory results. The proboscis, wings, and legs of the mosquito should be removed to enhance penetration of the various histological reagents. This may be done while the mosquitoes are immersed in the fixative. Embedding by means of the celloidin–paraffin double-embedding procedure has been reported to give satisfactory results (Shute and Maryon, 1966). However, this procedure is complicated and time-consuming, and it is rather difficult to obtain serial sections with it. A much simpler procedure involves embedding the mosquito in ester wax (1960 grade, manufactured by B.D.H. and distributed by Gallard-Schlesinger, Carle Place, New York). The fixed mosquitoes are brought to 70% ethanol and then, via several changes of ethylene glycol monoethyl ether (Cellosolve), into the ester wax. Serial sections of 4–10 μm are easily cut. The most satisfactory staining is with the Giemsa collophonium procedure (Shortt and Cooper, 1948; Bray and Garnham, 1962).

VII. HARVESTING, PURIFYING, AND MAINTAINING SPOROZOITES

A. General Considerations in Recovering Sporozoites from Mosquitoes

Sporozoites are formed within oocysts attached to the midgut wall of their mosquito vector. When the mature oocyst bursts, the sporozoites spill out into the surrounding hemolymph within the mosquito's abdomen and then spread throughout the hemocoel to form what has been described as a virtual "septicemia" within the hemolymph (Wenyon, 1926). Eventually, the sporozoites become concentrated within the salivary glands. Because the development of sporozoites is not always entirely synchronous, they may be found concurrently at three different sites within a mosquito during an infection: in oocysts, throughout the hemolymph, and within the salivary gland.

A number of studies have shown that there is a striking functional maturation of sporozoites between the time they are in the oocyst and the time they are found in the salivary gland. This maturation includes the attainment of normal infectivity (Vanderberg, 1975) and antigenicity (Vanderberg et al., 1972; Nussenzweig and Chen, 1974) by the sporozoite and a change in its motility (Vanderberg, 1974). Thus, in collecting sporozoites from mosquitoes, one must consider the site from which the sporozoites are obtained.

Another important consideration is the time of harvesting after the infective blood meal. Sporozoites appear to increase in infectivity during their residence within the salivary glands (Vanderberg, 1975), and an early harvest could result in a batch of sporozoites with suboptimal infectivity. On the other hand, too long a residence may result in a marked loss in infectivity (Porter et al., 1954; Fink, 1968).

Mosquitoes to be used for the harvesting of viable sporozoites are best anesthesized by light etherization or by chilling in a refrigerator. Overetherization or freezing of infected mosquitoes at temperatures below 0°C may damage sporozoite viability (Porter et al., 1952).

B. Salivary Gland Dissections

Clean suspensions of sporozoites are usually prepared by dissection and homogenization of salivary glands from infected mosquitoes (Shute and Maryon, 1966). Glands are generally removed as previously described (Section VI,C), though a procedure for mass isolation of salivary glands by squeezing them out of decapitated mosquitoes has been proposed by Bosworth et al. (1975). Once the glands are freed, virtually any type of homogenizing or grinding device is satisfactory. The use of a tight-fitting homogenizer driven by a motor should be avoided, however, so as not to damage or destroy the sporozoites that have been freed. Sporozoites from salivary gland dissections are generally clean enough for most experimental purposes. Further purification of the sporozoite suspension, if required, may be accomplished by subsequent gradient centrifugation or by column purification as described below. However, salivary gland dissection is tedious and time-consuming, and mass preparation of sporozoites by this technique demands a term of skilled dissectors.

C. Gradient Centrifugation Purification

An efficient method for the collection of large numbers of sporozoites from mosquitoes is to grind whole mosquitoes, or isolated thoraxes, and then to separate and concentrate the sporozoites in the resulting suspension. Grinding can be done with a chilled mortar and pestle and in the presence of one of the sporozoite harvesting media described in Section VII,E.

When whole mosquitoes infected with sporozoites are ground, the resulting suspension contains intact sporozoites as well as microorganisms and mosquito debris. Much of the mosquito material may be removed simply by filtration through a screen with openings large enough to permit passage of the sporozoites (Chen and Schneider, 1969), or by centrifugation at relatively slow speeds (25–100 g for 5 minutes). The sporozoites remaining in suspension may then be pelleted by centrifugation at about 700–1000 g for 20–30 minutes. A cleaner and more infective preparation of sporozoites can be obtained if the heads and abdomens of the mosquitoes are first removed, and the isolated thoraxes alone are ground (Vanderberg et al., 1972). Inclusion of the abdomen may cause another problem. The release of proteolytic enzymes of the midgut during grinding can have deleterious effects upon the sporozoites being collected. Thus, if whole mosquitoes are used, special precautions should be taken to keep the preparation at ice bath temperatures to reduce enzyme activity. Another shortcoming of the whole-mosquito homogenization procedure is that a large proportion of the sporozoites obtained may be noninfective, nonimmunogenic ones from the oocysts. For many types of experiments, however, this may not be a serious concern, and the reduced infectivity of the sporozoites thus obtained may be outweighed by the much greater ease of processing whole mosquitoes.

Both continuous and discontinuous gradients have been used for concentration of sporozoites from ground mosquitoes. Continuous gradients prepared with different concentrations of bovine serum albumin and a diatrizoate salt solution have been used for the separation of sporozoites by Schneider and Chen (1969) and Krettli et al. (1973). When the sporozoite suspension is layered on top of the gradient and centrifuged, the sporozoites are found to concentrate at a level of the gradient with a specific gravity of about 1.12. The fraction containing sporozoites can then be removed, and washed by further centrifugation. A discontinuous biphasic gradient prepared with the same components [bovine serum albumin and diatrizoate salt solution] was described by Beaudoin et al. (1977). After centrifugation, sporozoites were collected from the interface between the dense lower layer and the less dense upper layer. The sporozoites so collected were used for repeated experimental immunization, and the mice being immunized developed a concomitant hypersensitivity to the bovine serum albumin which could not be completely washed from the sporozoites. Thus, a later modification of this biphasic gradient substituted mouse serum for the serum albumin and simplified the gradient preparation procedure (Pacheco et al., 1979). However, for studies not employing repeated immunizations with sporozoites, bovine serum albumin is still preferred over whole serum. A modification that employs bovine serum albumin together with the simplified preparative procedure of Pacheco et al. (1979) has been described by Schulman et al. (1980). On the basis of a comparative assessment of all these gradient techniques, Vanderberg (1979) reported better and more consistent results with the discontinous than the continuous gradient procedure.

D. Column Purification

A DEAE-cellulose column procedure was described by Mack et al. (1978) for the separation of P. berghei sporozoites from other components of ground-up infected mosquitoes. The rationale for this was based on previous studies by Miller et al. (1973) that showed these sporozoites to be less negatively charged than the other components in the suspension, and thus susceptible to separation by charge. By use of this column, it was possible to obtain high yields of relatively clean viable sporozoites from ground-up whole mosquitoes or isolated thoraxes. Based on the success of this column, Moser et al. (1978) prepared a different type of DEAE-cellulose column that could be used to separate P. berghei sporozoites from dissected-out salivary glands.

Another column technique (Vanderberg, 1979) was based on the finding that P. berghei sporozoites had no detectable lectin-binding sites on their surface (Schulman et al., 1980). Thus, when a partially purified sporozoite suspension was applied to a column composed of Sepharose beads bound to concanavalin A, the sporozoites passed through, while most of the contaminating microorganisms were bound to the column.

E. Media and Conditions for Maintenance of Sporozoites

Saline and Ringer-type solutions by themselves are relatively unsatisfactory for maintaining the viability of isolated sporozoites. It is generally considered necessary to add a protein, usually in the form of serum or plasma, to obtain better sporozoite maintenance. Thus, Tonkin (1947) observed that P. gal-

linaceum sporozoites became practically noninfective after 1 hour in saline solution, whereas the addition of chicken plasma or serum permitted them to retain viability for several hours. Porter *et al.* (1952) had similar results with inactivated serum and with heparinized chicken whole blood as additives. Two other additives that have been used in lieu of serum have been chicken red cell extract for the maintenance of *P. gallinaceum* sporozoites (Whitman, 1948), and bovine serum albumin for the maintenance of *P. berghei* sporozoites (Vanderberg, 1974). In the latter case sporozoites were maintained in tissue culture medium 199 plus 3% bovine serum albumin at 4°C for 24 hours with virtually no loss of infectivity. Some degree of sporozoite infectivity could be retained under these conditions for periods up to 5 days.

There has been a tendency to replace the basic saline component of the suspension medium with more complex tissue culture media. Many workers now use tissue culture medium 199 with added serum (generally 10–50% serum homologous with the vertebrate host being used). Because fresh serum may have a deleterious effect on sporozoites (Porter *et al.*, 1952), the serum should be inactivated first at 56°C for 30 minutes. Fink and Schicha (1969) reported that Grace's insect tissue culture medium (with added serum) was more satisfactory than medium 199 for maintaining the viability of *P. berghei* and *P. cathemerium* sporozoites. This was confirmed for *P. berghei* by Verhave (1975).

The temperature at which sporozoite suspensions are maintained is also important. Viability is prolonged by chilling at ice bath temperatures (Brackett and Hughes, 1945; Davey, 1946; Vanderberg, 1974) and is rapidly lost at 37°C (Vanderberg, 1974). The pH of the maintenance medium should be adjusted close to neutrality; low pH may have a deleterious effect on sporozoite infectivity (Verhave, 1975).

F. Cryopreservation of Sporozoites

Though cryopreservation of the blood stages of plasmodia is a standard laboratory procedure, adequate cryopreservation of sporozoites has been far more difficult to achieve. Some small degrees of success were demonstrated by Jeffery and Rendtorff (1955) for *P. falciparum, P. ovale,* and *P. vivax;* Molinari (1961) for *P. gallinaceum* and *P. cynomolgi;* Weathersby and McCall (1967) for *P. gallinaceum;* and Bafort (1968, 1971) for *P. berghei* and *P. vinckei.* The quantitative work of Molinari (1961) demonstrated that less than 1% of the original viability of a batch of sporozoites was preserved by freezing. Studies by J. P. Vanderberg (unpublished results), who attempted to cryopreserve *P. berghei* sporozoites with glycerol or dimethyl sulfoxide as additives, gave similar poor results. However, Strome *et al.* (1977) have shown that the addition of serum enormously enhances recovery of the sporozoites. *Plasmodium berghei* sporozoites frozen in the presence of 7.5% dimethyl sulfoxide and 50% serum showed little loss of infectivity upon thawing, followed by challenge of susceptible mice.

G. Quantitation of Sporozoites in Suspension

In order to infect vertebrates with standardized doses of sporozoites, it is necessary to determine the concentration of sporozoites in a suspension and then to make appropriate dilutions. Several methods for quantitation have been described. Porter *et al.* (1952) mixed a sample volume of the sporozoite suspension with a known volume and concentration of chicken erythrocytes. By determining the ratio of sporozoites to erythrocytes in a Giemsa-stained smear, these authors were able to calculate the concentration of sporozoites in the original sample. Most workers, however, prefer to count the sporozoites directly in suspension in order to obtain results more rapidly. Standard hemocytometers for counting blood cells are commonly used for this purpose. Care must be taken to differentiate the sporozoites from mosquito bristles, muscle fibers, and strings of rod-shaped bacteria, all of which may superficially resemble sporozoites. Fink (1968) has advocated the use of phase-contrast microscopy for better differentiation. The Petroff–Hausser bacteria counting chamber is especially useful, because observations can be made with phase-contrast or dark-field microscopy and with higher magnifications than is possible with conventional blood cell counting chambers. A relatively simple counting procedure has been used by one of us (J. Vanderberg) for several years. A 10-μl sample drop of the sporozoite suspension is placed on a slide and covered with a 22 × 22 mm coverslip (total area of 484 mm^2). We have determined that, with our microscope, using a 40× phase-contrast objective, the total area of each field is 0.0855 mm^2 (this will obviously vary depending upon the microscope and the lenses used). By counting sporozoites in 100 fields at random, an area of 8.55 mm^2 of the coverslip is counted. This sample area is 8.55/484 (=1/56.6) of the total area under the coverslip. Thus, by multiplying the number of sporozoites counted in this 100-field sample area by 56.6, we obtain an estimate of the total number of sporozoites in the original 10-μl drop. Further multiplication by 100 gives the total sporozoite count per milliliter. When sporozoites are heavily concentrated, the sampling of fewer than 100 fields may be quite sufficient.

Sporozoites in suspension within a tube tend to settle and stick rather tenaciously to its bottom and sides. Thus, before specimens are taken from the tube for quantitation or for dilution, it should be vigorously agitated to resuspend the settled sporozoites. Siliconization of all glassware (Vanderberg *et al.*, 1968) may be helpful in reducing this problem. After sporozoite counts have been made they can be diluted to appropriate concentrations. If necessary, sporozoites can be sedimented by centrifugation (700–1000 g for 20–30 minutes) and then resuspended in a smaller volume of fluid.

VIII. INFECTING VERTEBRATES WITH SPOROZOITES

A. Infection by Mosquito Bite

The kinetics of sporozoite injection by mosquitoes during the act of feeding have been reviewed by Vanderberg (1977). In brief, only a very small percentage of the sporozoites in the salivary glands are actually injected during feeding. This appears to be due largely to the anatomy of the glands. Many of the sporozoites are within the cytoplasm of the gland cells, or "landlocked" within gland cells that have no access to the secretory duct of the salivary gland. Sporozoites that reach the lumen of the gland may have relatively little outward access because of the narrow dimensions of the salivary duct and the small amount of saliva actually injected by the feeding mosquitoes. Saliva and the sporozoites therein appear to be injected in two distinct ways. Some injection takes place within the skin and subcutaneous tissues of the host, while the mouthparts are probing for a blood source, and some injection takes place directly into capillaries. Sporozoites deposited in the extravascular tissues seem to be capable of leaving the injection site and reaching the circulatory system. Vanderberg (1974) has suggested that the sporozoite motility required for this translocation may be induced by albumin in the skin and subcutaneous tissues.

Most of the early experimental studies on infecting humans and experimental animals with sporozoites were done by allowing infected mosquitoes to feed. Often, this can be a highly efficient way of inducing infection. A single bite from an *A. aegypti* mosquito infected with *P. gallinaceum* will infect more than 85% of the chicks challenged, and more bites will ensure virtually 100% infection (Russell and Mohan, 1942; Coatney *et al.*, 1945a). However, one cannot easily quantitate the dose level the host is receiving (Fink, 1968). In addition, mosquito bites may not always be infective, even when apparently mature sporozoites are present in the gland (Laird, 1941).

B. Infection by Syringe

More uniformity in infective dose levels can be achieved by syringe inoculation. Generally, intravenous inoculation is the most efficient, though intramuscular and intraperitoneal inoculations are also useful (Porter *et al.*, 1952). Oral inoculation of sporozoites has been reported to be occasionally successful (Porter *et al.*, 1952; Yoeli and Most, 1971), though it has limited practical value.

The intramuscular inoculation of whole glands infected with *P. gallinaceum* was shown to infect close to 100% of chicks that received intact glands from one mosquito (Coatney *et al.*, 1945b). However, homogenizing the free glands and injecting the resulting suspension intramuscularly gave more consistent results (Coatney *et al.*, 1945c). The injection of each chick with the suspension volume obtained from one mosquito (Greenberg *et al.*, 1950) showed that high infection rates could be obtained with as little as 0.01 mosquito equivalents.

More workers currently inoculate with specific numbers of sporozoites rather than with mosquito equivalents. When sporozoite infectivity is high, few are needed. Fink (1968), working with the *P. cathemerium*–canary system, showed that the intravenous injection of 250 sporozoites per bird infected 100%, while two of four canaries were infected with inocula of as few as 5 sporozoites.

IX. QUANTITATION OF SPOROZOITE INFECTIVITY AND VIABILITY

A. Introduction

It is sometimes helpful to quantitate the infectivity of batches of sporozoites in order to compare the infectivity of one batch with that of another. The degree of parasitemia resulting from a sporozoite-induced infection is determined not by the total number of sporozoites injected but by the number of "successful" sporozoites able to complete development within the host. The size of this infective sporozoite inoculum may influence many characteristics of the ensuing parasitemia, including its duration and severity, its tendency to relapse, its response to drugs, and the possible development of immunity (reviewed by McGregor, 1965; Vanderberg, 1977). An accurate assessment of sporozoite infectivity is also necessary for studies on prophylaxis against sporozoite-induced malaria, either by drugs or by immunization. By assessing the infectivity of inocula to unprotected control animals and by comparing this with the infectivity of sporozoite inocula to immunized or drug-treated animals, one can quantitate the degree of protection raised against sporozoite challenge.

The infectivity of a sporozoite is generally measured by its ability to develop further within a susceptible host. This measurement may be made by assessing either the sporozoite's ability to transform itself into an EE form or its subsequent development into asexual blood stages. Two separate components of infectivity should be kept in mind: (1) All sporozoites are probably not equally infective, and a population of sporozoites may consist of individuals with a range of different infectivities, and (2) the innate infectivity of sporozoites may be modulated by the response of the host being challenged.

B. Assessment of Sporozoite Infectivity by Quantitation of Ensuing Parasitemia

The simplest way of assessing the infectivity of a batch of sporozoites is by determining the percentage of animals developing parasitemia after inoculation with a given dose of sporozoites. If a range of different doses is used, in general the higher the dose the greater the percentage of infections (Boyd, 1940; Vanderberg *et al.*, 1968). However, even if all animals develop patent blood infections after sporozoite inoculation, it is still possible to assess the degree of infectivity of the original sporozoite injection by noting the characteristics of the resulting blood infections. Not only are more animals infected with higher doses; in addition, the higher the dose the shorter the incubation period (Boyd, 1940; Greenberg *et al.*, 1950; Vanderberg *et al.*, 1968). All things being equal, the density of first-generation asexual parasites in the blood probably reflects the dose of sporozoites received by the host (McGregor, 1965). Light inocula will give rise to light initial parasitemia which may need several cycles of asexual development before the parasites can be found readily in blood smears. On the other hand, a heavy inoculum of infective sporozoites will be followed by corresponsingly dense parasitemia that is more readily observable at an earlier time. Typical results are shown in Table I.

However, one disadvantage of using the length of the prepatent period as an indicator of sporozoite viability is that the first day of patency for a given animal may depend upon the methods used to detect parasites. Because parasite density is normally quite low early in the infection, detection of the first parasite in a blood smear may be a chance occurrence, seen by one microscopist and not by another. Therefore, some workers have sought to assess the intensity of sporozoite-induced infections by examining the blood several days after the first day of patency. At this time, the parasitemia is higher and more readily measurable in an objective way. Thus, Porter *et al.* (1954) found that there was a relationship between the number of *P. gallinaceum* sporozoites inoculated and the degree of parasitemia reached on the sixth day of infection. This approach was put on firm mathematical grounds by Warhurst and Folwell (1968) who showed that asexual parasites of *P. berghei* increased in numbers logarithmically

TABLE I

Results of Intravenous Inoculation of A/J Mice with *Plasmodium berghei* Sporozoites[a]

Sporozoites per animal	Animals infected		Prepatent period in days ±SE
10,000	18/18	(100%)	4.0 ± 0.9
5,000	140/149	(94%)	4.6 ± 0.16
1,000	88/94	(94%)	5.1 ± 0.19
100	28/61	(46%)	5.8 ± 0.11
10	6/23	(26%)	6.8 ± 0.15

[a] Modified from Vanderberg *et al.*, 1968.

up to the time when about 2% of the erythrocytes were infected. Accordingly, the number of asexual parasites in the blood at any point up to this time can be regarded as a direct amplification of the number of infective sporozoites originally inoculated. Using this principle, Fink (1970) showed that within limits there was an inverse linear correlation between the log of the number of sporozoites injected and the log of the day on which the parasitemia reached a given level (2% parasitemia for *P. cathemerium* in canaries and 0.2% for *P. yoelii* in mice). A similar correlation procedure was used by Gregory and Peters (1970) for *P. berghei* (2% parasitemia level). Thus, one can determine the numbers of infective sporozoites injected by determining the mean day on which this standard parasitemia level is reached.

C. Assessment of Sporozoite Viability by Determining Rates of Conversion to Exoerythrocytic Forms

Differences in sporozoite inocula of about one-half of a log dilution are required before one can detect significant differences in the degree of the resulting parasitemias (Vanderberg *et al.,* 1968; Fink, 1970). A more sensitive way to distinguish differences between sporozoite inocula is to assess the percentage of sporozoites successfully developing into EE forms in a susceptible animal. This procedure is largely restricted to rodent malaria, as it is not possible to quantitate EE forms in avians and it is not a practical standard procedure with simians. Verhave (1975) and Vanderberg (1977) have shown that, within a given experiment, there is a proportional relationship between the number of sporozoites inoculated into an animal and the number of EE forms that develop. This establishes the validity of counting EE forms to determine the number of sporozoites that have successfully invaded the liver. The density of EE forms appears to be relatively uniform among the various liver lobes (Bray and Gunders, 1962; Verhave, 1975; Vanderberg, 1977). Thus, the density of these forms within a sample of any given lobe may be taken as the concentration for the liver as a whole. However, the distribution of EE forms within a small portion of a lobe is not always entirely uniform (Yoeli *et al.,* 1966; Verhave, 1975). Thus, a large sample is required for statistical validity.

Quantitation of EE forms of *P. berghei* has been described by Vanderberg *et al.* (1968) and Vanderberg (1977). A measured dose of sporozoites is injected intravenously into a young white rat (3–4 weeks old), which is killed approximately 42 hours later. (EE forms of this parasite begin to mature and burst at about 44 hours. Thus, some EE forms would be missed if the animal were killed much beyond this time.) The entire liver is removed, and its volume determined by volumetric displacement of water in a graduated cylinder. Entire lobes of liver are then fixed in Carnoy's (6:3:1) solution for 4 hours, after which cylinders of liver tissue of a constant diameter are punched out with a no. 2 cork borer. To count EE forms in the round sections subsequently cut at 7 μm thickness, slides are stained for 2 hours at 40°C in a solution of 0.25 mg of azure B per milliliter of 0.05 M potassium hydrogen phthalate at pH 4.0 (Flax and Himes, 1952). They are then rapidly dehydrated in tertiary butanol, cleared in xylol, and mounted in Permount. At least 100 sections should be examined from each experimental animal to determine the mean number of EE forms per section. The density of EE forms is estimated by the method of Garnham and Bray (as given in Wéry, 1966):

$$\begin{array}{cc} \text{Density of EE forms} \\ \text{in liver} \end{array} = \frac{\text{mean number of EE forms per section}}{\begin{array}{c}\text{mean EE form diameter times} \\ \text{surface area of each section}\end{array}}$$

The total number of EE forms per liver is calculated by multiplying the density of EE forms so obtained by the total liver volume previously estimated. As an alternative, slides may be stained with Giemsa–colophonium (Bray and Garnham, 1962) or any conventional histological stain. The advantage of azure B staining is that the EE forms stain darkly against a relatively light background and may be seen easily even at a relatively low scanning power. Vanderberg *et al.* (1968) have defined sporozoite viability as the percentage of sporozoites that develop into mature EE forms when inoculated into a given host. Another procedure for sampling liver and counting EE forms has been described by Verhave (1975).

D. Differential Host Susceptibility

Hosts may vary enormously in their susceptibility to a sporozoite challenge. In a comparative study of different species of rodents, Vanderberg *et al.* (1968) showed that, when *P. berghei* sporozoites were injected intravenously, the transformation rate of sporozoites into EE forms was 2% in the A/J mouse, 15% in the young white rat, and 48% in the tree rat, *Thamnomys,* the natural rodent host of this parasite.

Within a species, there may be considerable variability among strains. The Ippy strain of *Thamnomys* originating from the Central African Republic (Landau, 1973) has a much lower susceptibility to sporozoites than the strain studied by Vanderberg *et al.* (1968), which originated in Zaire (Verhave, 1975; J. P. Vanderberg, unpublished data). A wide range of differential susceptibilities exists among different inbred strains of mice (Most *et al.,* 1966). The age of the host may also influence its susceptibility to sporozoites. Vanderberg *et al.* (1968) used white rats 3–5 weeks old in their comparative susceptibility studies because prior studies (M. Yoeli, unpublished) had suggested that older rats were much less susceptible. However, rats develop an innate resistance to the blood stages of the parasite as they grow older. Thus, when one uses patent parasitemia as a measure of rat resistance to sporozoites, it may not be possible to distinguish between the host's resistance to sporozoites and its resistance to blood stages. Verhave (1975) showed, however, that 2-month-old rats developed significantly more EE forms than 4-month-old rats after sporozoite inoculation with *P. berghei*.

The susceptibility of individual animals to sporozoites may be reduced by a number of factors, including the physiological status of the host and prior or concurrent infections with malaria or other disease organisms. The EE forms of *P. berghei* do not develop properly in animals with fatty livers induced by ethionine treatment (Dunn *et al.*, 1972). Rats that have had a prior blood infection with rodent malaria show a marked reduction in EE forms when challenged with sporozoites of the same species (Bafort, 1971; Verhave, 1975). Verhave (1975) has suggested a number of possible mechanisms for this phenomenon, including circulating interferon, cross-reacting antibodies, activation of the complement system, increased nonspecific phagocytosis, and hepatic dysfunction. The severe pathogenic effects of malarial infection on the liver have been well documented by Maegraith (1968). Other infections that suppress malaria infections in rodents are *Eperythrozoon coccoides* (Peters, 1965) and viruses (Jahiel *et al.*, 1968). The latter may act through their ability to induce interferon production in rodents.

In some cases, treatment of the host may enhance its susceptibility to sporozoite challenge. It is a well-known phenomenon that splenectomizing a relatively insusceptible host significantly increases its susceptibility to sporozoites. Another treatment that has been suggested to enhance susceptibility to sporozoite challenge is pretreatment with phlorizen, a drug known to clear glycogen from the liver. Bray and Williamson (1953) found that one monkey so treated had five times as many EE forms of *P. cynomolgi* in its liver as a nontreated control monkey. However, J. P. Vanderberg (unpublished results) was not able to repeat these results with the *P. berghei*–young rat system. Still another suggested treatment has been administration of methionine. *Aotus* monkeys fed DL-methionine were reported to have enhanced susceptibility to *P. falciparum* sporozoites (Ward and Hayes, 1972; Hayes and Ward, 1977).

X. SPECIFIC HOST–PARASITE–VECTOR SYSTEMS IN MALARIA RESEARCH

A. Introduction

Research workers studying mosquito transmission of malaria may choose from four different groups of host–parasite systems, namely, avian, rodent, simian, and human malarias. Each has certain inherent advantages and disadvantages for research.

A primary consideration in selecting a host–parasite–vector combination for a laboratory study should be its potential for answering particular scientific questions. Whether an investigator is concerned with pharmacology, parasite genetics, oocyst development, sporozoite infectivity, vertebrate host immune responses, or a variety of host–parasite characteristics, there is usually a model system suited to the experimental design.

Ultimately, however, the choice of a laboratory model is determined by the availability of facilities for maintaining the vertebrate host of the malarial parasite. This choice is influenced by considerations such as availability of experimental animals, cost per animal, and the ease and cost of animal husbandry. Of the three main types of nonhuman animal models (rodent, avian, and primate) rodent malarias emerge as most suitable for most laboratory studies. Characteristics, advantages, and deficiencies of the three groups of malaria models will be considered below.

Many generalizations can be made about sporozoite transmission that appear to hold reasonably true for all the diverse species of malaria. Indeed, one of the aims of this chapter thus far has been to call attention to the fundamental similarities found in the different species. However, each species of malaria also has unique characteristics that distinguish it from other species. Knowledge gained from studies conducted on animal models may or may not be applicable to human malarias. Consequently, one must be cautious in applying information gained from animal models directly to human malarias. Ultimately, all findings must be verified with the human parasites in their human hosts.

B. Avian Malarias

1. Introduction and History

Progress in human malaria research has proceeded in parallel and with heavy dependence on research on the malarias of birds. Hewitt (1940) noted: "Were it not for the use of birds as experimental hosts it is doubtful whether the mosquito transmission of malaria would have been so early established."

Laveran described the protozoan parasite of malaria in human blood in 1880 and wrote soon thereafter that research could go no further until an animal model was developed. Without knowledge of Laveran's work or comments, Danilewsky in 1885 described protozoan parasites in the blood cells of birds. Research on bird malarias expanded rapidly, particularly in Italy. Grassi and Feletti (1890a) described two distinct species of bird malaria, later naming one *Haemamoeba relicta* (=*P. relictum*). Other European workers described a variety of avian malaria species and began work on the biology of the parasites. However, it fell to a young investigator at The Johns Hopkins University in Baltimore to unravel the mystery of the sexual cycle of malaria. W. G. MacCallum, working with *Haemoproteus* in the blood of crows, described exflagellation and fertilization and correctly interpreted the biological significance of these events (MacCallum, 1897, 1898). These studies permitted him to make similar observations with *P. falciparum* (MacCallum, 1897). MacCallum's discovery allowed Ross to complete his studies with bird malaria and demonstrate conclusively the role of the mosquito as definitive host and vector (Ross, 1898).

Thereafter avian malarias assumed a central role in malaria research. Koch (1899) and Ruge (1901) were the first to infect domestic canaries with avian parasites from wild-caught birds. The first synthetic antimalarial drugs were tested in the 1920s on bird malarias, and today *P. gallinaceum* in chickens remains a useful system for screening drugs. Significantly, the EE cycle in malaria was first demonstrated with an avian malaria (Raffaele, 1934).

In recent years, avian malarias have fallen from favor as regular tools for laboratory research. Although several species with unique features are maintained, only *P. gallinaceum* is routinely used in studies involving the sexual cycle of the parasite. *Plasmodium lophurae* is used for studies on *in vitro* culture, biochemistry, and immunology, but the only known isolate of this parasite has lost the capacity to produce gametocytes and is completely dependent on the hypodermic syringe for transmission.

2. *Plasmodium relictum*

a. Introduction.   The early history of research on the avian malaria parasite *P. relictum* is inextricably bound to the history of malaria research in general. The avian parasite Danilewsky described in 1885 was probably *P. relictum*, and the parasite was carefully described and named in a series of papers published by Grassi and Feletti (1890a,b, 1891, 1892). Ronald Ross' *Proteosoma* was in fact *P. relictum*, and his studies on this parasite in *Culex* mosquitoes, sparrows, and larks served to establish the mosquito transmission of malaria.

Plasmodium relictum was used in some of the earliest studies on the EE development of malaria (Raffaele, 1936). The concept of premunition in avian malarias was based on studies of this parasite in canaries (Sergent and Sergent, 1952). *In vitro* cultivation of the EE forms (Hawking, 1946) and sporogonic stages (Ball and Chao, 1960) of this parasite have received considerable attention.

Plasmodium relictum in canaries proved to be an invaluable tool for the screening of potential antimalarial compounds; one of the first synthetic antimalarials, Plasmochin (pamaquine) was derived from this avian screen (Roehl, 1926). Although *P. relictum* drug screens continued in use until the 1960s, the pharmaceutical industry in general has now converted to screens using *P. gallinaceum* or various rodent or primate malarias.

b. Vertebrate Hosts.   *Plasmodium relictum* naturally infects a wide variety of bird species and has a cosmopolitan distribution (Garnham, 1966). For the purposes of laboratory studies, however, the canary remains the standard host for studies on the EE and asexual cycles within the bird and for the production of gametocytes for the infection of mosquitoes. Although *P. relictum* has been studied in such common laboratory animals as ducks, pigeons, and doves, and in such exotic hosts as penguins, the canary remains the host of choice.

c. Mosquito Hosts. *Plasmodium relictum* will develop in a variety of mosquito species; members of the genera *Anopheles* and *Aedes* are usually poor hosts, while *Culex* mosquitoes are generally susceptible. There is also a wide range of susceptibility within this genus. Tested against a coindigenous strain of *P. relictum,* infection rates ranged from 100% in *C. stigmatasoma* to 98% in *C. tarsalis* to 50% in *C. pipiens fatigans* (Herman *et al.,* 1954). An extensive list of mosquito species susceptible or refractory to *P. relictum* and other avian malarias has been prepared by Huff (1965).

d. Experimental Procedures. As noted above, the normal laboratory model for *P. relictum* includes the canary and *Culex* mosquitoes (usually *C. pipiens* or *C. tarsalis*) as hosts. Canaries may be infected by the bite of sporozoite-carrying mosquitoes, by the injection of dissected sporozoites, or by the injection of parasitized blood from an infected bird. The prepatent period for sporozoite-induced infections lasts from 6 to 9 days (Sergent and Sergent, 1952), while prepatent periods for blood-induced infections depend on the number of parasites injected (Boyd, 1925). Once patent, parasitemias in canaries rise rapidly and peak 4–6 days after patency. The asexual cycle is usually asynchronous and lasts 30–36 hours. Birds frequently die at the peak of infection but, if the crisis period is survived, a state of premunition characterized by low-level, usually microscopically undetectable parasitemia is achieved. Canaries may remain infected but subpatent for years (Bishop *et al.,* 1938) and may serve as a source of infectious blood for subpassage into other birds at any time. While in a state of premunition, these birds cannot be reinfected.

Gametocytes may appear in the circulation at the same time as the first asexual parasites. Infectivity to mosquitoes increases with increasing gametocytemia, although mosquitoes can be infected early in an infection before the first gametocytes are detectable (Shah *et al.,* 1934). Mosquito infections are best achieved during the ascending phase of parasitemia; attempts to infect mosquitoes after the peak of asexual parasitemia are usually unsuccessful (Shah *et al.,* 1934).

The *P. relictum*–canary–*Culex* research model, although seldom used today, retains certain advantages. The parasite can be obtained from wild-caught birds and transferred to canaries. Canaries are easily obtained and maintained in small cages. Bird cages and feed can be purchased in local pet shops. *Culex* mosquitoes are not difficult to rear, and colonies are available from many laboratories.

The disadvantages of this model system are fairly obvious. Canaries are expensive and can be used only once. Their small size makes bleeding and intravenous injections difficult. They are sensitive to handling and frequently succumb to the infection. In spite of these drawbacks, the *P. relictum* malaria model remains a useful experimental tool with a potential for solving some of the still unanswered questions concerning malaria.

3. *Plasmodium cathemerium*

a. Introduction. The discovery of a new species of avian malaria in a house sparrow in Baltimore in 1924, and its eventual designation as *P. cathemerium* (Hartman, 1927), added an important new laboratory model for research. Hegner and Manwell (1927) used this species, by then established in canaries, as a screen for synthetic antimalarial compounds. At the same time, in an extended series of pioneering studies, Huff (1927, 1929, 1931, 1934, 1935) used this parasite to establish the genetic basis of mosquito susceptibility to the malaria parasite.

b. Vertebrate Hosts. *Plasmodium cathemerium* is a cosmopolitan infection of passerine birds. Canaries are readily infected with sporozoites or parasitized blood and are the typical laboratory hosts. *Plasmodium cathemerium* will infect ducks but not chickens.

c. Mosquito Hosts. The natural vector of *P. cathemerium* is unknown, but presumed to be one of the ornithophilic species of *Culex*. In the laboratory this parasite will infect a number of mosquito species (Huff, 1965; Garnham, 1966), but *C. pipiens* and *C. quinquefasciatus* (=*C. pipiens fatigans*) are particularly good vectors.

d. Experimental Procedures. Procedures for handling *P. cathemerium* in canaries are similar to those outlined for *P. relictum*. *Plasmodium cathemerium* has a synchronous asexual cycle lasting about 24 hours (Taliaferro, 1925). Parasitemias in canaries rise rapidly, and about one-third of infected birds die from an acute infection. The parasite exhibits a circadian cycle of gametocyte maturation with maximum infectivity to mosquitoes feeding in the evening (1800–2200 hours) (Shah *et al.*, 1934; Hawking and Gammage, 1970). Detailed descriptions for infecting mosquitoes and for challenging canaries with sporozoites have been given by Fink (1968, 1970).

Advantages and disadvantages of the *P. cathemerium*–canary–*Culex* model are similar to those described for *P. relictum*.

4. *Plasmodium gallinaceum*

a. Introduction. A new blood parasite was first seen in jungle fowl in 1910, but 25 years elapsed before it was described as *P. gallinaceum* (Brumpt, 1935). Soon thereafter it became a major tool in malaria research. Using this parasite in chickens, James and Tate (1937) unequivocally established the existence of an EE cycle for malaria. With the advent of World War II, it became evident that a more efficient drug-screening system was necessary for the development of new antimalarial compounds. Based on a number of criteria, the *P. gallinaceum*–chicken system was chosen as a replacement for the less selective *P. relictum* and *P. cathemerium* screens (Curd 1943). *Plasmodium gallinaceum* screens in one form or another continued in use into the 1970s and are still considered useful by some investigators. The parasite has been used extensively for studies on the physiology of gametogenesis (Bishop and McConnachie, 1956, 1960; Carter and Nijhout, 1977; Nijhout and Carter, 1978; Nijhout, 1979), immunity against the sexual stages of the infection (Eyles, 1952a,b; Huff *et al.*, 1958; Gwadz, 1976; Carter and Chen, 1976; Carter *et al.*, 1979a,b), and the first studies on immunity against sporozoites (Mulligan *et al.*, 1941).

Only one strain of *P. gallinaceum,* the 8A strain, is currently in use.

b. Vertebrate Hosts.   The natural hosts for *P. gallinaceum* are the jungle fowl of Asia. In the laboratory, the domestic chicken has proved a superb host. Passerine birds and canaries are generally refractory to infection.

c. Mosquito Hosts.   *Plasmodium gallinaceum* is less fastidious than most avian malarias and will infect a wide variety of mosquito species (Huff, 1965; Garnham, 1966). The parasite develops best in several species of *Aedes* and *Mansonia;* its natural vector in Sri Lanka is probably *M. crassipes* (Niles *et al.*, 1965). *Plasmodium gallinaceum* in the laboratory will infect representatives of *Armigeres, Culex, Culiseta,* and *Anopheles,* although none of these vectors are as efficient as *Aedes.*

Aedes aegypti is the usual mosquito host for laboratory studies with *P. gallinaceum*. This mosquito is easily reared and a good feeder. One can expect uniform infections when this mosquito is fed directly on chickens or through a membrane on blood with reasonable numbers of gametocytes. *Aedes aegypti* is genetically well defined (Craig and Hickey, 1967), and a number of studies have examined the genetic basis of vector competence in this species (Ward, 1963; Kilama and Craig, 1969).

d. Experimental Procedures.   Chickens may be infected by the bite of infectious mosquitoes, by the injection of dissected sporozoites, or by the injection of parasitized blood taken from a donor chicken with either patent parasitemia or a latent, subpatent infection.

The prepatent period following the injection of sporozoites lasts 72–75 hours, but the first significant wave of erythrocytic parasites does not appear until 7 days after infection, when the so-called flooding effect occurs (Huff and Coulston,

TABLE II

Schedule for Inoculation of *Plasmodium gallinaceum* into Chicks to Achieve Desired Parasitemia on Postinoculation Day Indicated

Inoculum (parasitized erythrocytes)[a]	Parasitemia on day postinoculation	
	1–10%	40–50%
2×10^8	2	3
4×10^7	3	4
8×10^6	4	5
1.6×10^5	5	6
3.2×10^4	6	7

[a] Blood from donor chicken with 5–15% rising parasitemia is inoculated intravenously into 500-g chicks.

1944). The prepatent period for blood-induced infections is directly dependent on the number of parasites injected. The predictability of patency in blood-induced infections is illustrated by the infection schedule used in the Malaria Section, Laboratory of Parasitic Diseases, National Institutes of Health (Table II) (D. Seeley and J. Edelin, personal communication). Fifty chicks (3 weeks old and weighing approximately 50 g each) are infected on Friday of each week by intravenous injection of infected blood to provide patent birds for the following week's research. Resulting parasitemias are fairly uniform. Ten birds will be at peak parasitemia on each of the 5 days. Investigators requiring lower parasitemias usually have a range of birds to choose from.

The asexual parasitemia in chickens is relatively synchronous, with a 36-hour cycle showing peaks of schizogony at midnight and midday on alternate days (Giovannola, 1938). Mortality in chickens is age-dependent; small chicks may suffer 100% mortality, while older birds usually survive even massive blood infections. After the initial peak of parasitemia, premunition is achieved and birds remain infected but subpatent for life.

Gametocytes appear in the circulation with the first asexual parasites and are infectious to mosquitoes at that time. Infectivity rises with rising gametocytemia, and maximum mosquito infections are achieved on the day prior to the peak of asexual parasitemia (Eyles, 1951, 1952a,b; Carter and Gwadz, 1980). After the peak of asexual parasitemia, gametocyte infectivity to mosquitoes is sharply reduced.

Sporozoite-induced infections are generally less virulent, and gametocyte infectivity persists a few days beyond the day of peak asexual parasitemia. Oocyst counts in mosquitoes fed on these chicks are usually lower than in those fed on birds infected by blood inoculation.

Advantages of the *P. gallinaceum*-chicken-*A. aegypti* laboratory model for the study of malaria are numerous. Chicks are inexpensive and readily obtainable from commercial hatcheries. Chicken caging and feed are easily obtained at reasonable prices. Chicks and chickens are large enough to allow easy infection and bleeding or direct mosquito feedings, and are easily restrained without anesthetic for bleeding or feeding. *Plasmodium gallinaceum* infections in chickens are predictable and consistently infectious to mosquitoes. *Aedes aegypti* is easy to rear, and its eggs can be stored dry for months and hatched when needed; the females avidly feed on chickens or through membranes and survive well beyond the time of sporozoite maturation. The chicken is a well-defined laboratory animal with regard to its physiology and immune responses.

The disadvantages of this model are few. Chickens are not particularly clean; they grow quickly, and long-term studies require large cages. The USDA has stringent quarantine and security requirements for the maintenance of *P. gallinacem* (standards not required for *P. relictum* or *P. cathemerium*). Details and forms for approval for the use of *P. gallinaceum* may be obtained from USDA/ APHIS, Veterinary Services, Import/Export Staff, Federal Building, Hyattsville, Maryland.

5. *Other Avian Malaria Parasites*

There is in addition a great variety of avian malarias that have been described and many that have been studied in the laboratory, some with exotic hosts and others with exotic vectors. Few of these parasites are in use or even available today; their details may be found in Huff (1965) and Garnham (1966).

C. Rodent Malarias

1. *Introduction and History*

The availability of a simple laboratory model for the study of mammalian malaria had long been a dream of malariologists, but it was not until 1948 that such a model became available. Two Belgian entomologists, Vincke and Lips (1948), described a new malaria parasite, *P. berghei,* from the blood of a tree rat, *Thamnomys surdaster,* collected in the Katanga region within the southeast portion of the former Belgian Congo (now known as Zaire). This discovery culminated years of research by Vincke during which time he elucidated the life cycle of the parasite while working virtually isolated in central Africa. Interestingly, the mosquito stages of the parasite were the first to be observed. During an antimalarial survey in December 1943, Vincke noted sporozoites in the salivary glands of the mosquito *A. dureni millecampsi,* collected from a gallery forest fringing a river near an important mining center, Elisabethville (now Kisangani). Entomological studies, including precipitin tests on the blood meal contents of the mosquitoes' midguts, conducted during the next several years led Vincke to the conclusion that the mosquito probably fed on rodents or insectivores. Upon the isolation of *P. berghei* from *Thamnomys* in 1948, Vincke postulated that the mosquito sporozoite infection and the rodent blood infection he had discovered were the same species. However, it was not until 1950 that he could show that sporozoites collected from these mosquitoes produced a typical *P. berghei* parasitemia when inoculated into laboratory mice. Thus, the life cycle was completed. The detailed history of this important discovery has been described by Bafort (1971) and Bruce-Chwatt (1978).

Subsequently, other species and subspecies of rodent malarias were isolated from a number of different sites throughout central Africa. The taxonomy and zoogeography of these species have been reviewed by Carter and Diggs (1977) and by Killick-Kendrick (1978). In brief, two groups are now recognized: the berghei group and the vinckei group, each being composed of two valid species. The berghei group contains *P. berghei* and *P. yoelii* (with three recognized subspecies of the latter). The vinckei group contains *P. vinckei* (with four subspecies) and *P. chabaudi* (with two subspecies). Cyclic passage through laboratory mosquitoes has been accomplished with all these species (and with most of the subspecies). However, not all are of equal value as laboratory models for experimental transmission of malaria by mosquitoes; some are more readily passaged than others.

During the 15 years that followed the discovery of *P. berghei*, many workers tried relatively unsuccessfully to transmit the parasite via a variety of anophelines (Raffaele and Baldi, 1950; Rodhain and Vincke, 1951, 1952; Yoeli and Wall, 1951, 1952; Box *et al.*, 1953; Perez-Reyez, 1953; Ramakrishnan *et al.*, 1953; Vincke, 1954; Bray, 1954; Rodhain *et al.*, 1955; Celaya *et al.*, 1956; Yoeli and Most, 1960). Several of these workers succeeded in obtaining various degrees of midgut infection, but only rarely were salivary gland infections produced, and these were invariably light. Because continued failure to transmit a strain in the laboratory was generally accompanied by a decreasing ability to produce gametocytes, it was necessary to isolate new strains from the wild or from the occasional successful mosquito passage in the laboratory.

The problem was resolved with the finding that *P. berghei* completes its sporogony in mosquitoes at relatively low optimal temperatures of 18°–21°C (Yoeli *et al.*, 1964; Vanderberg and Yoeli, 1964, 1966). This is the approximate temperature range that the natural vector, *A. dureni*, is subjected to in its microclimate within the gallery forests of central Africa during the summer transmission season of *P. berghei*. Previous laboratory studies had used higher maintenance temperatures based on our stereotype of the African tropics: hot and humid. By utilizing normal maintenance temperatures of 21°C and the efficient laboratory vector *A. stephensi*, the production of large numbers of sporozoites of *P. berghei* has become a routine laboratory procedure.

It is interesting to note that the long delay in establishing a laboratory system for mosquito transmission of rodent malaria was due largely to chance in the sequence of discovery of the different species of rodent malaria. The remaining three species, *P. vinckei, P. chabaudi,* and *P. yoelii,* were isolated from environments with relatively warmer temperatures during the transmission season, and these species complete their cyclic development in mosquitoes at temperatures above 24°C. As Carter and Diggs (1977) have pointed out, "It is ironic that *P. berghei* is the only murine malaria with low temperature requirements. If any of the other murine malaria plasmodia had been discovered first, it is probable that sporogony would have been achieved in the laboratory and the demonstration of the pre-erythrocytic stages of the parasites would have taken place many years earlier." This, however, is only partially true. *Plasmodium vinckei,* the second species to be isolated, was discovered only 4 years after the discovery of *P. berghei* (Rodhain, 1952). For various reasons it never received the full attention of laboratory workers enjoyed by *P. berghei* during the 1950s and early 1960s.

2. *Plasmodium berghei* and *Plasmodium yoelii*

a. Introduction.   In general, the berghei group parasites (*P. berghei* and *P. yoelii*) are more readily transmissible in the laboratory than those of the vinckei group (*P. vinckei* and *P. chabaudi*). Though *P. yoelii* can be as easily transmitted by mosquitoes under laboratory conditions as *P. berghei* (Landau and Killick-Kendrick, 1966; Wéry, 1968), a survey of the literature shows that most workers tend to use *P. berghei* for their studies. In view of the similarities between these two species, and the fact that techniques for their mosquito transmission are much the same, they will be discussed together.

Several strains of *P. berghei* are available. The NYU-2 strain (Yoeli and Most, 1960), one of the most commonly used strains in laboratories for biological studies on asexual stages, lost its ability to produce gametocytes several years ago and must be transmitted by serial blood passage via syringe. Three gametocyte-producing strains are in common use: (1) The KSP 11 was isolated in 1961 by J. Jadin from an infected *A. dureni* mosquito caught in the Kasapa gallery forest of the Katanga region. This strain produces the highest gametocytemia of all known strains and consequently has been used for a number of studies on exflagellation (Yoeli *et al.,* 1963; Garnham, 1964) and *in vitro* formation of ookinetes from gametocytes (Weiss and Vanderberg, 1977). (2) The NK-65 strain was isolated at New York University Medical School in New York from infected *A. dureni* sent by J. Bafort from the Kisanga gallery forest in 1965. (The NK-65 strain designation is thus derived from New York–Kisanga, 1965.) The cyclic passage of this strain has been described by Vanderberg *et al.* (1968) and Vanderberg (1977). (3) The ANKA strain was isolated at the Prince Leopold

Institute in Antwerp from infected mosquitoes sent by J. Bafort from the Kasapa gallery forest, also in 1965. (The ANKA strain designation is thus derived from Antwerp–Kasapa.) The cyclic passage of this strain has been described by Vincke *et al.* (1966) and Vincke and Bafort (1968).

One must be cautious in choosing a laboratory strain of rodent malaria to work with, and several admonitions are particularly relevant. First, the source of the strain must be carefully considered. Some species or strains may have been mixed up accidentally during laboratory transmission. In addition, some ''strains'' isolated from the wild have turned out in retrospect to be mixtures of different species of rodent malarias (Carter and Wallicker, 1975). Furthermore, it is best to use a strain that has been regularly passaged through laboratory mosquitoes over a period of several years. There appears to be a selection process whereby the investigator automatically selects for better sporozoite production under laboratory conditions.

b. Vertebrate Hosts. The natural hosts of rodent malarias are several species of African rodents, especially those of the genus *Thamnomys* (thicket or tree rats). In the laboratory, *P. berghei* and *P. yoelii* are usually studied in white mice, white rats, or hamsters. All of these are suitable for studies on the sporogonic stages of the parasites.

c. Mosquito Hosts. The natural vector of *P. berghei* is *A. dureni millecampsi,* a rodentophilic mosquito found in the highlands of central Africa. The natural vector of *P. yoelii* is still unknown. No worker has yet succeeded in laboratory colonization of *A. dureni;* virtually all studies with substitute laboratory vectors have shown *A. stephensi* to be the most satisfactory mosquito for laboratory transmission of all species of rodent malarias.

d. Experimental Procedures. Gametocytes of *P. berghei* and *P. yoelii* capable of infecting mosquitoes may be produced in hamsters, mice, or rats. Before giving specific details on the production of gametocytes in rodents, some general principles should be pointed out. (1) To avoid deterioration of gametocyte-producing ability in a malaria strain, the maintenance schedule should include periodic passages via sporozoites. Ideally, no more than three rodent-to-rodent passages of the parasite should be used before interposition of a sexual cycle by mosquito passage. (2) Gametocyte production patterns in sporozoite-induced infections are not always predictable. Thus, rodents used as sources of gametocytes for mosquito feedings are best infected with blood from another rodent. (3) Gametocyte infectivity is highest relatively early in the infection. The numbers of gametocytes found in the blood may continue to increase thereafter, but the infectivity to mosquitoes generally decreases. Thus, it is best to infect the rodent with a relatively high dose of parasites in order to obtain high gametocytemia as early as possible before gametocyte infectivity begins to decline.

A detailed protocol for producing infectious gametocytes of *P. berghei* in hamsters has been given by Vanderberg *et al.* (1968) and Vanderberg (1977). Laboratory-reared golden hamsters 3–5 weeks old were used for mosquito feedings. The hamsters were infected with an intraperitoneal inoculation of heparinized blood obtained by heart puncture from a donor hamster infected with the NK-65 strain of *P. berghei*. Blood from the donor animal (taken only after a parasitemia of 40% or more had been reached) was diluted 1:10 with 0.85% saline solution, and 1 ml was injected intraperitoneally into each recipient hamster. The parasite dose thus was generally between 2 and 3×10^8 infected red blood cells. The recipient hamsters, infected as described, were most infective to mosquitoes for the first few days of their gametocytemia, even though their gametocyte count usually continued to increase thereafter. The most satisfactory mosquito infections were obtained when the mosquitoes were permitted to feed 3 and 4 days after the blood inoculation from the donor hamster. At this time generally 1–4% of the erythrocytes are parasitized by gametocytes. Permitting the same mosquitoes to feed on two consecutive days was done for two purposes. First, mosquitoes which failed to take a blood meal at the initial feeding generally took one the next day. Second, many mosquitoes fed on both days, thus leading to superinfections. Mosquitoes permitted to fed on two consecutive days eventually developed significantly more sporozoites in their salivary glands than those that fed on either of the two separate days (Vanderberg and Nawrot, 1968). Similar procedures for raising infectious gametocytes of *P. berghei* and *P. yoelii* have been worked out independently and described by other workers, including Vincke and Bafort (1968) and Wéry (1968). Even higher gametocytemias can be produced in mice by intravenous inoculation of diluted or undiluted blood from the infected donor animal.

Procedures for feeding *A. stephensi* mosquitoes on infected hamsters have been described by Vanderberg (1977). Prior to use, hamsters were anesthetized with sodium pentobarbital (veterinary Nembutal, Abbott Laboratories), each hamster receiving 0.05–0.1 ml intraperitoneally. Each was placed on top of a cage containing about 400 female mosquitoes which had emerged several days previously. The mosquitoes had been starved overnight by removing sugar water from their cages and then fed through the wire screening on top of the cage. Infective feedings and subsequent maintenance of the infected mosquitoes took place in an insectary maintained at 21°C and at about 75% RH.

Some workers do not advocate the use of anesthesia and have suggested that the lowered skin temperature induced by anesthesia makes rodents less attractive to mosquitoes. These workers prefer to immobilize the rodent by taping it to a board and inserting the board in the mosquito cage (Wéry, 1966, 1968; Landau and Killick-Kendrick, 1966). However, starved *A. stephensi* mosquitoes feed quite well on anesthetized rodents (Vanderberg, 1977). Inserting the rodent into the mosquito cage cannot be recommended, as it is difficult to prevent large numbers of mosquitoes from escaping when the rodent is removed. Shaving the rodent's hair before feeding is also unnecessary. Killick-Kendrick (1971) suggests feeding no more than 150 mosquitoes per mouse. Because of their larger size, hamsters can support the feeding of several hundred mosquitoes apiece.

After feeding, mosquitoes should be supplied with 10% sucrose or glucose solution during their entire maintenance period. In addition, a normal blood meal from an uninfected rodent about 1 week after the initial infective blood meal appears to increase mosquito longevity and thus overall sporozoite recovery (Vanderberg and Nawrot, 1968). Placing a bowl of water or wet filter paper in the cage for oviposition is unnecessary. Indeed, higher sporozoite yields are obtained without oviposition (Vanderberg and Nawrot, 1968). Perhaps, the resorption of yolk material that occurs when oviposition is prevented aids in nutrition of the parasites developing within the mosquito. Some workers have reported enhanced sporogonic development when mosquitoes are fed on animals with p-aminobenzoic acid in their drinking water or when the mosquitoes are maintained on glucose to which p-aminobenzoic acid has been added (Peters and Howells, 1978).

Perhaps the most important consideration in the maintenance of infected mosquitoes is the insectary temperature. *Plasmodium berghei*-infected mosquitoes should be maintained at 21° ± 1°C. They should also receive their infective blood meal at this temperature, because the parasites are most sensitive to elevated temperatures early during their development. Even short exposures to high temperatures shortly after the infective blood meal may have a deleterious effect on sporogony (Vanderberg and Yoeli, 1966). Mosquitoes infected with *P. yoelii* are generally maintained at temperatures of about 24°–26°C.

When *A. stephensi* mosquitoes infected with *P. berghei* are maintained at 21°C, the first sporozoites invade the salivary glands 10–12 days after the mosquitoes' infective blood meal. Generally, the optimum time for recovery of infective salivary gland sporozoites is 15–18 days after the infective blood meal (Vanderberg, 1975). Methods for harvesting sporozoites and for maintaining them *in vitro* prior to challenging animals have already been discussed (Section VII).

Rodents are most effectively challenged by the intravenous inoculation of sporozoites into a tail vein. An inoculum of about 0.2 ml works well for both mice and rats. Vanderberg *et al.* (1968) have suggested using A/J mice for experiments in which relatively large numbers of rodents must be challenged (immunizations, chemotherapy, etc.), and young rats (3–5 weeks old) for experiments requiring the demonstration of EE forms in the liver (see Section IX,D).

The chief advantage of rodent malaria parasites for laboratory study is that they are useful models for the investigation of mammalian malaria. For the first time, it became possible to use small, inexpensive mammalian hosts in large numbers to investigate many aspects of mammalian malaria. Avian malaria differs from mammalian malaria in a number of significant ways. Nowhere do they differ more than in the biology of their EE forms. The discovery that the localization and the morphology of these forms in rodent malaria was similar to what had been demonstrated for simian and human malarias has made rodent malaria a prime investigative tool for the study of sporozoite invasion and differentiation in the mammalian host. A number of findings on sporozoite biology and immunization, first made with the rodent malaria model, were later extended to simian and human malarias.

The chief disadvantage of the rodent malaria model for studies on sporogony is that the standard laboratory vector is not as efficient as the natural one. Sporogonic development in the laboratory vector, *A. stephensi,* is often highly asynchronous, and sporozoite viability may vary considerably from one experiment to another. Most investigators working with the model have reported occasional periods of inexplicably low sporozoite viability. The minimum doses of sporozoites required for infection with rodent malaria are generally higher than for avian or primate malarias. In addition, rodent malarias have unfortunately not yet lived up to their potential as models for relapse malaria. Though chronicity and relapse seem to occur in nature (Landau and Boulard, 1978), no one has yet succeeded in demonstrating true relapse in laboratory rodent hosts under experimental conditions.

3. Other Rodent Malaria Parasites

The two remaining species, *P. vinckei* and *P. chabaudi,* are members of the vinckei group. These species do not ordinarily infect rats or hamsters and are commonly maintained in laboratory mice. Detailed procedures for cyclic transmission of *P. chabaudi* have been described by Wéry (1968), and for *P. vinckei* by Bafort (1969, 1971). However, both of these authors conclude that *P. berghei* is a more easily handled species for mosquito transmission in the laboratory. *Plasmodium chabaudi* and *P. vinckei* tend to give considerably lighter salivary gland infections than *P. berghei,* but the few sporozoites that reach the salivary glands seem to be more infectious than those of *P. berghei.* A novel way of efficiently infecting mosquitoes with *P. chabaudi* has been reported by D. Wallicker (personal communication). Blood from infected mice is transferred to splenectomized rats which then develop substantial gametocytemias. Mosquitoes can be infected by feeding on these rats.

D. Simian Malarias

1. Introduction and History

The description of three distinct human malarias, later called *P. vivax* and *P. malariae* (Grassi and Feletti, 1890b) and *P. falciparum* (Welch, 1897), was quickly followed by the description of a number of blood parasites of apes and monkeys. *Plasmodium kochi,* later placed in the genus *Hepatocystis,* was first seen in several African monkey species (Kossel, 1899; Laveran, 1899). Investigations with captive zoo animals led to the description of *P. pitheci* from the orangutan, and *P. cynomolgi* and *P. innui* from macaques, all in 1907. *Plasmodium brasilianum* was described from a New World monkey in 1908, and *P. knowlesi* was first seen in 1927 and given specific rank in 1932. Thereafter, parasites were described from the great apes of Africa and Asia, and from numerous monkey species throughout the tropics. The history of these searches and a compendium of current knowledge on primate malarias can be found in the classic monograph of Coatney *et al.* (1971).

As research tools, malarias of subhuman primates have proved invaluable. There are species which closely parallel the parasites affecting humans in their biology, pathology, and response to antimalarial drugs and, indeed, several of these species will infect humans. In this section the primate malarias most frequently used in the laboratory, which readily infect mosquitoes, will be considered in detail.

2. Plasmodium cynomolgi

a. Introduction. This vivaxlike parasite was first seen in imported Javanese macaques in Hamburg in 1907 and named *P. cynomolgi* a year later (Mayer, 1908). Since then, numerous isolates designated subspecies or strains from the Malaysian region, Java, and India have been characterized. Because *P. cynomolgi* (Mayer, 1907) closely resembles *P. vivax* in morphology and biology, it has been used as a model for studies relating to the human parasite. The EE stages of primate malarias in the liver were first demonstrated with this parasite (Shortt and Garnham, 1948), and it has been used extensively for studies on the mechanism of relapse (reviewed by Garnham, 1967). *Plasmodium cynomolgi* also plays an important role as a drug screen for antimalarials effective against the liver stages of the parasite (Schmidt *et al.,* 1948; Rossan *et al.,* 1964).

b. Vertebrate Hosts. The most common laboratory host for *P. cynomolgi* is the rhesus monkey, *Macaca mulatta,* but the parasite will infect several species of macaques and a wide range of New and Old World monkeys (Garnham, 1966; Coatney *et al.,* 1971). In addition, *P. cynomolgi* will infect humans (Eyles *et al.,* 1960).

c. Mosquito Hosts. The natural hosts of *P. cynomolgi* are probably forest-dwelling, monkey-biting members of the genus *Anopheles,* often of the leucosphyrus group of the subgenus *Cellia.* Good laboratory vectors are numerous, but *A. balabacensis, A. freeborni,* and *A. stephensi* are particularly supportive of the growth of oocysts and sporozoites (Coatney *et al.,* 1971).

d. Experimental Procedures. Monkeys are readily infected with sporozoites by mosquito bite or injection, or by the injection of parasitized blood. The prepatent period for sporozoite-induced infections ranges from 7 to 16 days, with a mean of 9.8 days (Coatney et al., 1971). The length of patency after injection of infected blood depends on the number of asexual parasites injected.

Plasmodium cynomolgi infections are seldom lethal; peak parasitemias in spleen-intact monkeys rarely exceed 10%. Infected animals will show repeated recrudescences and, if treated with a blood schizonticide such as chloroquine, sporozoite-induced infections will demonstrate a classic pattern of relapse (Coatney et al., 1971). The asexual parasites exhibit a vivaxlike, tertian, 48-hour maturation period.

Gametocytes appear early in both blood- and sporozoite-induced infections, usually coincident with the first asexual parasites, and are infectious at that time. Coatney and his co-workers have extensively studied the cycles of infectivity of *P. cynomolgi* to various mosquito species and have made the following observations. Gametocytes mature at about the same time as schizonts and are short-lived. Infectivity may be cyclic, showing a pattern of every-other-day infectivity to mosquitoes. *Plasmodium cynomolgi* may also show the so-called Hawking phenomenon (Section III,D,3) in which feedings at night produce heavy mosquito infections and day feedings produce very light infections (Hawking et al., 1968; Garnham and Powers, 1974; R. W. Gwadz, unpublished observations).

Mosquitoes feed best on monkeys which have been tranquilized. As noted above, ketamine hydrochloride is a particularly effective, rapid-acting, nonnarcotic anesthetic for use in primates. Once it has been determined that a monkey is or should be a gametocyte carrier, the animal can be anesthetized and restrained on a board, and prestarved caged mosquitoes can be applied to the abdomen of the animal. Mosquitoes will feed readily through the cage netting, and most will feed to repletion in 10–15 minutes. Alternatively, blood may be drawn from the monkey and fed to mosquitoes in a membrane feeder (Section IV). Again, mosquitoes will engorge in a few minutes.

Monkeys that have been repeatedly infected and cured develop immunity, show reduced asexual and sexual parasitemias when rechallenged, and are significantly less infectious to mosquitoes. However, if these monkeys are surgically splenectomized, they may be reinfected, will develop both asexual and sexual parasitemias, and will be highly infectious to mosquitoes. Splenectomized monkeys may be repeatedly infected, cured, and reinfected, and sustain good infectivity for mosquitoes.

The *P. cynomolgi*–rhesus monkey–*Anopheles* mosquito model demonstrates a number of significant features. *Plasmodium cynomolgi* closely resembles *P. vivax* in morphology, biology, and pathogenicity. The parasite shows a vivaxlike relapse pattern in the rhesus monkey and responds to the same drugs that affect the human parasite. *Plasmodium cynomolgi* infections are predictable and infectious to a wide range of colonized anopheline species.

The disadvantages of this model are associated with the need for a monkey host. Rhesus and other monkey species are expensive to buy and even more expensive to maintain. They are often in short supply and require elaborate caging, feeding, and watering systems. However, because of its homologies with human malarias, it remains an important tool in malaria research.

3. *Plasmodium knowlesi*

a. Introduction. *Plasmodium knowlesi* (Sinton and Mulligan, 1932) is a parasite of southeast Asian monkeys first seen in 1927 but not formally described for several years (Sinton and Mulligan, 1932). Soon thereafter it was adopted for the treatment of general paresis resulting from neurosyphilis in humans (Knowles and Das Gupta, 1932). In recent years, the parasite has been used extensively for laboratory studies on natural immunity (e.g., Voller and Rossan, 1969), antigenic variation (Brown and Brown, 1965), and immunization against merozoites (Mitchell *et al.,* 1974, 1975), sporozoites (Gwadz *et al.,* 1979), and gametes (Gwadz and Green, 1978). It has lent itself to numerous studies on the invasion of the erythrocyte by merozoites (see Chapter 4, Vol. 1) and has been successfully cultivated *in vitro* using the techniques of Trager and Jensen (1976) for continuous cultivation (R. Beach, personal communication).

b. Vertebrate Hosts. *Plasmodium knowlesi* naturally infects various macaques in Malaysia and the Philippines. In the laboratory, the host of choice is the rhesus monkey, *M. mulatta.* In addition, experimental infections will develop in a number of monkey species (Coatney *et al.,* 1971). Humans may be infected naturally (Chin *et al.,* 1965) or experimentally (Chin *et al.,* 1968).

c. Mosquito Hosts. *Plasmodium knowlesi* in nature infects members of the leucosphyrus group of *Anopheles* in peninsular Malaysia. In the laboratory, only *A. balabacensis,* a member of this group, is available to support effective development of sporozoites to maturity. *Anopheles freeborni* will sustain oocyst growth in numbers comparable to simultaneously fed *A. balabacensis,* but sporozoites seldom reach the salivary glands (R. Rosenberg, personal communication). *Anopheles stephensi* will support the growth of a few oocysts, sporozoites will mature, salivary glands will be invaded, and the bite of mosquitoes will be infectious, but this mosquito is considered a relatively poor laboratory host (Hawking *et al.,* 1957).

The major reservation regarding the general use of *A. balabacensis* is the requirement for forced copulation to maintain the colony. However, recent selection in Malaysia by Cheong and his co-workers has produced a self-mating strain of *A. balabacensis* which retains its high level of susceptibility to *P. knowlesi* (R. W. Gwadz and R. Rosenberg, unpublished data).

d. Experimental Procedures. *Plasmodium knowlesi* is unique among primate malarias in that it has a quotidian cycle of maturation; asexual parasites take 24 hours to develop. Moreover, the parasite is highly synchronous, with schizogony taking place at about noon. Blood-induced infections with *P. knowlesi* in the rhesus monkey are characteristically fulminating and usually result in the death of the animal if it is not treated with chloroquine. Sporozoite infections can be equally lethal (Coatney *et al.*, 1971), but infections induced by the bites of infected mosquitoes may run a sublethal course in 30–40% of rhesus monkeys (R. W. Gwadz, unpublished observations).

The prepatent period for sporozoite-induced infections is 6–7 days; thereafter the parasitemia rises rapidly, and animals may die of an acute infection 5–6 days later.

Gametocytes begin their development with the noontime schizogony and require 36 hours to mature. Consequently, a synchronous peak of gametocyte infectivity occurs at about midnight. Hawking *et al.* (1968) clearly demonstrated the cyclic nature of gametocyte infectivity, using *A. stephensi*, a poor vector of the parasite. Studies in the Malaria Section at the National Institutes of Health at Bethesda, Maryland, have consistently demonstrated that *P. knowlesi* infects mosquitoes best at about midnight ±2 hours. *Anopheles balabacensis* mosquitoes fed at noon are seldom infected, while mosquitoes fed at midnight support 100–1000 oocysts per gut (R. W. Gwadz, personal observations). Because *P. knowlesi* shows a 10-fold rise in parasitemia as a result of each afternoon's schizogony, only three nights can be used for mosquito feedings. Gametocyte infectivity on the night of peak asexual parasitemia is usually significantly depressed or completely absent (Carter and Gwadz, 1980).

Infected monkeys must be anesthetized prior to mosquito feedings and handled as described for *P. cynomolgi* infections. *Plasmodium knowlesi* will infect equally well by feeding mosquitoes directly on an infected monkey or by feeding mosquitoes on the same blood through a membrane. Splenectomized rhesus monkeys can be used repeatedly if cured at or before the peak of parasitemia, allowed to recover 8–12 weeks, and then reinfected with the same or a heterologous strain of *P. knowlesi*.

The *P. knowlesi*–rhesus monkey–*A. balabacensis* model shares many of the advantages of the *P. cynomolgi* system, although *P. knowlesi* is not a relapsing malaria. Because *P. knowlesi* is so predictably synchronous and lethal, it has been used for a number of studies of immunization against the various stages of the malaria cycle.

The disadvantages of the system are similar to those encountered with any other monkey malaria with regard to the problems associated with monkey husbandry. In addition, the lethal nature of this parasite requires extra attention to prevent the unnecessary deaths of vital research animals. Also, the difficulties associated with the rearing of *A. balabacensis* make studies requiring sporogonic stages of the cycle somewhat more demanding.

4. Other Simian Malaria Parasites

There are a number of other simian malarias which can be transmitted by mosquitoes in the laboratory. Many have erratic or unpredictable patterns of gametocyte production, while others such as *P. coatneyi* will infect best at night (W. Collins, personal communication; R. W. Gwadz, unpublished observations). None of these malarias are used regularly for studies on the sporogonic cycle. Details of the life cycles and hosts of these malarias may be found in Garnham (1966) and Coatney *et al.* (1971).

E. Human Malarias

1. Introduction and History

Studies with parasites of laboratory animals are usually done with the hope of ultimately transferring the knowledge thus gained to studies on human parasites. Studies on these human parasites are generally difficult to carry out because of ethical, safety, and practical considerations. Nevertheless, much has been learned about the sporogonic stages of the malaria parasites of humans. Indeed, many of the fundamental observations on the sporogony of malaria were first made with human malarias.

Most of the early progress was made by observations on patients naturally infected with malaria in endemic regions. Thus, the discovery of the exflagellation of microgametocytes was made by taking blood from a soldier infected with *P. falciparum* in Algeria (Laveran, 1880). The discovery by MacCallum (1897) of fertilization of the malaria parasite was accomplished with blood from a patient infected with *P. falciparum* at the Johns Hopkins Hospital in Baltimore not long after MacCallum had first observed this phenomenon in *Haemoproteus* (MacCallum, 1897, 1898). The oocyst was first discovered by Ross (1897) in mosquitoes that had fed on a patient infected with *P. falciparum* in India, though the further elucidation of the sporogonic stages of malaria was done by Ross using an avian malaria model. Many of the careful subsequent observations on the morphology and biology of the sporogonic stages were made with parasites from naturally infected patients by Grassi (1900) and his associates in Italy, and later by Schaudinn (1903) in Germany. Thus, by the first decade of the twentieth century much of what we know of the sporogonic stages of human malaria parasites had already been worked out.

An extraordinary impetus to experimental work on malaria was provided by the discovery that many syphylitic patients suffering from general paresis could be successfully treated by infecting them with malaria (Wagner-Jauregg, 1922). As a result of this discovery, for which Wagner-Jauregg later received the Nobel prize, "malaria fever therapy" for neurosyphilis and various chronic psychoses was initiated. For the first time it became ethically possible to infect humans deliberately with a known pathogen in order to cure a more serious illness. Because these observations could be made under carefully controlled conditions on already hospitalized patients, more has been learned about the dynamics of incubation periods, prepatent periods, patterns of infection, etc., for malaria than for any other disease of humans. Infections were generally induced by the transfer of infected blood from one patient to another. However, this was objected to and eventually forbidden in Great Britain on grounds that highly neurotropic strains of syphilis could thus be transferred between patients (James and Shute, 1926). Thereafter, a system was set up at the Horton Hospital near London for transmission by sporozoites (James, 1931; James *et al.,* 1932). Subsequently a number of similar facilities were established at hospitals throughout the world. In the United States, the most prominent such research was conducted at the South Carolina State Hospital in Columbia, South Carolina, by Coatney, Young, and their associates, and at the Florida State Hospital in Tallahassee, Florida, by Boyd and his associates. Studies conducted through the mid-1940s added much to our knowledge of sporozoite transmission of human malaria. One such facility, in Rumania, is still in operation (Shute *et al.,* 1976; Ungureanu *et al.,* 1976).

When better means of antisyphilitic therapy became available during the 1940s, many of the malaria fever therapy programs were phased out. However, much of the research in the United States continued at state and federal prison facilities with prisoner volunteers who agreed to become infected with malaria. The most prominent research on sporozoite-induced malaria at such facilities was carried out at the U.S. Penitentiary in Atlanta, Georgia, by Coatney, Young, and their associates, and at the Maryland House of Correction in Jessup, Maryland, by Clyde, McCarthy and their associates (Coatney *et al.,* 1948; Clyde *et al.,* 1973). Though these studies were generally conducted with a high regard for the safety and comfort of the volunteers, a controversy developed in the 1970s over the ethics of such research in prison facilities, and all the studies were eventually terminated.

The pendulum has now swung back again. At the present time, most of the research on sporozoite transmission and on the sporogonic stages of human malarias is being conducted with naturally infected patients in endemic areas. One such research facility is operated by the British Medical Research Council at Fajara in The Gambia, West Africa. At the same time, recent progress in the *in vitro* culture of *P. falciparum* gametocytes (see Chapters 5 and 6) may someday facilitate many studies on the sporogonic stages of this parasite without any need for human subjects.

2. Plasmodium vivax

a. Introduction. The sporogonic stages of *P. vivax* (Grassi and Feletti, 1890b) were first described by the Italian malariologists Grassi *et al.* (1898) and Bastianelli and Bignami (1899). Because the parasite was the most common of the malarias used for fever therapy among paretics, a great deal has been learned about its transmission under controlled conditions.

One of the characteristics of sporozoite-induced infections with *P. vivax* is the phenomenon of delayed prepatent periods and relapse, features which are best studied under controlled experimental conditions and which require the laboratory production of sporozoites. At least 10 different strains of the parasite have been characterized (Garnham, 1966). They vary in their average prepatent periods, their patterns of relapse, and in the relative ease or difficulty of infecting mosquitoes. Strains of temperate origin, such as the St. Elizabeth (Coatney and Young, 1941) and the North Korean (Shute *et al.*, 1976) strains, tend to be associated with periodic relapses. This has been suggested to be an adaptation designed to conserve the parasite within its human host during the winter and allow efficient infections of mosquitoes during a subsequent spring or summer relapse correlated with a mosquito biting season (James, 1931; Hackett, 1937). Many strains of tropical origin, such as the Chesson strain (Ehrman *et al.*, 1945), do not show this prolonged prepatency or relapse pattern (Ungureanu *et al.*, 1976, though some tropical strains do (Coatney *et al.*, 1971).

b. Vertebrate Hosts. Humans are the natural hosts of *P. vivax,* although a number of simians have been infected under experimental conditions. Parasitemias can be induced in chimpanzees (Rodhain, 1956) and in the *Aotus* monkey (Porter and Young, 1966). Infective gametocytes can be produced in chimpanzees (Bray, 1957), and sporozoites formed in mosquitoes that feed on such chimpanzees have been used to induce therapeutic malaria in humans (Shute *et al.*, 1976). Infective gametocytes can also be produced in *Aotus* monkeys (Young *et al.*, 1966; Baerg *et al.*, 1969; Ward *et al.*, 1969; Coatney *et al.*, 1971). Chimpanzees challenged with sporozoites have been used to study exoerythrocytic schizogony of *P. vivax* (Rodhain, 1956; Bray, 1957), and *Aotus* monkeys have been found to be susceptible to challenge with *P. vivax* sporozoites (Baerg *et al.*, 1969).

c. Mosquito Hosts. At least 40 different species of *Anopheles* are known to transmit *P. vivax* (Garnham, 1966). For the most part, studies on experimental transmission have tended to utilize geographically coindigenous mosquito and plasmodial species. Thus, studies in Europe (including England) have used mostly *A. maculipennis* and *A. labranchiae atroparvus,* studies in India have used *A. stephensi,* studies in the United States have used *A. quadrimaculatus* and *A. freeborni,* and studies in Central America have used *A. albimanus.* As mentioned previously in Section II,A, different strains of these species may vary in their susceptibility to malaria. On the basis of the ease with which it may be mass produced, and its general suitability as a vector, *A. stephensi* is one of the most favorable experimental hosts for *P. vivax.*

d. Experimental Procedures. Upon the introduction of *P. vivax* parasitemia, either by sporozoites or blood transfer, gametocytes appear relatively early from the first to the fifth day of patency and usually reach their maximum density about 4–6 days after the asexual parasites have reached a peak. Densities of about 5–10/mm³ of blood are usually required for minimal infections of mosquitoes, though infections may often be obtained at gametocyte levels so low as to be nondetectable microscopically (James, 1931). Generally though, gametocyte levels approaching several hundred per cubic millimeter are required for heavy infections (Boyd, 1949). It has long been known that blacks of West African origin are relatively insusceptible to *P. vivax* infection, and recent studies have related this insusceptibility to certain inherited blood group determinants (Miller *et al.,* 1975, 1976).

Sporogony within the mosquito proceeds more rapidly for *P. vivax* than for any of the other human malaria parasites. At maintenance temperatures of 20°–21°C sporogony takes about 15–16 days, at 24°–26°C it takes about 9–11 days, and at 28°–30°C only about 7–8 days (Stratman-Thomas, 1940; Knowles and Basu, 1943; Shute and Maryon, 1952). Sporozoites are highly infectious to humans. Generally the bite of a single infected mosquito is sufficient to induce parasitemia. The intravenous or intradermal injection of as few as 10 sporozoites is ordinarily sufficient to infect (Shute *et al.,* 1976; Ungureanu *et al.,* 1976). Detailed procedures for establishing facilities for experimental vivax malaria have been described by James (1931), Boyd and Stratman-Thomas (1933a), Boyd *et al.* (1936a), Mayne and Young (1941), and Coatney *et al.* (1948).

3. *Plasmodium falciparum*

a. Introduction. Fifteen years after Laveran discovered exflagellation of the gametocytes of *P. falciparum* (Welch, 1897) *in vitro* within blood taken from a patient, Ross (1895) observed that this process took place within the midgut contents of a mosquito that had just fed on a human sick with falciparum malaria. Not long after, Ross (1897) discovered the oocyst of this species. It was left to Grassi *et al.* (1899) to work out the complete sporogonic development of the parasite and to transmit the infection successfully by mosquito bite under experimental conditions.

Plasmodium falciparum is the most pathogenic of all the human plasmodial species, and consequently there has been much interest in its biology and transmission. Because of the low susceptibility of many blacks to *P. vivax*, it was necessary to use other species of malaria, especially *P. falciparum*, in malaria fever therapy of paretics (Boyd and Kitchen, 1937). It was also considered ethical to use *P. falciparum* therapy on patients who had already had induced attacks of *P. vivax* but had not benefitted therapeutically from this (James *et al.*, 1932).

Many different experimentally transmitted strains of *P. falciparum* have been described (Garnham, 1966). These vary in such characteristics as their prepatent period, their virulence, their sensitivity to drugs, and their infectivity to various species of mosquito.

b. Vertebrate Hosts. Humans are the only natural hosts of *P. falciparum*. Simian models have been used, however, with some degree of success. Splenectomized chimpanzees have been shown to produce infective gametocytes (Bray, 1958), and chimpanzees challenged with sporozoites have been used to study EE schizogony (Bray, 1958; Bray and Gunders, 1962, 1963). Infective gametocytes can also be produced in *Aotus* monkeys (Collins *et al.*, 1968; Ward *et al.*, 1972; Hayes and Ward, 1977). Sporozoites injected into *Aotus* monkeys can complete EE development and lead to parasitemia (Collins and Aikawa, 1977).

c. Mosquito Hosts. At least 66 different anopheline vector species for *P. falciparum* have been described (Garnham, 1966). For experimental purposes the African species, *A. gambiae,* is the vector par excellence. However, for purposes of safety this species should not be introduced into any endemic region outside Africa. In such cases, the vectors of choice have been *A. stephensi* and *A. freeborni,* based on their relatively high susceptibility to *P. falciparum* strains from a wide range of geographic regions, and because of the relative ease with which they may be mass-produced in insectaries.

Many species of anophelines are efficient vectors only for geographically coindigenous strains of *P. falciparum*. Thus, the European species *A. maculipennis* was found to be an efficient vector for European strains but not for Indian or African strains of *P. falciparum* (James *et al.*, 1932). Similarly, the European mosquito *A. labranchiae atroparvus* was found to be a good vector for European strains but not for African strains of this parasite (Shute and Maryon, 1951). Three strains of *P. falciparum* originating in the southeastern United States have been shown to be easily transmitted by the coindigenous mosquito *A. quadrimaculatus* but not by the Central American species *A. albimanus*. Conversely, a Panamanian strain of *P. falciparum* was satisfactorily transmitted by *A. albimanus* but not quite so efficiently by *A. quadrimaculatus* (Garnham, 1964). Several other similar examples have been presented by Coatney *et al.* (1971). In view of this, these authors have concluded: ''The results of comparative infectivity studies are so variable between different isolates of *P. falciparum* that it is often necessary to feed a number of species on the host of a 'new' isolate in order to determine which of the species available will serve as suitable experimental vectors.''

d. Experimental Procedures. One of the most unusual characteristics of *P. falciparum* is the prolonged period of time, approximately 10 days, required for gametocyte development. The gametocytes generally develop in blood spaces within internal organs and appear in the peripheral blood about 7–12 days after the asexual parasites are first seen in a primary infection (Jeffery, 1960; Kitchen and Putnam, 1942). The gametocytes often appear in a wave at about the same time the asexual parasitemia begins to decline. After the gametocytemia has risen to a peak it may remain at a relatively high level for a period of about 3 weeks and may recur thereafter throughout the infection. Further maturation of *P. falciparum* gametocytes continues even after their release into the peripheral circulation, as indicated by the lack of infectivity of these gametocytes to mosquitoes for several days after their appearance in adequate numbers in the peripheral blood (Jeffery and Eyles, 1955).

Densities of approximately 50–100 gametocytes/mm^3 of blood are usually required for minimal infections of susceptible mosquitoes (Boyd and Kitchen, 1937; Collins, 1962; James, 1931), whereas higher gametocytemias of up to about 1000/mm^3 are often required for heavy mosquito infection (Boyd *et al.*, 1935; McCarthy and Clyde, 1973). These levels are considerably higher than what is needed for infections with *P. vivax* gametocytes.

As the above data suggest, an individual infected with *P. falciparum* may have to withstand continual parasitemia for up to 2–3 weeks before attaining a gametocyte level sufficient to infect mosquitoes. In a nonimmune patient or volunteer, the levels of parasitemia reached during this extended period can easily become life-threatening. Thus, for ethical reasons it is necessary that the subject be under the strictest medical care and observation at all times and that antimalarial drugs be administered to control the asexual parasitemia. This approach is possible in view of the fact that quinine taken by a patient to control asexual parasitemia does not prevent mosquitoes from being infected by the gametocytes (Bastianelli and Bignami, 1900). An illustration of how this may be carried out in practice is shown in Fig. 4 (from McCarthy and Clyde, 1973). As can be seen, parasitemia was periodically "cooled off" by regular doses of quinine. During this treatment, gametocytes appeared on the eighth day of parasite patency, increased in number until day 18, and then slowly decreased. Mosquito infectivity commenced at a low level on day 14, peaked on day 17, and then declined. Chloroquine treatment may be used similarly (Wilkinson *et al.*, 1976). One of the chief problems in conducting experimental work on mosquito transmission of *P. falciparum* is the difficulty of obtaining individuals with sufficient numbers of infectious gametocytes. In a study conducted by Clyde *et*

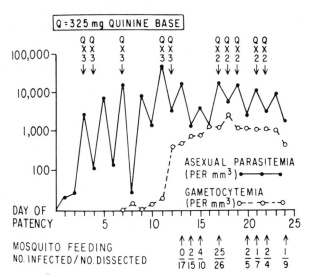

FIG. 4. Infection of *A. stephensi* mosquitoes fed at different times on a volunteer infected with *P. falciparum*. Parasitemia was controlled with repeated small doses of quinine as indicated (from McCarthy and Clyde, 1973).

al. (1973), for instance, only 6 of 33 volunteers infected with *P. falciparum* became useful as gametocyte donors. In hyperendemic areas such as Africa, much greater frequencies of gametocytes are found in young children than in adults (Bruce-Chwatt, 1951; Muirhead-Thomson, 1954; Wilson, 1936). The most practical and ethical way of infecting mosquitoes under these circumstances is to collect small quantities of blood from gametocyte bearers brought to a clinic for antimalarial therapy and to feed mosquitoes on the blood through a membrane.

After mosquitoes have ingested an infective blood meal, complete sporogony with sporozoite invasion of salivary glands takes about 11 days at 24°C, 10 days at 25°C, and 9 days at 30°C. Sporozoites are typically highly infective to humans. Clyde reported that, during the course of 7 years of work with *P. falciparum* in prison volunteers, all of 173 volunteers challenged by the bite of small numbers of infected mosquitoes developed parasitemia (Clyde *et al.*, 1973).

4. Other Human Malaria Parasites

Sporozoite transmission of *P. ovale* and *P. malariae* has been less frequently studied. During the studies on malaria fever therapy, it was found that *P. ovale* produced infections that were less severe and less therapeutic than other malarias. Consequently, relatively little work was done with this species. Procedures for infecting mosquitoes with *P. ovale* have been reviewed by Coatney *et al.* (1971).

Plasmodium malariae has always been much more difficult to transmit via mosquitoes than any of the other species, and no consistently good laboratory vector has ever been found. The parasite usually produces few gametocytes which tend to develop relatively late in the infection and, even when high gametocytemias are obtained, infection of mosquitoes has proved to be difficult. Sporogonic development within mosquitoes takes significantly longer than is the case with the other species. Consequently, the degree of mosquito survival may be quite low by the time infective sporozoites can be found within the salivary glands. The most successful cyclic transmission system for *P. malariae* has been reported by Ciucă *et al.* (1964) in Rumania. These workers used the VS strain of the parasite and the vector *A. labranchiae atroparvus* which fed on patients in psychiatric wards. These relatively good results were confirmed by Garnham (1966).

XI. CONCLUSIONS

In this brief review we have discussed a wide range of animal models available for laboratory studies requiring mosquito transmission of plasmodia. From these models an investigator should be able to select one that fits the experimental design and remains within certain limits of space, cost and availability of animal and insect husbandry.

The importance of the mosquito cycle in malaria has been but should not be minimized by the researcher. Sporozoite-induced infections differ markedly from infections induced by the injection of infected blood. Pre-patent periods, course and intensity of parasitemia, gametocyte production, immune responses and pathology all depend on the initial mode of infection. Total reliance on syringe passed parasites may give misleading results and bear little relationship to mosquito borne infections. Only mosquito-produced sporozoites can initiate an infection comparable to those experienced in nature.

REFERENCES

Adler, S., and Tchernomoretz, I. (1941). Continued passage of extraerythrocytic form of *Plasmodium gallinaceum* in the absence of erythrocytic schizogony. *Ann. Trop. Med. Parasitol.* **35**, 241–246.

Baerg, D. C., Porter, J. A., and Young, M. D. (1969). Sporozoite transmission of *Plasmodium vivax* to Panamanian primates. *Am. J. Trop. Med. Hyg.* **18**, 346–350.

Bafort, J. (1968). The effects of low temperature preservation on the viability of the sporozoites of *Plasmodium berghei*. *Ann. Trop. Med. Parasitol.* **62**, 301–304.

Bafort, J. (1969). Etude du cycle biologique du *Plasmodium v. vinckei*. *Ann. Soc. Belge Med. Trop.* **49**, 533-628.

Bafort, J. (1971). The biology of rodent malaria with particular reference to *P. vinckei*. *Ann. Soc. Belge Med. Trop.* **51**, 1-204.

Bafort, J., Vincke, I. H., and Timperman, G. (1965). Gametocytogenesis of *Plasmodium vinckei*. *Nature (London)* **208**, 1230-1231.

Ball, G. H., and Chao, J. (1960). *In vitro* development of the mosquito phase of *Plasmodium relictum*. *Exp. Parasitol.* **9**, 47-55.

Bano, L. (1958). Partial inhibitory effect of *Plistophora culicis* on the sporogonic cycle of *Plasmodium cynomolgi* in *Anopheles stephensi*. *Nature (London)* **181**, 430.

Barzilai-Vivaldi, G., and Kauders, O. (1924). Die Impf-Malaria-experimentall durch Anophelen nicht übertragbar. *Wien. Klin. Wochenschr.* **37**, 1055-1057.

Bastianelli, G., and Bignami, A. (1899). Sullo svillupo dei parassiti della terzona nell *Anopheles claviger*. *Atti Soc. Studi Malar.* **1**, 28-49.

Bastianelli, G., and Bignami, A. (1900). Malaria and mosquitoes. *Lancet* **1**, 79-83.

Basu, B. C. (1939). Studies on the biology of the malaria parasite, *Plasmodium falciparum*. *J. Malar. Inst. India* **2**, 155-157.

Beaudoin, R. L., Strome, C. P. A., Mitchell, F., and Tubergen, T. A. (1977). *Plasmodium berghei*: Immunization of mice against the ANKA strain using the unaltered sporozoite as an antigen. *Exp. Parasitol.* **42**, 1-5.

Bennett, G. F., Warren, M., and Cheong, W. H. (1966). Biology of the simian malarias of Southeast Asia. II. The susceptibility of some Malaysian mosquitoes to infection with five strains of *Plasmodium cynomolgi*. *J. Parasitol.* **52**, 625-631.

Bignami, A., and Bastianelli, G. (1890). Observations on aestivo-autumnal malarial fevers. (Cited by Marchiafava and Bignami, 1894.)

Bishop, A. (1943). Variation in gametocyte production in a strain of *Plasmodium relictum* in canaries. *Parasitology* **35**, 82-87.

Bishop, A. (1955). Problems concerned with gametogenesis in Haemosporidiidea with particular reference to the genus *Plasmodium*. *Parasitology* **45**, 163-185.

Bishop, A., and Gilchrist, B. M. (1946). Experiments upon the feeding of *Aedes aegypti* through animal membranes with a view to applying this method to the chemotherapy of malaria. *Parasitology* **37**, 85-100.

Bishop, A., and McConnachie, E. W. (1956). A study of the factors affecting the emergence of the gametocytes of *Plasmodium gallinaceum* from the erythrocytes and the exflagellation of the male gametocytes. *Parasitology* **46**, 192-215.

Bishop, A., and McConnachie, E. W. (1960). Further observations on the *in vitro* development of the gametocytes of *Plasmodium gallinaceum*. *Parasitology* **50**, 431-448.

Bishop, A., Tate, P., and Thorpe, M. (1938). The duration of *Plasmodium relictum* infection in canaries. *Parasitology* **30**, 388-391.

Blacklock, D. B., and Wilson, C. (1942). Appartus for the collection of mosquitoes in ships, with notes on methods of salivary gland dissection. *Ann. Trop. Med. Parasitol.* **36**, 53-62.

Bosworth, A. B., Schneider, I., and Freier, J. E. (1975). Mass isolation of *Anopheles stephensi* salivary glands infected with malarial sporozoites. *J. Parasitol.* **61**, 769-772.

Box, E. D., Celaya, B. L., and Gingrich, W. (1953). Development of *Plasmodium berghei* in *Anopheles quadrimaculatus*. *Am. J. Trop. Med. Hyg.* **2**, 624-627.

Boyd, G. (1925). The influence of certain experimental factors upon the course of infections with *Plasmodium praecox*. *Am. J. Hyg.* **5**, 818-838.

Boyd, M. F. (1940). The influence of sporozoite dosage in vivax malaria. *Am. J. Trop. Med.* **20**, 279-286.

Boyd, M. F. (1942). On the varying infectiousness of different patients infected with vivax malaria. *Am. J. Trop. Med.* **22**, 73-81.

Boyd, M. F. (1949). "Malariology," 2 vols. Saunders, Philadelphia, Pennsylvania.

Boyd, M. F., and Kitchen, S. F. (1937). On the infectiousness of patients infected with *Plasmodium vivax* and *Plasmodium falciparum*. *Am. J. Trop. Med.* **17**, 253–262.

Boyd, M. F., and Russell, J. C. (1943). Preliminary observations on the inheritance of susceptibility to malaria infection as a character of *Anopheles quadrimaculatus*. *Am. J. Trop. Med.* **23**, 451–457.

Boyd, M. F., and Stratman-Thomas, W. (1933a). A controlled technique for the employment of naturally induced malaria in the therapy of paresis. *Am. J. Hyg.* **17**, 37–54.

Boyd, M. F., and Stratman-Thomas, W. (1933b). Studies on benign tertian malaria. II. The clinical characteristics of the disease in relation to the dosage of sporozoites. *Am. J. Hyg.* **17**, 666–685.

Boyd, M. F., Stratman-Thomas, W. K., and Kitchen, S. F. (1935). On the relative susceptibility of *Anopheles quadrimaculatus* to *Plasmodium vivax* and *Plasmodium falciparum*. *Am. J. Trop. Med.* **15**, 485–493.

Boyd, M. F., Stratman-Thomas, W. K., and Kitchen, S. F. (1936a). Modifications in a technqiue for the employment of naturally induced malaria in the therapy of paresis. *Am. J. Trop. Med.* **16**, 323–329.

Boyd, M. F., Stratman-Thomas, W. K., and Muench, H. (1936b). The occurrence of gametocytes of *Plasmodium vivax* during the primary attack. *Am. J. Trop. Med.* **16**, 133–138.

Boyd, M. F., Christophers, R., and Coggeshall, L. T. (1949). Laboratory diagnosis of malaria infections. *In* "Malariology" (M. F. Boyd, ed.), Vol. 1, pp. 155–204. Saunders, Philadelphia, Pennsylvania.

Brackett, S., and Hughes, C. O. (1945). Chilling as a means of retaining the viability of the sporozoites of *Plasmodium gallinaceum*. *J. Parasitol.* **31**, 288–289.

Bray, R. S. (1954). The mosquito transmission of *Plasmodium berghei*. *Indian J. Malariol.* **8**, 263–274.

Bray, R. S. (1957). Studies on malaria in chimpanzees. II. *Plasmodium vivax*. *Am. J. Trop. Med. Hyg.* **6**, 514–520.

Bray, R. S. (1958). Studies on malaria in chimpanzees. VI. *Laverania falciparum*. *Am. J. Trop. Med. Hyg.* **7**, 20–24.

Bray, R. S., and Garnham, P. C. C. (1962). The Giemsa-colophonium method for staining protozoa in tissue sections. *Indian J. Malariol.* **16**, 153–155.

Bray, R. S., and Gunders, A. E. (1962). Studies on malaria in chimpanzees. IX. The distribution of the pre-erythrocytic forms of *Laverania falcipara*. *Am. J. Trop. Med. Hyg.* **11**, 437–439.

Bray, R. S., and Gunders, A. E. (1963). Studies on malaria in chimpanzees. XI. The early forms of the pre-erythrocytic phase of *Laverania falcipara*. *Am. J. Trop. Med. Hyg.* **12**, 13–18.

Bray, R. S., and Williamson, J. (1953). The development of the pre-erythrocytic cycle of *Plasmodium cynomolgi* in normal and glycogen-depleted monkey livers. *Trans. R. Soc. Trop. Med. Hyg.* **47**, 263–264.

Bray, R. S., McCrae, A. W. R., and Smalley, M. E. (1976). Lack of circadian rhythm in the ability of the gametocytes of *Plasmodium falciparum* to infect *Anopheles gambiae*. *Int. J. Parasitol.* **6**, 399–401.

Brown, K. N., and Brown, I. N. (1965). Immunity to malaria: Antigenic variations in chronic infections of *Plasmodium knowlesi*. *Nature (London)* **208**, 1286–1288.

Bruce-Chwatt, L. J. (1951). Malaria in Nigeria. *Bull. W.H.O.* **4**, 301–327.

Bruce-Chwatt, L. J. (1978). Introduction. *In* "Rodent Malaria" (R. Killick-Kendrick and W. Peters, eds.), pp. xi–xxv. Academic Press, New York.

Brumpt, E. (1935). Paludisme aviaire: *Plasmodium gallinaceum* n.sp. de la poule domestique. *C. R. Hebd. Seances Acad. Sci.* **200**, 783–786.

Brumpt, E. (1949). The human parasites of the genus *Plasmodium*. *In* "Malariology" (M. Boyd, ed.), Vol. 1, pp. 65–121. Saunders, Philadelphia, Pennsylvania.

Burgess, R. W. (1960). Comparative susceptibility of *Anopheles gambiae* and *Anopheles melas* to infection by *Plasmodium falciparum* in Liberia, West Africa. *Am. J. Trop. Med. Hyg.* **9,** 652–655.

Cantrell, W., and Jordan, H. B. (1946). Changes in the infectiousness of gametocytes during the course of *Plasmodium gallinaceum* infections. *J. Infect. Dis.* **78,** 153–159.

Carter, R., and Chen, D. H. (1976). Malaria transmission blocked by immunization with gametes of the malaria parasite. *Nature (London)* **263,** 57–58.

Carter, R., and Diggs, C. (1977). Plasmodia of rodents. *In* "Parasitic Protozoa" (J. P. Kreier, ed.), Vol. 3, pp. 359–465. Academic Press, New York.

Carter, R., and Miller, L. H. (1979). Evidence for environmental modulation of gametocytogenesis in *Plasmodium falciparum* in continuous culture. *Bull. W.H.O.* **57**(Suppl. 1), 37–52.

Carter, R., and Nijhout, M. M. (1977). Control of gamete formation (exflagellation) in malaria parasites. *Science* **195,** 407–409.

Carter, R., and Walliker, D. (1975). New observations on the malaria parasites of rodents of the Central African Republic—*Plasmodium vinckei petteri* subsp. nov. and *Plasmodium chabaudi* Landau, 1965. *Ann. Trop. Med. Parasitol.* **69,** 187–196.

Carter, R., Gwadz, R. W., and McAuliffe, F. M. (1979a). *Plasmodium gallinaceum:* Transmission-blocking immunity in chickens. I. Comparative immunogencity of gametocyte- and gamete-containing preparations. *Exp. Parasitol.* **47,** 185–193.

Carter, R., Gwadz, R. W., and Green, I. (1979b). *Plasmodium gallinaceum:* Transmission-blocking immunity in chickens. II. The effect of antigamete antibodies *in vitro* and *in vivo* and their elaboration during infection. *Exp. Parasitol.* **47,** 194–208.

Celaya, B. L., Box, E. D., and Gingrich, W. D. (1956). Infectivity of *Plasmodium berghei* for *Anopheles quadrimaculatus* and other mosquitoes. *Am. J. Trop. Med. Hyg.* **5,** 168–182.

Chen, D. H., and Schneider, I. (1969). Mass isolation of malaria sporozoites from mosquitoes by density gradient centrifugation. *Proc. Soc. Exp. Biol. Med.* **130,** 1318–1321.

Chin, W., Contacos, P. G., Coatney, G. R., and Kimball, H. R. (1965). A naturally acquired quotidian-type malaria in man transferable to monkeys. *Science* **149,** 865.

Chin, W., Contacos, P. G., Collins, W. E., Jeter, M. H., and Alpert, E. (1968). Experimental mosquito-transmission of *Plasmodium knowlesi* to man and monkey. *Am. J. Trop. Med. Hyg.* **17,** 355–358.

Christophers, S. R. (1924). The mechanism of immunity against malaria in communities living under hyperendemic conditions. *Indian J. Med. Res.* **12,** 273–294.

Christophers, S. R. (1960). *Aedes aegypti.* The Yellow Fever Mosquito. Its Life History, Bionomics and Structure." Cambridge Univ. Press, London and New York.

Ciucă, M., Lupaşcu, G., Negulici, E., and Constantinescu, P. (1964). Recherches sur la transmission expérimentale de *P. malariae* à l'homme. *Arch. Roum. Pathol. Exp. Microbiol.* **23,** 763–776.

Clements, A. N. (1963). "The Physiology of Mosquitoes." Pergamon, Oxford.

Clyde, D., Most, H., McCarthy, V., and Vanderberg, J. (1973). Immunization of man against sporozoite-induced falciparum malaria. *Am. J. Med. Sci.* **266,** 169–177.

Coatney, G. R., and Young, M. D. (1941). The taxonomy of the human malaria parasites with notes on the principal American strains. *In* "Human Malaria," Publ. No. 15, pp. 19–24. Am. Assoc. Adv. Sci., Washington, D.C.

Coatney, G. R., Cooper, W. C., and Miles, V. I. (1945a). Studies on *Plasmodium gallinaceum.* I. The incidence and course of the infection in young chicks resulting from single mosquito bites. *Am. J. Hyg.* **41,** 109–118.

Coatney, G. R., Cooper, W. C., and Trembley, H. L. (1945b). Studies on *Plasmodium gallinaceum*. II. The incidence and course of the infection in young chicks following the inoculation of infected salivary glands. *Am. J. Hyg.* **41,** 119-122.

Coatney, G. R., Cooper, W. C., and Trembley, H. L. (1945c). Studies on *Plasmodium gallinaceum*. III. The incidence and course of the infection in young chicks following the subcutaneous inoculation of pooled sporozoites. *Am. J. Hyg.* **42,** 323-329.

Coatney, G. R., Cooper, W. C., and Ruhe, D. S. (1948). Studies in human malaria. VI. The organization of a program for testing potential antimalarial drugs in prisoner volunteers. *Am. J. Hyg.* **47,** 113-119.

Coatney, G. R., Collins, W. E., Warren, M., and Contacos, G. (1971). "The Primate Malarias." U. S. Dept. of Health, Education, and Welfare, Washington, D. C.

Coggeshall, L. T. (1938). *Plasmodium lophurae,* a new species of malaria parasite pathogenic for the domestic fowl. *Am. J. Hyg.* **27,** 615-618.

Collins, W. E. (1962). Comparative infectivity of *Plasmodium falciparum* (Colombia strain) to *Anopheles quadrimaculatus* and *Anopheles albimanus. Mosq. News* **22,** 257-259.

Collins, W. E., and Aikawa, M. (1977). Plasmodia of nonhuman primates. *In* "Parasitic Protozoa" (J. Kreier, ed.), Vol. 3, pp. 467-492. Academic Press, New York.

Collins, W. E., Contacos, P. G., Gunn., E. G., Jeter, M. H., and Sodeman, T. M. (1968). Monkey to man transmission of *Plasmodium falciparum* by *Anopheles freeborni* mosquitoes. *J. Parasitol.* **54,** 1166-1170.

Collins, W. E., Warren, M., Skinner, J. C., Richardson, B. B., and Kearse, T. S. (1977). Infectivity of the Santa Lucia (El Salvador) strain of *Plasmodium falciparum* to different anophelines. *J. Parasitol.* **63,** 57-61.

Collins, W. E., Warren, M., Skinner, J. C., Richardson, B. B., and Kearse, T. S. (1979). Effect of sequential infections with *Plasmodium vivax* and *P. falciparum* in the *Aotus trivirgatus* monkey. *J. Parasitol.* **65,** 605-608.

Covell, G. (1960). Relationship between malarial parasitaemia and symptoms of the disease. *Bull. W.H.O.* **22,** 605-619.

Craig, G. B., Jr., and Hickey, W. A. (1967). Genetics of *Aedes aegypti. In* "Genetics of Insect Vectors of Diseases" (J. W. Wright and R. Pal, eds.), pp. 67-131. Elsevier, Amsterdam.

Craige, B., Jr., Alving, A., Jones, R., Jr., Whorton, C., Pullman, T., and Eichelberger, L. (1946). The Chesson strain of *Plasmodium vivax* malaria. II. Relationship between prepatent period, latent period, and relapse rate. *J. Infect. Dis.* **80,** 228-236.

Crandall, M. (1977). Mating-type interactions in micro-organisms. *In* "Receptors and Recognition" (P. Cuatrecasas and M. F. Greaves, eds.), Ser. A Vol. 3, pp. 45-100. Wiley, New York.

Cuboni, E. (1926). Gametenfreie *Plasmodium vivax*-Stämme. *Wein. Klin. Wochenschr.* **39,** 1475-1476.

Curd, F. H. S. (1943). The activity of drugs in the malaria of man, monkeys and birds. *Ann. Trop. Med. Parasitol.* **37,** 115-143.

Danilewsky, B. (1885). Zur Lehre von der Malaria-infection bei Menschen und Vögeln. *Arch. Hyg.* **25,** 227.

Darling, S. T. (1910). Factors in the transmission and prevention of malaria in the Panama Canal Zone. *Ann. Trop. Med. Parasitol.* **4,** 179-223.

Davey, D. G. (1946). The use of avian malaria for the discovery of drugs effective in the treatment and prevention of human malaria. II. Drugs for causal prophylaxis and radical care or the chemotherapy of exoerythrocytic forms. *Ann. Trop. Med. Parasitol.* **40,** 453-471.

De Arruda-Mayr, M., Cochrane, A. H., and Nussenzweig, R. S. (1979). Enhancement of a simian malarial infection (*Plasmodium cynomolgi*) in mosquitoes fed on rhesus (*Macaca mulatta*) previously infected with an unrelated malaria (*Plasmodium knowlesi*). *Am. J. Trop. Med. Hyg.* **28,** 627-633.

Dunn, M. A., Quinn, T. C., and Terwedow, H. A. (1972). Pre-erythrocytic rodent malaria, *Plasmodium berghei*—Prevention of development in the ethionine fatty liver. *Am. J. Trop. Med. Hyg.* **21**, 288–292.

Ehrman, F. C., Ellis, J. M., and Young, M. D. (1945). *Plasmodium vivax* Chesson strain. *Science* **101**, 377.

Eyles, D. E. (1951). Studies on *Plasmodium gallinaceum*. I. Characteristics of the infection in the mosquito, *Aedes aegypti*. *Am. J. Trop. Med. Hyg.* **54**, 101–112.

Eyles, D. E. (1952a). Studies on *Plasmodium gallinaceum*. II. Factors in the blood of the vertebrate host influencing mosquito infection. *Am. J. Trop. Med. Hyg.* **55**, 276–290.

Eyles, D. E. (1952b). Studies on *Plasmodium gallinaceum*. III. Factors associated with the malaria infection in the vertebrate host which influence the degree of infection in the mosquito. *Am. J. Trop. Med. Hyg.* **55**, 386–391.

Eyles, D. E., Coatney, G. R., and Getz, M. E. (1960). Vivax-type parasite of macaques transmissible to man. *Science* **132**, 1812–1813.

Findlay, G. M., Maegraith, B. G., Markson, J. L., and Holden, J. R. (1946). Investigations in the chemotherapy of malaria in West Africa. V. Sulphonamide compounds. *Ann. Trop. Med. Parasitol.* **40**, 358–367.

Fink, E. (1968). Experimentelle infecktion von Kanarien mit *Plasmodium cathemerium* durch den Stitch infizierter Mücken *(Culex pipiens)* und durch Inokulation isolierter Sporozoiten. *Z. Parasitenkd.* **31**, 232–253.

Fink, E. (1970). Die quantitative Bestimmung der Wirkung exogener und endogener Faktoren auf Sporozoiten und Gewebsformen der Kleintiermalaria. *Tropenmed. Parasitol.* **21**, 357–372.

Fink, E., and Schicha, E. (1969). Influence of synthetic insect T. C. medium on the survival of malaria sporozoites *in vitro*. *(Plasmodium berghei yoelii* and *P. cathemerium.) Z. Parasitenkd.* **32**, 93–94.

Flax, M., and Himes, M. (1952). Microspectrophotometric analysis of metachromatic staining of nucleic acids. *Physiol. Zool.* **25**, 297–311.

Freyvogel, T. A. (1966). Shape, movement *in situ* and locomotion of plasmodial ookinetes. *Acta Trop.* **23**, 201–222.

Galun, R., Avi-Dor, Y., and Bar-Zeev, M. (1963). Feeding response in *Aedes aegypti* stimulated by adenosine triphosphate. *Science* **142**, 1674–1675.

Gambrell, W. E. (1937). Variations in gametocyte production in avian malaria. *Am. J. Trop. Med.* **17**, 689–726.

Garnham, P. C. C. (1931). Observations on *Plasmodium falciparum* with special reference to the production of crescents. *Kenya East Afr. Med. J.* **8**, 2–21.

Garnham, P. C. C. (1956). Microsporidia in laboratory colonies of *Anopheles*. *Bull. W.H.O.* **15**, 845–847.

Garnham, P. C. C. (1964). The structure of the early sporogonic stages of *Plasmodium berghei*. *In* "International Colloquium on *Plasmodium berghei*" (J. Jadin, ed.), pp. 15–21. Inst. Méd. Trop. Prince Léopold, Antwerp.

Garnham, P. C. C. (1966). "Malaria Parasites and Other Haemosporidia." Blackwell, Oxford.

Garnham, P. C. C. (1967). Relapses and latency in malaria. *Protozoology* **2**, 55–64.

Garnham, P. C. C., and Powers, K. G. (1974). Periodicity of infectivity of plasmodial gametocytes: The "Hawking phenomenon." *Int. J. Parasitol.* **4**, 103–106.

Gerberg, E. J., Richard, L. T., and Poole, J. B. (1966). Standardized feeding of *Aedes aegypti* (L.) mosquitoes on *Plasmodium gallinaceum* Brumpt-infected chicks for mass screening of antimalarial drugs. *Mosq. News* **26**, 359–363.

Giovannola, A. (1938). II *Plasmodium gallinaceum* Brumpt, 1935: I cositti corpi *Toxoplasma*—Simili el alcune inclusioni di probabile natura parassitaria ni globuli bianchi del *Gallus gallus*. *Riv. Parassitol.* **2**, 129–142.

Gordon, R. M., and Lumsden, W. H. R. (1939). A study of the behavior of the mouthparts of mosquitoes when taking up blood from living tissue, together with some observations on the ingestion of microfilariae. *Ann. Trop. Med. Parasitol.* **33,** 259–278.

Grassi, B. (1900). Studi di uno zoologo sulla malaria. *Atti R. Accad. Naz. Lincei, Mem. Cl. Sci. Fis., Mat. Nat.* **3,** 299–505.

Grassi, B., Bastianelli, G., and Bignami, A. (1898). Ulteriori recerche sul ciclo dei parassiti malarici umani sul corpo del zanzarone. *Atti Accad. Naz. Lincei, Cl. Sci. Fis., Mat. Nat., Rend.* **8,** 21–28.

Grassi, B., Bignami, A., and Bastianelli, G. (1899). Ciclo evolution delle semilone nell' *Anopheles claviger. Atti Soc. Studi Malar.* **1,** 14–27.

Grassi, R., and Feletti, B. (1890a). Parasites malariques chez les oiseaux. *Boll. Mens. Accad. Gioenia Sci. Nat. Catania* **13,** 297–300.

Grassi, R., and Feletti, B. (1890b). Parassiti malarici negli uccelli: Nota preliminarie. *Boll. Mens. Accad. Gioenia Sci. Nat. Catania* **13,** 3–6.

Grassi, R., and Feletti, B. (1891). Nuova contribuzione allo studi della malaria. *Boll. Mens. Accad. Gioenia Sci. Nat. Catenia* **16,** 16–20.

Grassi, R., and Feletti, B. (1892). Contribuzione allo studio dei parassiti malarici. *Atti Accad. Gioenia Sci. Nat. Catania* [4] **5,** 1–80.

Greenberg, J., Trembley, H. L., and Coatney, G. R. (1950). Effects of drugs on *Plasmodium gallinaceum* infections produced by decreasing concentrations of a sporozoite inoculum. *Am. J. Hyg.* **51,** 194–199.

Gregory, K. G., and Peters, W. (1970). The chemotherapy of rodent malaria. IX. Causal prophylaxis. Part 1: A method for demonstrating drug action on exoerythrocytic stages. *Ann. Trop. Med. Parasitol.* **64,** 15–24.

Griffiths, R. B., and Gordon, R. M. (1952). An apparatus which enables the process of feeding by mosquitoes to be observed in the tissues of a live rodent, together with an account of the ejection of saliva and its significance in malaria. *Ann. Trop. Med. Parasitol.* **46,** 311–319.

Gwadz, R. W. (1976). Malaria: Successful immunization against the sexual stages of *Plasmodium gallinaceum. Science* **193,** 1150–1151.

Gwadz, R. W., and Green, I. (1978). Malaria immunization in rhesus monkeys: A vaccine effective against both the sexual and asexual stages of *Plasmodium knowlesi. J. Exp. Med.* **148,** 1311–1323.

Gwadz, R. W., Cochrane, A. H., Nussenzweig, V., and Nussenzweig, R. S. (1979). Preliminary studies on vaccination of rhesus monkeys with irradiated sporozoites of *Plasmodium knowlesi* and characterization of surface antigens of these parasites. *Bull. W.H.O.* **57**(Suppl. 1), 165–173.

Hackett, L. W. (1937). "Malaria in Europe: An Ecological Study." Oxford Univ. Press, London and New York.

Hartman, E. (1927). Three species of bird malaria, *Plasmodium praecox, P. cathemerium* n.sp., and *P. inconstans* n.sp. *Arch. Protistenkd.* **60,** 1–18.

Hawking, F. (1946). Growth of protozoa in tissue culture. II. *Plasmodium relictum,* exoerythrocytic forms. *Trans. R. Soc. Trop. Med. Hyg.* **40,** 183–188.

Hawking, F. (1972). Unsuccessful attempts to stimulate the production of gametocytes in *Plasmodium berghei. Trans. R. Soc. Trop. Med. Hyg.* **66,** 513–514.

Hawking, F. (1975). Circadian and other rhythms of parasites. *Adv. Parasitol.* **13,** 123–182.

Hawking, F., and Gammage, K. (1970). The timing of the asexual cycles of *Plasmodium lophurae* and of *P. cathemerium. J. Parasitol.* **56,** 17–26.

Hawking, F., Mellanby, H., Terry, R. J., and Winfrith, A. F. (1957). Transmission of *Plasmodium knowlesi* by *Anopheles stephensi. Trans. R. Soc. Trop. Med. Hyg.* **51,** 397–402.

Hawking, F., Worms, M. J., and Gammage, K. (1968). 24 and 48 hour cycles of malaria parasites in the blood: Their purpose, production and control. *Trans. R. Soc. Trop. Med. Hyg.* **62,** 731–760.

Hawking, F., Wilson, M. D., and Gammage, K. (1971). Evidence for cyclic development and short-lived maturity in the gametocytes of *Plasmodium falciparum*. *Trans. R. Soc. Trop. Med. Hyg.* **65**, 549–559.

Hayes, D. E., and Ward, R. A. (1977). Sporozoite transmission of falciparum malaria (Burma-Thau. strain) from man to *Aotus* monkey. *Am. J. Trop. Med. Hyg.* **26**, 184–185.

Hegner, R., and Manwell, R. (1927). The effects of Plasmochin on bird malaria. *Am. J. Trop. Med.* **7**, 279–285.

Herman, C. M., Reeves, W. C., McClure, H. E., French, E. M., Hannam, W., Herrold, R. C., Rosen, L., and Brookman, B. (1954). Studies on avian malaria in vectors and hosts of encephalitis in Kern County, California. *Am. J. Trop. Med. Hyg.* **3**, 704–708.

Hewitt, R. (1940). "Bird Malaria," *Am. J. Hyg.* Monogr. Ser. No. 15. Johns Hopkins Press, Baltimore, Maryland.

Huff, C. G. (1927). Studies on the infectivity of plasmodia of birds for mosquitoes with special reference to the problem of immunity in the mosquito. *Am. J. Hyg.* **7**, 706–734.

Huff, C. G. (1929). The effects of selection upon susceptibility to bird malaria in *Culex pipiens* L. *Ann. Trop. Med. Parasitol.* **23**, 427–442.

Huff, C. G. (1930). Individual immunity and susceptibility of *Culex pipiens* to various species of bird malaria as studied by means of double infectious feeding. *Am. J. Hyg.* **12**, 425–441.

Huff, C. G. (1931). The inheritance of natural immunity to *Plasmodium cathemerium* in two species of *Culex*. *J. Prev. Med.* **5**, 249–259.

Huff, C. G. (1934). Comparative studies on susceptible and insusceptible *Culex pipiens* in relation to infection with *Plasmodium cathemerium* and *P. relictum*. *Am. J. Hyg.* **19**, 123–147.

Huff, C. G. (1935). Natural immunity and susceptibility of culicine mosquitoes to avian malaria. *Am. J. Trop. Med.* **15**, 427–434.

Huff, C. G. (1965). Susceptibility of mosquitoes to avian malaria. *Exp. Parasitol.* **16**, 107–132.

Huff, C. G., and Coulston, F. (1944). The development of *Plasmodium gallinaceum* from sporozoite to erythrocytic trophozoite. *J. Infect. Dis.* **75**, 231–249.

Huff, C. G., and Gambrell, E. (1934). Strains of *Plasmodium cathemerium* with and without gametocytes. *Am. J. Hyg.* **19**, 404–415.

Huff, C. G., and Marchbank, D. F. (1955). Changes in infectiousness of malarial gametocytes. I. Patterns of oocyst production in seven host-parasite combinations. *Exp. Parasitol.* **4**, 256–270.

Huff, C. G., Marchbank, D. F., and Shiroishi, T. (1958). Changes in infectiousness of malarial gametocytes. II. Analysis of the possible causative factors. *Exp. Parasitol.* **7**, 399–417.

Hulls, R. H. (1971). The adverse effects of a microsporidian on sporogony and infectivity of *Plasmodium berghei*. *Trans. R. Soc. Trop. Med. Hyg.* **65**, 421–422.

Hunter, G. W., Weller, T. H., and Jahnes, W. G. (1946). An outline for teaching mosquito stomach and salivary gland dissection. *Am. J. Trop. Med.* **26**, 221–228.

Jadin, J., Yoeli, M., and Pierreux, G. (1959). Réapparition du processus d'extraflagellation chez une souche de *Plasmodium berghei* régulièrement entretenue par passage mécanique. *Ann. Soc. Belge Med. Trop.* **39**, 847–850.

Jahiel, R. I., Nussenzweig, R. S., Vanderberg, J. P., and Vilček, J. (1968). Antimalarial effect of interferon inducers at different stages of development of *Plasmodium berghei* in the mouse. *Nature (London)* **220**, 710–711.

James, S. P. (1931). Some general results of a study of induced malaria in England. *Trans. R. Soc. Trop. Med. Hyg.* **24**, 477–538.

James, S. P. (1934). The Shute method of making preparations of exflagellating gametocytes and ookinetes of malarial parasites. *Trans. R. Soc. Trop. Med. Hyg.* **28**, 104–105.

James, S. P., and Shute, P. G. (1926). "Report on the First Results of Laboratory Work on Malaria in England." Malaria Commission of the League of Nations Health Organization, Geneva.

James, S. P., and Tate, P. (1937). New knowledge of the life cycle of malaria parasites. *Nature (London)* **139**, 545.

James, S. P., Nicol, W. D., and Shute, P. G. (1932). A study of induced malignant tertian malaria. *Proc. R. Soc. Med.* **25**, 1153–1186.

James, S. P. Nicol, W. D., and Shute, P. G. (1936). Clinical and parasitological observations on induced malaria (with notes on their application to the study of malaria epidemics). *Proc. R. Soc. Med.* **29**, 879–894.

Jeffery, G. M. (1960). Infectivity to mosquitoes of *Plasmodium vivax* and *Plasmodium falciparum* under various conditions. *Am. J. Trop. Med. Hyg.* **9**, 315–320.

Jeffery, G. M., and Eyles, D. E. (1955). Infectivity to mosquitoes of *Plasmodium falciparum* as related to gametocyte density and duration of infection. *Am. J. Trop. Med. Hyg.* **4**, 781–789.

Jeffery, G. M., and Rendtorff, R. C. (1955). Preservation of viable human malaria sporozoites by low-temperature freezing. *Exp. Parasitol.* **4**, 445–454.

Jeffery, G. M., Young, M. D., and Eyles, D. E. (1956). The treatment of *Plasmodium falciparum* infection with chloroquine with a note on infectivity to mosquitoes in primaquine and pyrimethamine-treated cases. *Am. J. Hyg.* **64**, 1–11.

Kilama, W. L., and Craig, G. B., Jr. (1969). Monofactorial inheritance of susceptibility to *Plasmodium gallinaceum* in *Aedes aegypti*. *Ann. Trop. Med. Parasitol.* **63**, 419–432.

Killick-Kendrick, R. (1971). The collection of strains of murine malaria parasites in the field and their maintenace in the laboratory by cyclical passage. *Symp. Br. Soc. Parasitol.* **9**, 39–64.

Killick-Kendrick, R. (1978). Taxonomy, zoogeography and evolution. *In* "Rodent Malaria" (R. Killick-Kendrick and W. Peters, eds.), pp. 1–52. Academic Press, New York.

Killick-Kendrick, R., and Warren, M. (1968). Primary exoerythrocytic schizonts of a mammalian *Plasmodium* as a source of gametocytes. *Nature (London)* **220**, 191–192.

Kitchen, S. F., and Putnam, P. (1942). Observations on the mechanism of the parasite cycle in falciparum malaria. *Am. J. Trop. Med.* **22**, 361–386.

Knowles, R., and Basu, B. C. (1943). Laboratory studies on the infectivity of *Anopheles stephensi*. *J. Malar. Inst. India* **5**, 1–29.

Knowles, R., and Das Gupta, B. M. (1932). A study of monkey-malaria and its experimental transmission to man. *Indian Med. Gaz.* **67**, 301–320.

Koch, R. (1898). Berichte über die Ergebnisse der Forschungen in Deutsch Ost Africa. *Arb. Gesundheits amte, Berlin* **14**, 292–308.

Koch, R. (1899). Über die Entwickelung der Malariaparasiten. *Z. Hyg. Infektionskr.* **32**, 1–24.

Korteweg, P. C. (1930). Zur Frage des Gametengehaltes bei verschiendenen Plasmodien stämmen und ihres Rückganges bei mehreren Menschenpassagen. *Wien. Klin. Wochenschr.* **43**, 801–803.

Kossel, H. (1899). Über einen malariaähnlichen Blutparasiten bei affen. *Z. Hyg. Infektions kra.* **32**, 25–32.

Krettli, A., Chen, D. H., and Nussenzweig, R. S. (1973). Immunogenicity and infectivity of sporozoites of mammalian malaria isolated by density-gradient centrifugation. *J. Protozool.* **20**, 662–665.

Laird, R. (1941). Observations on mosquito transmission of *Plasmodium lophurae*. *Am. J. Hyg.* **34C**, 163–167.

Landau, I. (1973). Diversité des méchanisms assurant la pérennité de l'infection chez les sporozoaires cocciomorphes. *Mem. Mus. Natl. Hist. Nat., Ser. A* [N.S.] **77**, 1–62.

Landau, I., and Bouland, Y. (1978). Life cycles and morphology. *In* "Rodent Malaria" (R. Killick-Kendrick and W. Peters, eds.), pp. 53–84. Academic Press, New York.

Landau, I., and Killick-Kendrick, R. (1966). Rodent plasmodia of the République Centrafricaine: The sporogony and tissue stages of *Plasmodium chabaudi* and *P. berghei yoelii*. *Trans. R. Soc. Trop. Med. Hyg.* **60**, 633–649.

Laveran, A. (1880). Note sur un nouveau parasite trouvé dans le sang de plusieurs malades atteints de fièvre palustre. *Bull. Acad. Med., Paris* **9**, 1235–1236.

Laveran, A. (1899). Les hématozoaires endoglobulaires (Haemocytozoa). *Cinquantenaire Soc. Biol.* pp. 124–133.

Lumsden, W. H. R., and Bertram, D. S. (1940). Observations on the biology of *Plasmodium gallinaceum* in the domestic fowl, with special reference to the production of gametocytes and their development in *Aedes aegypti*. *Ann. Trop. Med. Parasitol.* **34,** 135–160.

MacCallum, W. G. (1897). On the flagellated form of the malaria parasite. *Lancet* **2,** 1240–1241.

MacCallum, W. G. (1898). On the haematozoan infections of birds. *J. Exp. Med.* **3,** 117–136.

McCarthy, V. C., and Clyde, D. F. (1973). Influence of sulfalene upon gametocytogenesis of *Plasmodium falciparum* and subsequent infections patterns in *Anopheles stephensi*. *Exp. Parasitol.* **33,** 73–78.

MacDonald, W. W. (1967). The influence of genetic and other factors on vector susceptibility to parasites. *In* "Genetics of Insect Vectors of Disease" (J. W. Wright and R. Pal, eds.), p. 567. Elsevier, Amsterdam.

McGhee, R. B. (1951). The adaptation of the avian malaria parasite *Plasmodium lophurae* to a continuous existence in infant mice. *J. Infect. Dis.* **88,** 86–97.

McGregor, I. A. (1965). Consideration of some aspects of human malaria. *Trans. R. Soc. Trop. Med. Hyg.* **59,** 145–152.

Mack, S. R., and Vanderberg, J. P. (1978). *Plasmodium berghei:* Energy metabolism of sporozoites. *Exp. Parasitol.* **46,** 317–322.

Mack, S. R., Vanderberg, J. P., and Nawrot, R. (1978). Column separation of *Plasmodium berghei* sporozoites. *J. Parasitol.* **64,** 166–168.

Maegraith, B. (1968). Liver involvement in acute mammalian malaria with special reference to *Plasmodium knowlesi* malaria. *Adv. Parasitol.* **6,** 189–231.

Manson, P. (1896). The life-history of the malaria germ outside the human body. *Lancet* **1,** 831–833.

Marchiafava, E., and Bignami, A. (1894). "On Summer-Autumnal Fevers," p. 51. New Sydenham Soc., London.

Marchiafava, E., and Bignami, A. (1900). Malaria. *In* "Twentieth Century Practice, an International Encyclopedia of Modern Medical Science" (T. L. Stedman, ed.), Vol. XIX, pp. 1–522. Wm. Wood, New York.

Marchoux, E. (1922). Multiplicité des races dans les trois formes de parasites du paludisme. *Bull. Soc. Pathol. Exot.* **15,** 108–109.

Mashadeni-Al, H. M., and Davidson, G. (1978). A study of the genetics of the susceptibility of *Anopheles gambiae* species A, to malaria infection. *Heredity* **37,** 457.

Mayer, M. (1907). Über Malaria beim Affen. *Med. Klin. Berlin* **3,** 579–580.

Mayer, M. (1908). Über Malariaparasiten bei Affen. *Arch. Protistenkd.* **12,** 314–321.

Mayne, B., and Young, M. D. (1941). The technic of induced malaria as used in the South Carolina State Hospital. *Vener. Dis. Inf.* **22,** 271–276.

Mendis, K. N., and Targett, G. A. T. (1979). Immunisation against gametes and asexual erythrocytic stages of a rodent malaria parasite. *Nature (London)* **277,** 389–391.

Micks, D. W. (1949). Investigations on the mosquito transmission of *Plasmodium elongatum*. *J. Natl. Malar. Soc.* **8,** 206–218.

Miller, L. H., Powers, K., Finerty, J., and Vanderberg, J. P. (1973). Difference in surface charge between host cells and malarial parasites. *J. Parasitol.* **59,** 925–927.

Miller, L. H., Mason, S., Dvorak, J. A., McGinniss, M. H., and Rothman, I. K. (1975). Erythrocyte receptors for (*Plasmodium knowlesi*) malaria: Duffy blood group determinants. *Science* **189,** 561–563.

Miller, L. H., Mason, S., Clyde, D. F., and McGinniss, M. H. (1976). The resistance factor to *Plasmodium vivax* in blacks: The Duffy-blood-group genotype, $F_y F_y$. *N. Engl. J. Med.* **295,** 302–304.

Mitchell, G. H., Butcher, G. A., and Cohen, S. (1974). A merozoite vaccine effective against *Plasmodium knowlesi* malaria. *Nature (London)* **252**, 311-313.

Mitchell, G. H., Butcher, G. A., and Cohen, S. (1975). Merozoite vaccination against *Plasmodium knowlesi* malaria. *Immunology* **29**, 397-407.

Molinari, V. (1961). The action of low temperatures on plasmodia. *J. Trop. Med. Hyg.* **64**, 225-232.

Moser, G., Brohn, F. H., Danforth, H. D., and Nussenzweig, R. S. (1978). Sporozoites of rodent and simian malaria, purified by anion exchangers, retain their immunogenicity and infectivity. *J. Protozool.* **25**, 119-124.

Most, H., Nussenzweig, R. S., Vanderberg, J., Herman, R., and Yoeli, M. (1966). Susceptibility of genetically standardized (JAX) mouse strains to sporozoite- and blood-induced *Plasmodium berghei* infections. *Mil. Med.* **131**, Suppl., 915-918.

Mühlens, P., and Kirschbaum, W. (1924). Weitere parasitologische Beobachtungen bei künstlichen Malaria-infektionen von Paralytikem. *Arch. Schiffs.-Trop.-Hyg.* **28**, 131-144.

Muirhead-Thomson, R. C. (1954). Factors determining the true reservoir of infection of *Plasmodium falciparum* and *Wuchereria bancrofti* in a West African village. *Trans. R. Soc. Trop. Med. Hyg.* **48**, 208-225.

Muirhead-Thomson, R. C., and Mercier, E. C. (1952). Factors in malaria transmission by *Anopheles albimanus* in Jamaica. *Ann. Trop. Med. Parasitol.* **46**, 103-116.

Mulligan, H. W., Russell, P. F., and Mohan, B. N. (1941). Active immunization of fowls against *P. gallinaceum* by injections of killed homologous sporozoites. *J. Malar. Inst. India* **4**, 25-34.

Nijhout, M. M. (1979). *Plasmodium gallinaceum:* Exflagellation stimulated by a mosquito factor. *Exp. Parasitol.* **48**, 75-80.

Nijhout, M. M., and Carter, R. (1978). Gamete development in malaria parasites: Bicarbonate-dependent stimulation by pH *in vitro. Parasitology* **76**, 39-53.

Niles, W. J., Fernando, M. A., and Dissanaike, A. S. (1965). *Mansonia crassipes* as the natural vector of filarioides, *Plasmodium gallinaceum* and other plasmodia of fowls in Ceylon. *Nature* (London) **205**, 411-412.

Nussenzweig, R. S., and Chen, D. (1974). The antibody response to sporozoites of simian and human malaria parasites: Its stage and species specificity and strain cross-reactivity. *Bull. W.H.O.* **50**, 293-297.

Pacheco, N. D., Strome, C. P. A., Mitchell, F., Bawden, M. P., and Beaudoin, R. L. (1979). Rapid, large-scale isolation of *Plasmodium berghei* sporozoites from infected mosquitoes. *J. Parasitol.* **65**, 414-417.

Perez-Reyes, R. (1953). *Anopheles aztecus,* a new definitive host for the cyclical transmission of *Plasmodium berghei. J. Parasitol.* **39**, 603-604.

Peters, W. (1965). Competitive relationship between *Eperythrozoon coccoides* and *Plasmodium berghei* in the mouse. *Exp. Parasitol.* **16**, 158-166.

Peters, W., and Howells, R. E. (1978). Chemotherapy. *In* "Rodent Malaria" (R. Killick-Kendrick and W. Peters, eds.), pp. 345-391. Academic Press, New York.

Peters, W., Chance, M. L., Lissner, R., Momen, H., and Warhurst, D. C. (1978). The chemotherapy of rodent malaria. XXX. The enigmas of the "NS lines" of *P. berghei. Ann. Trop. Med. Parasitol.* **72**, 23-36.

Porter, J. A., and Young, M. D. (1966). Susceptibility of Panamian primates to *Plasmodium vivax. Mil. Med.* **131**, 952-958.

Porter, R. J., Laird, R. L., and Dusseau, E. M. (1952). Studies on malarial sporozoites. I. Effect of various environmental conditions. *Exp. Parasitol* **1**, 229-244.

Porter, R. J., Laird, R. L., and Dusseau, E. M. (1954). Studies on malarial sporozoites. II. Effect of age and dosage of sporozoites on their infectiousness. *Exp. Parasitol.* **3**, 267-274.

Pringle, G. (1966). A quantitative study of naturally-acquired malaria infections in *Anopheles gam-*

biae and *Anopheles funestus* in a highly malarious area of East Africa. *Trans. R. Soc. Trop. Med. Hyg.* **60,** 626–632.

Raffaele, G. (1934). Un ceppo italiano du *Plasmodium elongatum. Riv. Malariol.* **13,** 3–8.

Raffaele, G. (1936). Presumibili forme iniziale di evoluzione di *P. relictum. Riv. Malariol.* **15,** 318–324.

Raffaele, G., and Baldi, A. (1950). Sulla morfologia e sulla transmissione di *Plasmodium berghei. Riv. Malariol.* **29,** 314.

Ramakrishnan, S. P., Young, M. D., Jeffery, G. M., Burgess, R. W., and McLendon, S. B. (1952). The effect of single and multiple doses of Paludrine upon *Plasmodium falciparum. Am. J. Hyg.* **55,** 239–245.

Ramakrishnan, S. P.,Prakash, S., and Krishnaswami, A. K. (1953). Studies on *Plasmodium berghei.* X. A critical analysis of experimental mosquito transmission. *Indian J. Malariol.* **7,** 67–81.

Ramkaran, A. E., and Peters, W. (1969). Infectivity of chloroquine resistant *Plasmodium berghei* to *Anopheles stephensi* enhanced by chloroquine. *Nature (London)* **223,** 635–666.

Robertson, J. D. (1945). Notes on gametocyte threshold for infection of *Anopheles gambiae* and *Anopheles melas* in West Africa. *Ann. Trop. Med. Parasitol.* **39,** 8–10.

Rockefeller Foundation (1948). Malaria, genetic studies. *In* "The Rockefeller Foundation, International Health Division, Anu Rep., pp. 6–8. Rockefeller Found., New York.

Rockefeller Foundation (1950). Malaria, genetic studies. *In* "The Rockefeller Foundation, International Health Division, Annu. Rep., pp. 29–31. Rockefeller Found., New York.

Rodhain, J. (1952). *Plasmodium vinckei* n.sp.: Un deuxième *Plasmodium* parasite de rongeurs sauvages au Katanga. *Ann. Soc. Belge Med. Trop.* **32,** 275–280.

Rodhain, J. (1956). Les formes préérythrocytaires du *Plasmodium vivax* chez le chimpanzé. *Ann. Soc. Belge Med. Trop.* **36,** 99–103.

Rodhain, J., and Vincke, I. H. (1951). Essai d'évolution de *Plasmodium berghei* chez *Anopheles maculipennis* var. *arthroparvus. Ann. Soc. Belge Med. Trop.* **31,** 297–301.

Rodhain, J., and Vincke, I. H. (1952). Note au sujet de l'évolution de *Plasmodium berghei* chez *Anopheles maculipennis* var. *arthroparvus. Ann. Soc. Belge Med. Trop.* **32,** 165–167.

Rodhain, J., Pons, C., Vandenbraden, J., and Bequaert, J. (1912). Contribution au mécanisme de la transmission des trypanosomes par les glussinen. *Arch. Schiffs-Trop.-Hyg.* **16,** 732–739.

Rodhain, J., Wanson, M., and Vincke, I. H. (1955). Nouveaux essais d'évolution de *Plasmodium berghei* chez diverses espèces d'anophèles. *Ann. Soc. Belge Med. Trop.* **35,** 203–217.

Roehl, W. (1926). Die Wirkung des Plasmochins auf die Vogelmalaria. *Arch. Schiffs-Trop.-Hyg.* **30,** 311–318.

Ross, R. (1895). The crescent-sphere-flagella metamorphosis of the malaria parasite in the mosquito. *Trans. S. Indian Branch Br. Med. Assoc.* **6,** 334–350.

Ross, R. (1896). Letter to Patrick Manson, 1895. (Cited Manson, 1896.)

Ross, R. (1897). On some peculiar pigmented cells found in two mosquitoes fed on malarial blood. *Br. Med. J.* **2,** 1786–1788.

Ross, R. (1898). "Report on the Cultivation of *Proteosoma* Labbé in Grey Mosquitoes." Govt. Press, Calcutta.

Ross, R. (1923). "Memoirs." Murray, London.

Rossan, R. N., Fisher, K. F., Greenland, R. D., Genther, C. S., and Schmitt, L. H. (1964). The localization of infective pre-erythrocytic forms of *Plasmodium cynomolgi. Trans. R. Soc. Trop. Med. Hyg.* **58,** 159–163.

Ruge, R. (1901). Untersuchungen über das deutsche *Proteosoma. Centralb. Bakteriol.* **29,** 187–191.

Russell, P. F., and Mohan, B. N. (1942). The immunization of fowls against mosquito-borne *Plasmodium gallinaceum* by injections of serum and of inactivated homologous sporozoites. *J. Exp. Med.* **76,** 477–495.

Rutledge, L. C., Ward, R. A., and Gould, D. J. (1964). Studies on the feeding response of mosquitoes to nutritive solutions in a new membrane feeder. *Mosq. News* **24**, 407–419.

Rutledge, L. C., Hayes, D. E., and Ward, R. A. (1970). *Plasmodium cynomolgi:* Sources of variation in susceptibility of *Anopheles quadrimaculatus, A. balabacensis,* and *A. stephensi. Exp. Parasitol.* **27**, 53–59.

Schaudinn, F. (1903). Studien über krankheitserregende Protozoen. *Kaiserl. Gesundhamt.* **19**, 169–250.

Schmidt, L. H., Fradkin, R., Squires, W., and Genther, C. S. (1948). Malaria chemotherapy. II. The response of sporozoite-induced infections with *Plasmodium cynomolgi* to various antimalarial drugs. *Fed. Proc., Am. Soc. Exp. Biol.* **7**, 253–254.

Schneider, I., and Chen, D. H. (1969). Isolation of malaria sporozoites on Renografin-serum albumin gradients. *Am. Zool.* **9**, 501.

Schüffner, W. A. P. (1919). Two subjects relating to the epidemiology of malaria. *Meded. Burgerl. Geneeskd. Dienst. Ned.-Ind.* **9**, 1–52; reprinted in English translation in *J. Malar. Inst. India* **1**, 221–256 (1938).

Schulman, S., Oppenheim, J. D., and Vanderberg, J. P. (1980). *Plasmodium berghei* and *Plasmodium knowlesi:* Serum binding to sporozoites. *Exp. Parasitol.* **49**, 420–429.

Schulze, F. (1925). Die Malariabehandlung der Paralyse. *Dtsch. Med. Wochenschr.* **51**, 1856–1858.

Sergent, Ed., and Sergent, Et. (1952). Recherches expérimentals sur l'infection latente et la prémunition dans le paludisme. *Arch. Inst. Pasteur Alger.* **30**, 203–239.

Shah, K. (1934). The periodic development of sexual forms of *Plasmodium cathemerium* in the peripheral circulation of canaries. *Am. J. Hyg.* **19**, 392–403.

Shah, K., Rozeboom, L., and Del Rosario, F. (1934). Studies on the infectivity of *Plasmodium cathemerium* of canaries for mosquitoes. *Am. J. Hyg.* **20**, 502–507.

Shortt, H. E., and Cooper, W. (1948). Staining of microscopical sections containing protozoal parasites by modification of McNamara's method. *Trans. R. Soc. Trop. Med. Hyg.* **41**, 427–428.

Shortt, H. E., and Garnham, P. C. C. (1948). The pre-erythrocytic development of *Plasmodium cynomolgi* and *Plasmodium vivax. Trans. R. Soc. Trop. Med. Hyg.* **41**, 785–795.

Shortt, H. E., Fairley, N. H., Covell, G., Shute, P. G., and Garnham, P. C. C. (1949). The pre-erythrocytic stage of *Plasmodium falciparum:* A preliminary note. *Br. Med. J.* **2**, 1006–1008.

Shute, P. G., and Maryon, M. (1951). A study of gametocytes in a West African strain of *Plasmodium falciparum. Trans. R. Soc. Trop. Med. Hyg.* **44**, 421–438.

Shute, P. G., and Maryon, M. (1952). A study of human malaria oocysts as an aid to species diagnosis. *Trans. R. Soc. Trop. Med. Hyg.* **46**, 275–292.

Shute, P. G., and Maryon, M. (1966). "Laboratory Technique for the Study of Malaria," 2nd ed. Churchill, London.

Shute, P. G., and Maryon, M. (1968). Some observations on true latency and long-term relapses in *Plasmodium vivax* malaria. *Arch. Roum. Pathol. Exp. Microbiol.* **27**, 893–898.

Shute, P. G., Maryon, M. E., and Pringle, G. (1965). A method for estimating the number of sporozoites in the salivary glands of a mosquito. *Trans. R. Soc. Trop. Med. Hyg.* **59**, 285–288.

Shute, P. G., Lupascu, G., Branzei, P., Maryon, M., Constantinescu, P., Bruce-Chwatt, L. J., Draper, C. C., Killick-Kendrick, R., and Garnham, P. C. C. (1976). A strain of *Plasmodium vivax* characterized by prolonged incubation: The effects of numbers of sporozoites on the length of the prepatent period. *Trans. R. Soc. Trop. Med. Hyg.* **70**, 474–481.

Sinden, R. E., and Croll, N. A. (1975). Cytology and kinetics of microgametogenesis and fertilization in *Plasmodium yoelii nigeriensis. Parasitology* **70**, 53–65.

Sinden, R. E., and Smalley, M. E. (1976). Gametocytes of *Plasmodium falciparum:* Phagocytosis by leucocytes *in vivo* and *in vitro. Trans. R. Soc. Trop. Med. Hyg.* **70,** 344–345.

Sinden, R. E., Canning, E. V., and Spain, B. (1976). Gametogenesis and fertilization in *Plasmodium yoelii nigeriensis:* A transmission electron microscope study. *Proc. R. Soc. London, Sec B* **193,** 55–76.

Sinton, J. A., and Mulligan, H. W. (1932). A critical review of the literature relating to the identification of the malarial parasites recorded from monkeys of the families Cercopithecidae and Colobidae. *Rec. Malar. Surv. India* **3,** 357–380.

Sinton, J. A., Baily, J. D., and Chand, D. (1926). Studies in malaria with special reference to treatment. The occurrence of sexual forms of *P. falciparum* in the peripheral circulation. *Indian J. Med. Res.* **13,** 895–916.

Smalley, M. E., and Sinden, R. E. (1977). *Plasmodium falciparum* gametocytes: Their longevity and infectivity. *Parasitology* **74,** 1–8.

Sodeman, T. M., Jumper, J. R., Contacos, P. G., and Smith, C. S. (1970). A technique for splenectomy of non-human primates. *J. Trop. Med. Hyg.* **73,** 33–35.

Spielman, A., and Kitzmiller, J. B. (1967). Genetics of populations of medically-important arthropods. *In* "Genetics of Insect Vectors of Disease" (J. W. Wright and R. Pal, eds.), pp. 459–485. Elsevier, Amsterdam.

Stephens, J. W. W., and Christopers, S. R. (1908). "The Practical Study of Malaria," 3rd ed. Univ. of Liverpool Press, Liverpool.

Stratman-Thomas, W. K. (1940). The influence of temperature on *Plasmodium vivax. Am. J. Trop. Med.* **20,** 703–715.

Strome, C. P. A., Tubergen, T. A., Leef, J. L., and Beaudoin, R. L. (1977). A quantitative long-term cryobiological study of malarial parasites. *Bull. W.H.O.* **55,** 305–308.

Taliaferro, L. G. (1925). Infection and resistance in bird malaria with special reference to periodicity and rate of reproduction of the parasites. *Am. J. Hyg.* **5,** 742–789.

Thompson, P. E., and Huff, C. G. (1944). A saurian malarial parasite, *Plasmodium mexicanum,* n.sp, with both elongatum- and gallinaceum types of exoerythrocytic stages. *J. Infect. Dis.* **74,** 48–67.

Thomson, D. (1911). A research into the production and death of crescents in malignant tertian malaria in treated and untreated cases by an enumerative method. *Ann. Trop. Med. Parasitol.* **6,** 57–82.

Tonkin, I. M. (1947). Influence of suspending fluid on survival of sporozoites *in vitro. Trans. R. Soc. Trop. Med. Hyg.* **41,** 259–262.

Trager, W. (1942). A strain of the mosquito *Aedes aegypti* selected for susceptibility to the avian malarial parasite *Plasmodium lophurae. J. Parasitol.* **28,** 457–465.

Trager, W., and Jensen, J. B. (1976). Human malaria parasites in continuous culture. *Science* **193,** 673–675.

Ungureanu, E., Killick-Kendrick, R., Garnham, P. C. C., Branzei, P., Romanescu, C., and Shute, P. G. (1976). Prepatent periods of a tropical strain of *Plasmodium vivax* after inoculations of tenfold dilutions of sporozoites. *Trans. R. Soc. Trop. Med. Hyg.* **70,** 482–483.

Vanderberg, J. P. (1974). Studies on the motility of *Plasmodium* sporozoites, *J. Protozool.* **21,** 527–537.

Vanderberg, J. P. (1975). Development of infectivity by the *Plasmodium berghei* sporozoite. *J. Parasitol.* **61,** 43–50.

Vanderberg, J. P. (1977). *Plasmodium berghei:* Quantitation of sporozoites injected by mosquitoes feeding on a rodent host. *Exp. Parasitol.* **42,** 169–181.

Vanderberg, J. P. (1979). Isolation and purification of sporozoites of the malaria parasites: A review. *Bull. W.H.O.* (in press).

Vanderberg, J. P., and Nawrot, R. (1968). Mosquito maintenance procedures for increased yields of sporozoites in the *Plasmodium berghei-Anopheles stephensi* system of rodent malaria. *Proc. Int. Congr. Trop. Med. Malaria, 8th, 1968 pp. 1277-1278.*

Vanderberg, J. P., and Yoeli, M. (1964). Some physiological and metabolic problems related to the *Plasmodium berghei* cycle in *Anopheles quadrimaculatus*. *In* "International Colloquium on *Plasmodium berghei*" (J. Jadin, ed.), pp. 171-178. Inst. Méd. Trop. Prince Léopold, Antwerp.

Vanderberg, J. P., and Yoeli, M. (1966). The effects of temperature on the sporogonic development of *Plasmodium berghei*. *J. Parasitol.* **52,** 559-564.

Vanderberg, J. P., Yoeli, M., and Rhodin, J. (1967). Electron microscopic and histochemical studies of sporozoite formation in *Plasmodium berghei*. *J. Protozool.* **14,** 82-103.

Vanderberg, J. P., Nussenzweig, R. S., and Most, H. (1968). Further studies on the *Plasmodium berghei-Anopheles stephensi*-rodent system of experimental malaria. *J. Parasitol.* **54,** 1009-1016.

Vanderberg, J., Nussenzweig, R. S., Sanabria, Y., Nawrot, R., and Most, H. (1972). Stage specificity of antisporozoite antibodies in rodent malaria and its relationship to protective immunity. *Proc. Helminthol. Soc. Wash.* **39,** 514-525.

Van der Kaay, H. J., Sikkema, A. C. L., and Boorsma, E. G. (1978). Observations on the development of *Plasmodium berghei berghei* (ANKA) in a susceptible and a refractory strain of *Anopheles atroparvus*. *Parasitology* **77** (3), xlvii.

Verhave, J. (1975). Immunization with sporozoites. An experimental study of *Plasmodium berghei* malaria. Ph.D. Thesis, Katholieke Universiteit te Nijmegen, The Netherlands.

Vincke, I. H. (1954). Experimental transmission of *Plasmodium berghei*. *Indian J. Malariol.* **8,** 257-263.

Vincke, I. H., and Bafort, J. (1968). Résultats de deux ans d'observation sur la transmission cyclique de *Plasmodium berghei*. *Ann. Soc. Belge Med. Trop.* **48,** 439-454.

Vincke, I. H., and Lips, M. (1948). Un nouveau plasmodium d'un rongeur sauvage du Congo, *Plasmodium berghei* n. sp. *Ann. Soc. Belge Med. Trop.* **28,** 97-104.

Vincke, I. H., Scheepers-Biva, M., and Bafort, J. (1965). Conservation de gamétocytes de *Plasmodium berghei* viables et transmissibles à basse température. *Ann. Soc. Belge Med. Trop.* **45,** 151-160.

Vincke, I. H., Bafort, J., and Scheepers-Biva, M. (1966). Observations récentes sur la transmission cyclique de *Plasmodium berghei*. *Ann. Soc. Belge Med. Trop.* **46,** 327-336.

Voller, A., and Rossan, R. N. (1969). Immunological studies on simian malaria. III. Immunity to challenge and antigenic variation in *P. knowlesi*. *Trans. R. Soc. Trop. Med. Hyg.* **63,** 507-523.

Wagner-Jauregg, J. (1922). Treatment of general paresis by inoculation of malaria. *J. Nerv. Ment. Dis.* **55,** 369-375.

Walliker, D., Carter, R., and Morgan, S. (1973). Genetic recombination in *Plasmodium berghei*. *Parasitology* **66,** 309-320.

Ward, R. A. (1962). Preservation of mosquitoes for malarial oocyst and sporozoite dissections. *Mosq. News* **22,** 306-307.

Ward, R. A. (1963). Genetic aspects of the susceptibility of mosquitoes to malarial infection. *Exp. Parasitol.* **13,** 328-341.

Ward, R. A., and Hayes, D. E. (1972). Sporozoite transmission of falciparum malaria (Vietnam, Smith strain) from monkey to monkey. *Trans. R. Soc. Trop. Med. Hyg.* **66,** 670-671.

Ward, R. A., and Savage, K. E. (1972). Effects of microsporidian parasites upon anopheline mosquitoes and malarial infection. *Proc. Helminthol. Soc. Wash.* **39,** 434-438.

Ward, R. A., Rutledge, L. C., and Hickman, R. L. (1969). Cyclical transmission of Chesson vivax malaria in sub-human primates. *Nature (London)* **224,** 1126-1127.

Ward, R. A., Hayes, D. E., Hembree, S. C., Rutledge, L. C., Anderson, S. J., and Johnson A. J. (1972). Infectivity of *Plasmodium falciparum* gametocytes from *Aotus trivirgatus* to anopheline mosquitoes. *Proc. Helminthol. Soc. Wash.* **39**, 33–46.

Ward, R. D., Lainson, R., and Shaw, J. J. (1978). Some methods for membrane feeding of laboratory reared, neotropical sandflies. (Diptera: Psychodidae). *Ann. Trop. Med. Parasitol.* **72**, 269–276.

Warhurst, D. C., and Folwell, R. O. (1968). Measurement of the growth rate of the erythrocytic stages of *Plasmodium berghei* and comparisons of the potency of inocula after various treatments. *Ann. Trop. Med. Parasitol.* **62**, 349–360.

Warren, M., Collins, W. E., Richardson, B. B., and Skinner, J. C. (1977). Morphological variants of *Anopheles albimanus* and susceptibility to *Plasmodium vivax* and *P. falciparum. Am. J. Trop. Med. Hyg.* **26**, 607–611.

Weathersby, A. B., and McCall, J. W. (1967). Survival of sporozoites of *Plasmodium gallinaceum* for 767 days in liquid nitrogen (−197 C°). *J. Parasitol.* **53**, 638–640.

Weiss, M. M., and Vanderberg, J. P. (1976). Studies on *Plasmodium* ookinetes. 1. Isolation and concentration from mosquito midguts. *J. Protozool.* **23**, 547–551.

Weiss, M. M., and Vanderberg, J. P. (1977). Studies on *Plasmodium* ookinetes. 2. *In vitro* development. *J. Parasitol.* **63**, 932–934.

Welch, W. H. (1897). Malaria: Definition, synonyms, history, and parasitology. *In* "Systematic Practice of Medicine" (Loomis and Thompson, ed.), Vol. 1, pp. 17–76. Lea Bros., New York.

Wenyon, C. M. (1926). "Protozoology," Vol. II. Wm. Wood, New York.

Wéry, M. (1966). Etude du cycle de *Plasmodium berghei yoelii* en vue de la production massive de sporozoites viables et de formes exoérythrocytaires. *Ann. Soc. Belge Med. Trop.* **46**, 755–788.

Wéry, M. (1968). Studies on the sporogony of rodent malaria parasites. *Ann. Soc. Belge Med. Trop.* **48**, 1–138.

Whitman, L. (1948). The prolonged viability of sporozoites of *Plasmodium gallinaceum* in extracts of washed chicken erythrocytes. *J. Immunol.* **59**, 285–294.

Wilkinson, R. N., Noeypatimanondh, S., and Gould, D. J. (1976). Infectivity of falciparum malaria patients for anopheline mosquitoes before and after chloroquine treatment. *Trans. R. Soc. Trop. Med. Hyg.* **70**, 306–307.

Wilson, D. B. (1936). Rural hyper-endemic malaria in Tanganyika territory. *Trans. R. Soc. Trop. Med. Hyg.* **29**, 583–618.

Yoeli, M. (1973). *Plasmodium berghei:* Mechanisms and sites of resistance to sporogonic development in different mosquitoes. *Exp. Parasitol.* **34**, 448–458.

Yoeli, M., and Most, H. (1960). The biology of a newly isolated strain of *Plasmodium berghei* in a rodent host and in experimental mosquito vectors. *Trans. R. Soc. Trop. Med. Hyg.* **54**, 549–555.

Yoeli, M., and Most, H. (1971). Sporozoite-induced infections of *Plasmodium berghei* administered by the oral route. *Science* **173**, 1031–1032.

Yoeli, M., and Wall, W. J. (1951). Complete sporogonic development of *Plasmodium berghei* in experimentally infected *Anopheles* sp. *Nature (London)* **168**, 1078.

Yoeli, M., and Wall, W. J. (1952). Cyclic transmission of *P. berghei* in the laboratory, *Nature (London)* **169**, 881.

Yoeli, M., Upmanis, R. S., and Most, H. (1963). Gametogony and sporogony of *Plasmodium berghei* preserved at low temperature. *J. Parasitol.* **49**, 926–929.

Yoeli, M., Most, H., and Boné, G. (1964). *Plasmodium berghei:* Cyclical transmissions by experimentally infected *Anopheles quadrimaculatus. Science* **144**, 1580–1581.

Yoeli, M., Upmanis, R. S., Vanderberg, J., and Most, H. (1966). Life cycles and patterns of development of *Plasmodium berghei* in normal and experimental hosts. *Mil. Med.* **131,** Suppl., 900–914.

Young, M. D., Hardman, N. F., Burgess, R. W., Frohne, W. C., and Sabrosky, C. W. (1948). The infectivity of native malarias in South Carolina to *Anopheles quadrimaculatus*. *Am. J. Trop. Med.* **28,** 303–311.

Young, M. D., Porter, J. A., and Johnson, C. M. (1966). *Plasmodium vivax* transmitted from man to monkey to man. *Science* **153,** 1006–1007.

Culture of the Invertebrate Stages of Plasmodia and the Culture of Mosquito Tissues

Imogene Schneider and Jerome P. Vanderberg

I. INTRODUCTION

Despite the acknowledged potential value of a culture system capable of supporting the growth and development of the insect stages of malaria parasites, significant advances toward this end have been few. In a recent review, Vander-

Malaria, Vol. 2

berg *et al.,* (1977) attributed this limited progress to the difficulty of designing a culture system (or systems) which would sequentially simulate or replace four different environments; namely, an intraerythrocytic milieu for gametocytes, the lumen of the mosquito midgut for ookinete formation, the mosquito hemocoel for oocyst and sporozoite development, and the salivary glands for sporozoite maturation. How fully these presumptive requirements of the parasites eventually coincide with the actual culture requirements remains to be seen but, given past history, the chances of a prompt and definitive answer seem rather remote.

Since the pioneering studies of Ball (1947, 1948), very few investigators have attempted to culture any of the sporogonic stages. Moreover, rarely has more than one individual or group been engaged in such research concurrently, effectively precluding a much needed exchange of information. Yet another factor impeding progress has been the use of several different host–parasite combinations, making it difficult to compare previous findings, as well as to assess the reliability of the different techniques and media employed.

Current reluctance to work with the insect stages stems in part from an appreciation of the obstacles (tedious dissection or isolation procedures, bacterial and fungal contamination from mosquito tissues, and inadequate media) previous investigators encountered as measured against their modest successes. For in no instance has it been possible to culture the entire sporogonic phase of any malarial parasite; rather, only by placing overlapping successive stages of the parasite *in vitro* for limited periods can development from gametocyte to sporozoite be followed.

Within the past few years, however, a number of developments have occurred which should improve chances for the successful cultivation of these stages. Continuous cycling of the erythrocytic stages has been achieved by Trager and Jensen (1976), including the formation of gametocytes capable of exflagellation (Carter and Beach, 1977). In addition, a number of reports have described conditions under which ookinetes may be formed *in vitro* (Rosales-Ronquillo and Silverman, 1974; Rosales-Ronquillo *et al.,* 1974; Weiss and Vanderberg, 1977; Chen *et al.,* 1977). These techniques not only permit culture to be initiated with younger stages but with far more parasites than was formerly possible and without concomitant bacterial or fungal contamination. Then too, primary cell cultures as well as continuous lines of insect origin, if required in a supportive role, are now readily available, thanks to advances in insect tissue culture methodology.

The demonstration that sporozoites are effective immunizing antigens against sporozoite-induced malaria (Nussenzweig *et al.,* 1967, 1972; Clyde *et al.,* 1973, 1975; Rieckmann *et al.,* 1974) provides the most recent incentive for culturing the insect stages of these parasites. Since a fundamental prerequisite for any practical application of a sporozoite vaccine is the availability, on demand, of massive numbers of sporozoites free of extraneous host material, a reliable culture system should provide the most feasible means of obtaining them.

In subsequent sections of this chapter, previous attempts to culture the sporogonic stages of various plasmodia are reviewed, as are current methods of initiating primary cell or organ cultures and continuous lines from mosquito species. The merits and possible drawbacks of designing a culture medium based on the composition of adult anopheline hemolymph rather than on an empirical basis are also discussed. Finally, a realistic assessment of future prospects for culturing the sporogonic stages is given.

II. ATTEMPTS TO CULTURE THE INVERTEBRATE STAGES OF PLASMODIA

A. Gametocytogenesis *in Vitro*

Studies on *in vitro* development of the sporogonic stages of malaria have generally been carried out by initiating the cultures with parasites that have already differentiated to some degree within the mosquito host. Ball and Chao (1960) were unable to obtain development of gametocytes to ookinetes when gametocyte-containing blood from canaries infected with *Plasmodium relictum* was transferred directly to a culture system. They noted, however, that this conversion could take place *in vitro* if the blood was first ingested by susceptible mosquitoes and either the entire blood-filled midgut or the removed clotted blood, by itself, was transferred to a culture vessel. This requirement of initiating cultures with partially developed sporogonic stages posed a number of different problems. There are several reasons why it is advantageous to bypass the mosquito entirely and to initiate *in vitro* sporogony with gametocytes taken directly from the vertebrate host.

Bypassing the mosquito vector eliminates the requirement for a regular supply of infected mosquitoes. Well-run insectaries are expensive operations, beyond the financial capabilities of many laboratories that might otherwise become involved in *in vitro* culture studies. Gametocytes taken directly from the vertebrate host can be obtained without the bacterial and fungal contaminants almost invariably present in material harvested from mosquitoes. The microorganisms can sometimes be controlled with antibiotics, though the possibility of toxicity to the malaria parasite must also be kept in mind. Taking parasites directly from the vertebrate host eliminates the concomitant introduction of mosquito tissue into the culture system. Mosquito midgut tissue, which is generally the tissue transferred, contains high levels of proteolytic secretory enzymes. In addition, subsequent autolysis of the tissue may have toxic effects on the culture. A number of different mechanisms may act to abort normal gametocyte-to-ookinete transformation within the mosquito midgut. These include the lethal action of antigamete antibodies taken in with the blood meal (Gwadz, 1976; Carter and Chen, 1976), the ingestion of gametocytes by leukocytes, a process which occurs in the mosquito midgut after the release of gametocytes from their host red blood cells (Sinden and Smalley, 1976), and the possible deleterious action of mosquito midgut enzymes. These abortive mechanisms can be operationally eliminated or controlled by bypassing the mosquito. It thus may ultimately be possible to obtain more efficient gametocyte-to-ookinete conversion *in vitro* than *in vivo*. Finally, it may eventually be possible to eliminate *in vivo* hosts for the parasite entirely. Gametocytes could theoretically be produced from a self-perpetuating *in vitro* cycle into which uninfected erythrocytes are inoculated and from which mature gametocytes are harvested.

In view of the obvious advantages of initiating sporogonic cultures with gametocytes rather than stages taken from the mosquito, it would be helpful to consider the following questions. (1) How are gametocytes formed *in vivo,* and how may this process be controlled under *in vitro* conditions? (2) How can the growth and differentiation of gametocytes be supported *in vitro* until they reach a state of functional maturity? (3) What are the factors that control gamete formation, fertilization, and ookinete differentiation, and how can these processes be controlled in an *in vitro* system?

1. Induction of Gametocyte Formation

The formation of gametocytes and the process of growth and differentiation leading to their maturity are known as gametocytogenesis. The factors that influence and control gametocytogenesis of malaria parasites within their vertebrate hosts is reviewed in this volume, Chapter 4. In brief, it is well established that gametocytes are differentiated from asexual parasites; that the ability to form gametocytes is both an inherent genetic character of the parasite strain and a response to the environmental influences encountered by the parasite; that the ability of a strain to form gametocytes tends to deteriorate with repeated serial blood passages by syringe; and that the formation and maturation of gametocytes, of some species at least, may occur synchronously and in coordination with the synchronicity of the asexual cycle.

That mature gametocytes could be formed under *in vitro* conditions was first clearly shown by Trager (1941, 1943) with *P. lophurae*. This parasite, which has since lost its ability to form gametocytes, was found to produce gametocytes on a regular basis when placed in culture. Over a period of several successive days increasing numbers of microgametocytes became capable of undergoing exflagellation. Trager interpreted this as indicating the continued survival and development of these gametocytes *in vitro*.

Several investigators have shown that *P. falciparum* gametocytes will undergo growth and development *in vitro* when blood from an infected patient or *Aotus* monkey is used to initiate the culture (Row, 1929; Trager, 1971; Mitchell *et al.*, 1976; Haynes *et al.*, 1976; Phillips *et al.*, 1976, 1978; Smalley, 1976). Although the clear morphological development of these gametocytes was noted *in vitro*, none of the parasites developed to complete functional maturity, i.e., acquired the ability to exflagellate or infectivity to susceptible mosquitoes. Since none of these were long-term continuously replicating cultures, it is difficult to determine whether any of the gametocytes seen actually initiated their development *in vitro*, although Haynes *et al.* (1976) found young gametocytes as long as 22 days after the initiation of culture. However, it seems likely that most of the gametocytes developed from ring forms that had already been genetically committed to become gametocytes in the humans or simians from which they were taken. Smalley (1976) showed that the numbers of gametocytes observed in his cultures varied considerably with the times during an infection that blood was taken from a given patient. Thus, the factors responsible for initiating the formation of gametocytes from asexual parasites appeared to reside within the patient from whom the parasites were taken rather than the culture environment into which they were placed.

A more convincing demonstration of the direct induction of gametocytes from asexual parasites *in vitro* requires a long-term continuously cycling system. That gametocytes of *P. falciparum* could be regularly produced and cultured in such a system was first shown by Trager and Jensen (1976) and confirmed with the same system by Vanderberg *et al.* (1977) and with a somewhat different culture system by Carter and Beach (1977).

Complete development of *P. falciparum* gametocytes within humans is considered to take approximately 10 days (Kitchen and Putnam, 1942; Jeffrey, 1960). During this time, the gametocyte differentiates from a parasite similar in structure to an asexual ring form to a morphologically mature "crescent." Various workers have arbitrarily classified the stages of development the gametocyte passes through during this process (Field and Shute, 1956; Hawking *et al.*, 1971). This classification system of five developmental stages has become generally accepted for descriptive studies of gametocyte development and has been illustrated in color plates by Carter and Miller (1979). Several workers have shown that gametocytes developing *in vitro* similarly go through this developmental sequence in an approximately 10-day period (Smalley, 1976; Jensen, 1979; Phillips *et al.*, 1978; Carter and Miller, 1979).

The present availability of *in vitro* systems in which *P. falciparum* gametocytes can be induced to form and subsequently to mature makes it possible to analyze experimentally the factors that control gametocytogenesis. As previously shown with *in vivo* studies, the induction of gametocyte production seems to depend upon inherent characteristics of the parasite strain, as well as undefined inducing factors within the environment. Some strains appear to be inherently better gametocyte producers than others. In some cases, strains that are initially good gametocyte producers in culture may lose this ability with continued culture. Jensen (1979) reported loss of gametocyte production by the FCR-1 strain after 3–4 months in continuous culture, but whether this represented a deficiency of the strain itself or was due to culture techniques is not yet clear. Conversely, one strain studied at the National Institutes of Health (the Z isolate of *P. falciparum*) has been observed to retain fully its gametocyte-producing potential over 1½ years in continuous culture, while another (the G isolate) appears to have increased its production potential in culture (Carter and Miller, 1979). Thus, in choosing an experimental system in which to study gametocyte development *in vitro*, one must select an appropriate parasite strain to work with as well as attempt to understand the environmental factors that modulate gametocyte production.

Recent studies by Carter and Miller (1979) have begun to elucidate these factors. To assess the relative rates of gametocyte formation in different culture vessels, they developed a method for estimation of the percentage of ring forms developing into gametocytes at any given time in the life of a culture. This was done by counting the ring forms at a particular time and then counting the stage II gametocytes into which these rings presumably developed 48 hours later. The actual conversion rates obtained were considered estimates because, as the authors noted, precise conversion rates could be calculated only if the precise "residence time" for each of the parasite stages was known with certainty. At the time of the study, these periods of residence could only be estimated. However, the ability to determine actual conversion rates is not as important as the ability to compare relative conversion rates in different cultures under different conditions. Using this procedure, Carter and Miller concluded that the process of dilution of an old culture with fresh erythrocytes and medium was responsible for turning off the production of gametocytes from asexual parasites, whereas conditions associated with a maintenance period of close to a week in culture induced renewed gametocytogenesis, generally on the order of a 5–20% conversion rate. This established that environmental conditions, as yet unspecified, directly modulated the rate of gametocyte production by *P. falciparum* in culture. The chief value of this study lies in its presentation of a quantitative approach to measuring the rate of gametocytogenesis, thereby opening up an experimental approach to assess the factors that may influence this process.

2. Maturation of Gametocytes

The development of gametocytes to functional maturity can be assessed either *in vitro* by noting the ability of the gametocytes to form gametes under appropriate conditions, or *in vivo* by testing the infectivity of the gametocytes in susceptible mosquitoes. Thus far, the only successes reported for the maturation of *P. falciparum* gametocytes formed *in vitro* have been by Carter and Beach (1977) and Carter and Miller (1979). On several occasions, microgametocytes were seen to exflagellate when removed from culture and placed under conditions that stimulated this process. The specific factors responsible for permitting complete gametocyte maturation in the isolated cases could not be determined, although a consistent feature of the production of such mature gametocytes has been a fall in hematocrit to very low levels (<0.5%) prior to full maturation and the maintenance of cultures for 2–3 weeks without the addition of fresh erythrocytes. Other workers have been unsuccessful in culturing gametocytes to full functional maturity (Vanderberg *et al.*, 1977; Jensen, 1979).

It has been pointed out by Carter and Miller (1979) and R. Carter (personal communication) that exflagellation of cultured gametocytes was observed only in instances when healthy stage V (the most mature stage) gametocytes were identifiable in a culture. Because stage IV and stage V gametocytes are essentially the same size, the cytological details of these parasites must be carefully observed before determining that complete morphological maturation has occurred. An important character that distinguishes these stages is the centralization of chromatin and pigment granules that occurs with the transition to stage V. Carter and Miller (1979) have used polarized light to visualize better the distribution and shape of the pigment granules, thus allowing a clearer differentiation of the developmental stages. Another procedure, used by Shute and Maryon (1951), involves partial destaining of already stained thin smears. Their technique allows excellent resolution of chromatin and pigment distribution, thereby permitting the sex of the gametocytes as well as the stage of development to be more readily distinguished.

It is extremely helpful to determine, as Carter and his co-workers have done, that *P. falciparum* gametocytes formed *in vitro* have the inherent capability to attain functional maturity. What is needed now is the formulation of culture conditions that will support this full maturation on a regular and repeatable basis. The solution of this problem would constitute an important breakthrough, as it would ensure the availability of large numbers of infective gametocytes without any requirement for a human or simian host. Studies on *in vitro* culture of *P. falciparum* sporogonic stages could then move on to the next stage: the development of ookinetes and beyond. *In vitro* support of complete gametocyte maturation appears to be mostly a matter of creating more favorable culture conditions. The culture medium commonly used, RPMI-1640, is a relatively simple tissue culture medium that, together with a small amount of serum, seems to supply all nutritional requirements for asexual parasites. All that is required of an infected erythrocyte is survival in culture for the 48 hours needed by the parasite to develop. Fresh, uninfected erythrocytes can then be added to the culture on a regular basis. The gametocyte, however, requires that its host erythrocyte survive for almost 2 weeks *in vitro,* a requirement that makes more stringent demands on a culture system.

An additional problem associated with support of gametocytes for the long maturation period required is competition from asexual parasites which tend to reach high parasitemias and eventually degenerate. Problems may thus arise from rapid depletion of nutrients by the growing parasites, from accumulation of toxic metabolic products in the culture, and from the toxic consequences of parasite death and degeneration. This problem may be resolved by (1) separation and concentration of gametocytes by gradients or other means, so that they may subsequently be cultured without competition, (2) a regular substitution of fresh culture medium by perfusion to maintain better homeostasis in the culture, (3) a reduction in the hematocrit to reduce competition, and (4) the use of small quantities of antimalarial drugs to control asexual parasites while at the same time permitting normal gametocyte maturation.

B. Gametogenesis *in Vitro*

After complete maturation of gametocytes in the vertebrate host, further developmental changes normally cease until the gametocytes are ingested by a suitable vector mosquito. Then, gametogenesis (gamete formation) occurs within the lumen of the mosquito's midgut. The macrogametocyte emerges from its host red blood cell to become a macrogamete, while flagellated microgametes emerge from the microgametocyte in a dramatic process known as exflagellation.

The ability to induce and control gametogenesis of mature gametocytes *in vitro* is of obvious importance. First, gametogenesis (especially exflagellation) is one of the important parameters used to determine successful maturation of gametocytes. Second, gametogenesis is a developmental step en route to the next task in development: fertilization and ookinete formation. Several separate factors that appear to play a role in the induction of exflagellation have now been identified; namely, reduction in temperature, elevation of pH, and an unidentified mosquito factor.

Immediately upon ingestion by a mosquito, gametocytes experience a drop in temperature from that of the homeothermic environment of the vertebrate bloodstream to that existing in the poikilothermic environment of the mosquito midgut. Sir Ronald Ross (1897) held that this temperature drop could not be the environmental stimulus triggering exflagellation, as exflagellation of *P. falciparum* occurred in his laboratory in India even at ambient temperatures close to that of the human body. Other studies, however, have suggested that a temperature drop is required (Boyd *et al.*, 1949; Sinden and Cross, 1975; Sinden and Smalley, 1976). It also seems clear that there are optimal temperatures for exflagellation *in vitro*. Below these optima, the time required for exflagellation increases with lowering of the temperature until it ceases entirely at unfavorably low temperatures. Thus, Shute and Maryon (1966) have shown that for human malarias exflagellation takes 12–15 minutes at 25°C, close to 30 minutes at 16°–20°C, and does not occur at all below 15°C. With rodent malaria, exflagellation does not occur at temperatures of 30°C or above and takes about 15 minutes at 25°C, about 30 minutes at 15°C, and over 1 hour at 12°C (Sinden and Croll, 1975).

Another physical change that occurs within blood once in the mosquito midgut is an elevation in pH (Micks *et al.*, 1948; Bishop and McConnachie, 1956). The work of several investigators has suggested that there is a loss of carbon dioxide from blood when it is removed from a host and exposed to air, or taken in by mosquitoes, and that the concomitant rise in pH due to the reduction in carbon dioxide tension may act to stimulate gametogenesis (Marchoux and Chorine, 1932; Chorine, 1933; Bishop and McConnachie, 1956, 1960). More recent studies by Carter and Nijhout (1977) and Nijhout and Carter (1978) have confirmed and extended these observations. These workers have rigorously demonstrated that gametogenesis in *P. gallinaceum* is controlled by the rise in pH that occurs rather than by the loss of carbon dioxide in itself. They have also confirmed the prior observations of Bishop and McConnachie (1960) that bicarbonate is needed for gametogenesis and discovered, in addition, that gametogenesis requires a continuous source of glucose (presumably as an energy source). The general applicability to mammalian malaria of these findings with avian malaria has yet to be determined.

Micks *et al.* (1948) suggested that gametogenesis and fertilization of *P. elongatum* and *P. cathemerium* gametocytes were stimulated by a chemical factor released from the midgut of the vector mosquito after its ingestion of blood. Similar suggestions have been made by other authors (Ball and Chao, 1960). The possible role of a mosquito factor in their system was suggested by the fact that gametogenesis and ookinete formation proceeded only after the gametocytes had been taken into the midgut of the vector mosquito and subsequently placed in culture. Similarly, Yoeli and Upmanis (1968) were unable to observe direct gametocyte-to-ookinete transformation when *P. berghei*-infected blood was removed from hamsters and transferred directly to their culture system. However, if the blood was first ingested by the vector mosquito, *Anopheles stephensi,* and then collected a few minutes later after ejection from the anus of the fed mosquito, ookinete formation subsequently occurred *in vitro*. These authors also found that infected blood taken directly from hamsters and mixed with an aqueous extract of the mosquito midgut supported the *in vitro* development of ookinetes. Although a mosquito secretory factor was postulated as being involved in the control of the overall process of gametocyte-to-ookinete differentiation, no attempts were made to determine at what point the factor might exercise its control, i.e., gametogenesis, fertilization, or differentiation of the ookinete. That such a factor may actually be involved in the control of gametogenesis itself has been suggested by the work of Nijhout (1977). Material extracted from *Aedes aegypti* or *A. stephensi* mosquitoes induced exflagellation of *P. gallinaceum* gametocytes over a wide pH range (7.4–8.4). Normally, exflagellation does not take place at the lower pH values (below 7.8) if the mosquito factor is absent. This factor, which has been named mosquito exflagellation factor (MEF) is heat-stable and dialyzable.

Thus, several different factors seem capable of stimulating gametocytes to undergo gametogenesis. If the malaria parasite is to be successful and maintain itself in nature, it will require a dependable adaptive mechanism for sexual reproduction and transmission via the mosquito. Premature gamete formation in the vertebrate bloodstream or excessively delayed gamete formation in the mosquito midgut would be suicidal to the parasite's existence. The mature gametocytes circulating in the blood must be in a developmental state capable of almost instant response under appropriate conditions. At the same time, factors inhibitory to gamete formation must be present in the vertebrate's blood, while stimulating factors must be present in the mosquito midgut.

How these different factors act upon the gametocyte to induce gametogenesis is not clear. Perhaps these diverse external stimuli are all capable of acting upon an intracellular process which in itself is the direct mediator of gametogenesis. Several inhibitors of phosphodiesterase were found to stimulate gametogenesis in *P. gallinaceum* (Martin *et al.*, 1978). These agents are known to elevate intracellular concentrations of cyclic nucleotides by preventing their hydrolysis. It was thus proposed that cyclic nucleotides may be involved in the intracellular control of gamete formation.

C. Demonstration of Exflagellation

Induction of exflagellation in gametocytes that have developed *in vitro* requires that they be placed under different environmental conditions than those they developed under. This may involve merely removing a sample from culture and placing it at a lower environmental temperature, as was done by Trager (1941, 1943) for *P. lophurae*. In addition, MEF may be added (as suggested by R. Carter, personal communication) or the gametocytes may have to be resuspended in a new medium that allows a more effective rise in pH. Carter and Beach (1977) have pointed out that the Trager–Jensen medium commonly used to culture *P. falciparum* at pH 7.3–7.4 contains a powerful buffer [25mM *n*-2-hydroxyethylpiperazine-*n'*-2-ethanesulfonic acid (HEPES)] that may prevent the pH from rising sufficiently rapidly to initiate gametogenesis. These authors were able to demonstrate exflagellation of *P. falciparum* successfully only after the parasites were removed from the original culture medium, washed, and resuspended in serum adjusted to pH 8.0 with bicarbonate (Carter and Beach, 1977; Carter and Miller, 1979).

Exflagellation is commonly demonstrated *in vitro* and quantified either by allowing it to proceed within a drop on a microscope slide, after which the preparation is dried, fixed, and stained for microscopic observation at leisure

(James, 1934; Shute and Maryon, 1966), or by preparing a wet mount slide and observing the process directly *in vitro* while it is occurring. Direct observation of exflagellation while it is occurring may be easier and more accurate, because the activity of the event calls attention to itself. The initial events of gametogenesis can be easily observed as a center of activity disturbing surrounding erythrocytes, while it might readily be missed in a fixed and stained slide. Observations are best made with phase-contrast illumination at magnifications approximating 40×. The cells should be diluted so that exflagellation can be readily seen and not obscured by overlying erythrocytes (Sinden and Croll, 1975; Carter and Nijhout, 1977).

D. Ookinete Formation

Though exflagellation and the process of fertilization of *Plasmodium* were observed *in vitro* as early as the late 1800s (Laveran, 1880; MacCallum, 1898), *in vitro* formation of ookinetes was not so readily demonstrated. MacCallum (1898) was able to observe *in vitro* ookinete formation from gametocytes of *Haemoproteus,* but not from *Plasmodium* gametocytes (MacCallum, 1897). As noted in Section II, A and B, neither Ball and Chao (1960) nor Yoeli and Upmanis (1968) were able to obtain gametocyte-to-ookinete transformation *in vitro* unless the infected blood utilized was first ingested by a mosquito.

Direct *in vitro* formation of ookinetes from *P. berghei* gametocytes removed from a rodent and transferred directly into culture was described by Alger (1968) and Rosales-Ronquillo *et al.* (1974). However, these methods gave results that were either unrepeatable or yielded small numbers of ookinetes (Shapiro *et al.,* 1975; Vanderberg *et al.,* 1977).

A technique for *in vitro* production of *P. berghei* ookinetes on a regular and repeatable basis was presented by Weiss and Vanderberg (1977). Gametocyte-containing blood was removed aseptically from hamsters and added to Eagle's minimum essential medium (MEM) containing 15% fetal calf serum. Incubation at 21°–22°C for 18–24 hours resulted in the formation of motile ookinetes. Typically from 1000 to 2000 ookinetes could be produced per cubic millimeter of infected hamster blood inoculated into culture. The most important element in the successful production of ookinetes was the presence of a high gametocytemia. Cocultivation of the gametocytes with mosquito or fish cell lines, as suggested by Rosales-Ronquillo *et al.* (1974), did not increase the yield of ookinetes obtained by Weiss and Vanderberg (1977).

Another method for *in vitro* production of *P. berghei* ookinetes was subsequently described by Chen *et al.* (1977). Infected blood from hamsters was mixed with a medium made up of 1:1 Hanks' basic salt solution and fetal bovine serum. After filtering the preparation through a cellulose paper column to remove leukocytes, the mixture was further diluted with the 1:1 medium and allowed to incubate at 19°C for 1–2 hours. The zygotes so formed were concentrated by gradient centrifugation and then returned to culture at 19°C for ookinete formation. Comparative studies have indicated that this procedure results in a cleaner, more concentrated preparation of ookinetes than the Weiss and Vanderberg (1977) procedure, but that the latter procedure results in a higher overall recovery of ookinetes (M. M. Weiss and J. P. Vanderberg, unpublished results). Both procedures give repeatable and consistent results, provided large numbers of viable gametocytes are available. The Chen *et al.* (1977) procedure has been successfully adapted for use in the *in vitro* production of *P. gallinaceum* ookinetes (Carter *et al.*, 1979).

E. Differentiation of Oocysts and Subsequent Development of Sporozoites

The ookinete, formed by elongation of the zygote, traverses the epithelial wall of the midgut and, while remaining in direct contact with the basement membrane, begins to assume the spherical shape of the oocyst. This process, followed in detail at the ultrastructural level, has been estimated to take between 18 and 72 hours for completion (Garnham *et al.*, 1969; Canning and Sinden, 1973; Davies, 1974). The subsequent stages of oocyst development leading to the formation of sporozoites has been studied at this level even more extensively (Terzakis *et al.*, 1966; Vanderberg and Rhodin, 1967; Vanderberg *et al.*, 1967; Terzakis, 1971). In brief, differentiation of the solid, spherical oocyst is signaled by the onset of both vacuolation and cleft formation which subdivides the cytoplasm into a number of subunits termed sporoblasts or sporoblastoid bodies. Incipient sporozoites then emerge from the surface of the sporoblasts and elongate into definitive sporozoites after the transfer of both nuclear and cytoplasmic components from the large central bodies. Depending upon the species, the oocyst under optimum conditions reaches maturity 4–21 days after an infective blood meal (Shute and Maryon, 1966).

Until recently, the great majority of studies involving culture of the sporogonic stages centered around parasites which had already developed *in vivo* to the point of being recognizable as oocysts. Thus Ball (1947, 1948) placed intact *Culex tarsalis* midguts with visible *P. relictum* oocysts in culture between 6 and 10 days after the mosquitoes had ingested infected blood (the sporogonic phase requires 10 days *in vivo* at 27°C). The viability of the mosquito tissue was judged on the basis of contractility of the hindgut, while oocyst development was assessed histologically. Despite modifications in medium, serum supplements, and gas content of the flasks, the oocysts failed to develop further, although the hindgut continued to contract for as long as 7 days.

Attempts by Ragab (1949) to culture *P. gallinaceum* oocysts attached to *A. aegypti* midguts in either perfusion chambers or hanging drops met a similar fate even more quickly, with survival of the mosquito tissues not exceeding 96 hours.

In subsequent studies, Ball (1954, 1964) and Ball and Chao (1957, 1960) resorted to far more complex media, based in part on analysis of whole-body homogenates of the vector mosquito (Clark and Ball, 1952, 1954, 1956) and in part on synthetic media which other investigators had found capable of supporting the growth of vertebrate cells. The mosquito tissue continued to contract *in vitro* for as long as 34 days, but degeneration of the midgut wall epithelium and connective tissue was apparent within 5–7 days. Although some of the oocysts increased to three times their original diameter by day 4 or 5, the true extent of parasite development in these studies is difficult to assess. The percentage of oocysts that showed some growth as compared to those which either showed no change or even decreased in size was not stated, nor were any details of the changes in internal development of the parasites given. The effectiveness of the more complex media is also difficult to assess, since other modifications in technique, perhaps of equal importance, were made simultaneously; namely, reducing the temperature of the cultures to 17°–18°C for the initial 24 hours and reducing the ratio of the volume of medium to the mass of tissue. Unquestionably, a somewhat more favorable *in vitro* environment was provided in these studies, but it should be emphasized that both the rate and the extent of oocyst development never approached that of the *in situ* controls.

Since Weathersby (1952) had shown that *P. gallinaceum* oocysts could develop in the hemocoel of a mosquito vector without benefit of attachment to the midgut wall, Ball and Chao (1957) dissected *P. relictum* oocysts away from the wall before placing them in a number of culture media supplemented with chick serum and embryo extract. Once again, the result was a limited amount of growth and development.

Despite repeated attempts by these investigators, little progress was made in defining the conditions required for long-term cultivation of the parasites. All but the most mature oocysts ceased development *in vitro* after 4 or 5 days, regardless of modifications in the medium or changes involving the type of culture chamber, extent of aeration, or method of medium exchange (Ball and Chao, 1963a,b, 1964; Ball, 1964). *In vitro* maturation and liberation of sporozoites from oocysts was possible only if the latter had undergone considerable development in the mosquito before being explanted (Ball and Chao, 1961).

Essentially similar results were obtained by Schneider (1968a) who cultured *P. gallinaceum* oocysts, usually along with small fragments of *A. aegypti* midgut, in a modification of Grace's culture medium (1962) supplemented with chick or fetal bovine serum. Other supplements (rabbit sera, chick embryo extract, and heterologous hemolymph), as well as mosquito tissue, were incorporated into some of the cultures. In general, the more mature the oocysts when placed in culture, the greater both the number of oocysts developing and the extent of that development. Thus, 9-day oocysts (the sporogonic phase of *P.*

gallinaceum in vivo is completed in 10 days at 25°C), containing immature sporozoites, required an additional 24 hours *in vitro* before rupturing. In contrast, 6-, 7- and early 8-day oocysts, which were still quite immature, showed no detectable growth or differentiation. However, in 8-day oocysts where the process of sporoblast formation and the budding of incipient sporozoites had occurred prior to explantation, the development of motile but noninfectious sporozoites took place in about 60% of the cultures.

The availability of a purported cell line from the mosquito *A. aegypti* (Grace, 1966) prompted Schneider (1968b) to test whether such cells could be used as a supportive substrate for parasite growth. Despite the presence of the cells, the same pattern of development was seen with 8- and 9-day oocysts as in medium alone, although a somewhat higher percentage of oocysts underwent development. The behavior of the younger oocysts appeared to depend upon the concentration of cells in the culture. Initial concentrations of 10^5/ml had a positive effect on the oocysts, as evidenced by the partitioning of the oocyst cytoplasm. However, at this concentration, the cells overgrew the flasks within 72 hours to the detriment of both cells and parasites. Removal of cells followed by partial renewal of the medium had no beneficial effect. Attempts to suppress cell multiplication with mitomycin C, in effect providing a "feeder layer" for the parasites (Puck and Marcus, 1955), were equally unsuccessful. The failure of the cells to provide a more adequate milieu than medium alone was attributed at the time to modifications in the cells' properties which had inevitability accrued during the long interval between initiation of the primary culture and establishment of the line. About 4 years later, however, Greene and Charney (1971) unequivocally demonstrated that the cells were of lepidopteran rather than mosquito origin.

Rather surprisingly, the presence of this same cell line was reported by Ball and Chao (1971) to enhance the growth of *P. relictum* oocysts when compared to medium alone or when the parasites were cultured with a bona fide line of *A. aegypti* cells (Singh, 1967). Within 1 week, a two- to threefold increase in diameter was noted in 3- and 4-day-old oocysts, while apparently mature sporozoites developed from 5-day-old oocysts after 6–8 days of culture. In comparing the results of culturing *P. gallinaceum* versus *P. relictum* with these lepidoteran cells, Schneider (1972) suggested that the latter plasmodial species, which tolerates a broad host–vector association in nature, might be less demanding of a culture system than the more restrictive *P. gallinaceum* parasite. Such an explanation, however, fails to account for the lack of any positive response on the part of *P. relictum* to an authentic mosquito cell line.

The probability that cells from any continuous insect cell line differ fundamentally from those in the intact insect, as a result of selective, adaptive, or genetic mechanisms (Brooks and Kurtti, 1971), led Schneider (1972) to compare the relative merits of primary cultures versus an established line of *A. stephensi* cells in supporting *P. cynomolgi* oocysts. While the oocysts invariably survived for a longer time *in vitro* when mosquito cells were present, there were no obvious differences in the extent of support, as measured by oocyst growth and/or development, between the two types of culture. In addition, cells from adult tissues in primary culture were no more effective than those from larval tissues.

In contrast to the above studies, in which identifiable oocysts were placed in culture, there are a few reports of oocysts or oocystlike structures developing *in vitro* following explantation of intact midguts containing *P. relictum*-infected blood (Ball and Chao, 1960; Ball, 1972) or of *P. berghei* gametocytes transferred to a nonvector (fathead minnow) cell line (Rosales-Sharp and Silverman, 1976). In the former studies, oocysts were seen developing on the midgut wall by day 4 *in vitro*, the largest attaining sizes of up to 31 μm in diameter. In the latter study, oocystlike structures were first seen on day 8 but apparently did not retain their morphological integrity for any length of time. Unfortunately, adequate documentation that these structures were indeed oocysts was not given in any of the above studies. Cultures such as these often contain substantial numbers of degenerating cells that superficially resemble oocysts. Such cells may originate from the explanted mosquito tissue, from the vertebrate host blood meal, or from the cocultured cell line. Careful morphological and histological study is required to distinguish these nonparasite cells from actual oocysts that have presumably developed *in vitro*. An even more rigorous procedure, as yet untried, for authenticating oocysts is the use of a fluorescent antibody test employing antibodies that react specifically with the parasite and not with the other cells in the culture.

At the opposing end of the sporogonic phase, differentiation of cultured oocysts to the point of releasing apparently mature sporozoites was reported for three species of malaria. Although the oocysts were well advanced developmentally when placed in culture, additional development, as with the younger stages, almost invariably lagged behind that of their counterparts *in vivo*. In the first study, both intact oocysts containing sporozoites and released sporozoites from ruptured oocysts of *P. relictum* were injected into parasite free canaries after 24–96 hours *in vitro*. Ten to 11 days later, sporozoites were found in the salivary glands of mosquitoes that had fed on 2 of the 11 injected canaries. Although additional oocysts from these same cultures continued to release sporozoites for up to 120 hours, none proved to be infectious. Indeed, the freed sporozoites lost both their motility and normal morphology within 24–48 hours (Ball and Chao, 1961).

Schneider (1968a) reported similar results when virtually mature *P. gallinaceum* oocysts were placed in culture. Four out of five chicks developed parasitemias after the injection of sporozoites released from oocysts less than 24 hours earlier. Once again, free sporozoites that remained *in vitro* for longer intervals were no longer infectious and became progressively more sluggish in their movements. Interestingly, sporozoites retained within oocysts that failed to rupture continued to show very active flexing movements for up to 7 days in culture. However, none of these "encapsulated" sporozoites were tested for infectivity.

In the third study, the infectiousness of cultured *P. berghei* sporozoites proved even more tenuous; only those injected within 3 hours of their release were infective to *Thamnomys surdaster*. The most successful cultures, defined as showing both oocyst growth and sporozoite release, were those that also included salivary glands (Walliker and Robertson, 1970).

In the interval between release from oocysts and eventual residence in the salivary glands, sporozoites undergo a maturation process which has been documented at the ultrastructural level (Vanderberg *et al.,* 1967; Vanderberg and Rhodin, 1967; Sterling *et al.,* 1973; Sinden and Garnham, 1973). Gradual changes in motility and increases in infectivity and antigenicity also take place (Vanderberg *et al.,* 1969, 1972; Vanderberg, 1974, 1975; Nussenzweig and Chen, 1974). Vanderberg (1975) suggested that this maturation process may be time-dependent rather than site-dependent. This seems to be true for at least two of the properties listed above. Once discrete sporozoites are seen in the intact oocyst, they become increasingly motile and upon rupture of the oocyst display not only active flexing and thrusting movements but also a kind of circular gliding motion similar to that described for mature sporozoites removed from salivary glands (Vanderberg, 1974). However, these movements gradually decline and cease altogether within 24–72 hours. Infectivity of recently released sporozoites has likewise been documented, but this property is also lost after, at most, 24 hours in the free state. Thus, residence in the salivary glands is not essential for either the acquisition of infectivity or for the appearance of a mature sporozoite gliding pattern. Apparently, the longer interval required for development within the cultured oocysts, sometimes a matter of hours, but often a matter of days, is sufficient for the sporozoites to acquire these two properties. Unfortunately, no attempts have been made to test whether such cultured sporozoites have any immunogenic potential, nor have any studies been made at the ultrastructural level. Of clear concern, however, is the loss of both motility and infectivity and probably viability so shortly after the sporozoites attain an extracellular state *in vitro*.

As discussed in previous sections, there have been a number of successes in recent years in the support *in vitro* of gametogenesis, fertilization, and ookinete formation by the malaria parasite. This is not too surprising in view of the fact that these developmental processes take place in the relatively unspecialized environment of the mosquito midgut during digestion of a blood meal. Subsequent sporogonic development, however, takes place in the much more specialized environment of the mosquito hemocoel. As detailed in the present section, progress in supporting the *in vitro* differentiation of these later stages has been less notable. This lack of progress can be attributed principally to two interrelated factors. With few exceptions, the oocysts were cultured in association with host tissue, sometimes because of technical considerations but more often either in the belief that the parasites were incapable of development without such tissue or with the expectation that the tissue would provide additional support over that of medium alone. However, until the late 1960s insect tissue culture tended to be a rather mystifying and inexact science. Hence investigators had to confront two different sets of unknowns when attempting to culture both parasite and host tissue simultaneously. The other salient and related shortcoming has been the lack of genuinely adequate culture media for both cells and parasites. Although some media have been patterned after the composition of the hemolymph of a particular insect, most have been assembled empirically, with components included or excluded on the basis of trial and error. Also, rather frequently, media designed for cells of one species have been utilized for culturing those of another. The fact that insect cells can adapt and grow under such culture conditions attests to their plasticity *in vitro,* a property malaria parasites apparently lack.

Fortunately, advances have been made on both fronts in recent years. If a cell substrate is found necessary for the additional development of parasites, standardized procedures are now available for initiating cell lines at will from a wide variety of insects, including many species of mosquitoes. In addition, it should now be possible to design culture media which more closely simulate the internal milieu of the mosquito vector based on recently completed analyses of adult anopheline hemolymph. Both of these topics are addressed more thoroughly in the following two sections.

III. CURRENT METHODS OF INITIATING PRIMARY CELL AND ORGAN CULTURES FROM MOSQUITO SPECIES WITH EMPHASIS ON ANOPHELINES

Throughout this section, the term "primary culture" implies that the culture was initiated from cells, tissues, or organs taken directly from one or more mosquitoes and from any stage of development. A continuous cell line arises from a primary culture after repeated subculturings, demonstrating the potential to be maintained indefinitely *in vitro* (Federoff, 1967).

A. Primary Cell Cultures and the Evolution of Continuous Cell Lines

With few exceptions, primary cultures from mosquito species initiated for the purpose of establishing continuous cell lines have been restricted to minced, trypsinized neonate larvae. This preference is due to four advantages the younger stages have over the older; namely, they can usually be collected in large numbers and in fairly synchronous development, their surfaces are easily sterilized to eliminate the possibility of contamination, the cells are in a very active stage of division and such stages are unable to synthesize tyrosinase (phenol oxidase), an enzyme which produces melanin via intermediary quinones that are toxic to cell cultures. Generally, about 200 larvae are required to initiate a culture vessel containing 1.25 ml of medium. A number of media have been used for culturing anopheline species (Singh and Bhat, 1969; Schneider, 1969; Pudney and Varma, 1971; Rosales-Ronquillo *et al.,* 1972; Stone and Hink, 1973), but adequate comparisons of their relative merits have not been made. All the media are supplemented with 10–20% fetal bovine serum.

Surface sterilization is accomplished by immersion of embryos having red eyespots (or a comparable developmental stage) in a 1:1 solution of bleach (approximately 5% sodium hypochlorite) and distilled water for 1–2 minutes followed by two changes of either 70% ethanol or 0.5% mercurous chloride in 70% ethanol for 5 minutes each. The eggs are washed several times in distilled water and then transferred to a petri dish having several layers of sterile, moistened filter paper. The larvae, after hatching in a 25°–28°C incubator, are cut into two or three pieces and incubated in 0.2–0.25% trypsin in Rinaldini's salt solution (Rinaldini, 1954) for 40–60 minutes at room temperature or for 5–10 minutes at 35°C. The pieces are washed a few times with complete medium (medium containing serum) and transferred to a suitable culture flask. Antibiotics are not routinely added to the cultures. [Additional technical details on maintaining the primary cultures until sufficient growth has occurred for successful subculturing may be found in papers by Schneider (1973) and Schneider and Blumenthal (1978).]

After a lag of 1–3 weeks, growth within the cultures takes place in one of two ways. In some instances, the cell clumps or larval pieces attach to the floor of the culture vessel and cells begin to migrate and divide, forming colonies of various sizes around the central mass. Equally likely, or in addition, hollow, cellular vesicles arise from the ends of the larval fragments as the latter remain floating in the medium. The vesicles, which are quite characteristic of dipteran primary cultures, enlarge by cell division and eventually tend to attach to the vessel bottom, break open, and continue growth as cell sheets. The interval between initiation of the primary culture and the initial subculture for anopheline species varies from 10 weeks (Marhoul and Pudney, 1972) to 3–4 months (Schneider, 1969; Pudney and Varma, 1971). Such an extensive adaptation period tends to be characteristic of insect cell culture in general and may well reflect inadequacies of the culture media rather than refractoriness on the part of the cells themselves (Brooks and Kurtti, 1971; Schneider and Blumenthal, 1978). Of the more than 30 continuous cell lines thus far established from mosquitoes, only two species, *A. gambiae* and *A. stephensi,* from the genus *Anopheles* are represented (Schneider, 1969; Pudney and Varma, 1971; Marhoul and Pudney, 1972); the remainder and great majority of lines have come from the genera *Aedes* and *Culex* (Hink, 1976).

Regardless of the source of the explants or the medium in which they are grown, a number of generalizations hold true for all the current mosquito cell lines. The cells grow in ambient air at optimum temperatures between 24° and 29°C, can withstand fairly wide ranges of pH and osmolality, and have a doubling time approaching that of vertebrate cell lines, even though the latter are grown at higher temperatures. The diploid number of chromosomes ($2n = 6$) predominates in the majority of cell lines, although heteroploidy becomes increasingly common as the time in culture increases. Most of the cells are readily pipetted off the bottom of the flask, so that it is rarely necessary to use any enzymatic treatment to detach them prior to subculturing. At least for the early passages, such enzymatic treatment tends to be detrimental to the cells. Finally, the cells are very sensitive to the quality of the serum supplement, tending to round up and float when subjected to unsuitable lots and being unable to reattach to a glass or plastic substrate upon subculturing.

B. Organ Cultures

Reports on primary explants of intact mosquito organs have been quite limited. The dissection of organs other than pupal or adult ovaries often results in bacterial and/or fungal contamination. Starving the mosquitoes 24–48 hours prior to dissection, as well as feeding them antibiotics to eliminate the microbes in the digestive tract, has been tried with varying degrees of success (Micks and Ferguson, 1961; Chao and Ball, 1964; Schneider, 1972). This contamination can be reduced by surface sterilization and by taking care not to rupture the diverticula during dissection, as the lumen of this fluid-filled sac contains large numbers of microbial contaminants. The use of axenically grown mosquitoes as a source for explants is very appealing, and a number of simple as well as very complex media have been devised for several species (Akov, 1962; Boorman, 1967, Wallis and Lite, 1970; Rosales-Ronquillo *et al.*, 1973). Unfortunately, the culture conditions are often difficult to duplicate, and the mosquitoes produced tend to be less vigorous than those raised under normal insectary conditions. Thus far, only Rosales-Ronquillo *et al.* (1972) have cultured organs from axenically reared *A. stephensi*. No obvious deterioration of the explants was apparent for up to 30 days *in vitro*.

Entire midguts with (Ragab, 1949; Ball, 1972) or without the peritrophic membrane (Gubler, 1968), as well as portions of midgut (see Section II), have been cultured for periods ranging from 2 days to 12 weeks. As the time in culture increases, maintenance of the structural and functional integrity of the organ becomes increasingly difficult, as evidenced by central necrosis. Inadequate oxygen or carbohydrate supplies and the accumulation of toxic metabolic products may hasten this process. Hence organ cultures tend to be short-lived. Occasionally, however, before any necrosis is visible or when it is still relatively minimal, migratory cells may issue from what appears to be a fully intact organ. These cells may proceed to divide and form growing cell sheets which gradually transform an organ culture into a cell culture. Although no continuous cell lines from mosquito midgut are available, all three existing cell lines from adult ovaries evolved in this manner (Kitamura, 1970; Hsu *et al.*, 1970, 1972). There is a good possibility, however, that these cells are not of ovarian origin; rather, they probably consist of one or more types of hemocytes or blood cells which normally circulate in the hemolymph and adhere to many, if not all, of the organs within the insect body (Smith, 1968). Thus far, five different hemocyte types (prohemocytes, plasmatocytes, granular cells, adipocytes, and spherule cells, according to the classification of Jones, 1970) have been described from the hemolymph of *A. stephensi* adults (D. A. Foley and J. P. Vanderberg, unpublished).

With one exception, salivary glands from mosquitoes have been incubated for 48 hours or less rather than placed under true long-term culture conditions (Walliker and Robertson, 1970; I. Schneider, unpublished results). In the study of Gavrilov and Cowez (1941), glands of both aedine and anopheline mosquitoes were cultured for up to 20 days in a medium consisting of chick plasma, chick embryo extract, and mosquito extract. Surface sterilization of the adults, followed by 6–10 rinses of the extirpated glands, was apparently sufficient to avoid contamination of the cultures. Both cell migration and division were reported, but here again, the surviving cells may well have been hemocytes rather than integral components of the glands themselves. Most surprising was the assertion that cultures held at 37°C, a temperature approaching the thermal limits of mosquitoes (Bates, 1949), gave better results than those held at 24°–26°C. Other adult mosquito organs that have been cultured for short periods of time have been the fat body and thoracic muscle (Hagedorn and Judson, 1972).

C. Some Limiting Factors of Mosquito Substrates for the Growth and Development of the Sporogonic Stages of Malaria Parasites

As seen in Section II, E, oocyst viability and development were enhanced to some extent by the presence of a cell substrate. Two questions have yet to be fully answered, however: (1) Why are the cells of the mosquito host, either in the form of continuous cell lines or as organ cultures, unable to support complete development of the parasites *in vitro* (2) Why are cell lines from nonvector sources sometimes more effective as substrates than those from the natural vectors? As stated previously, most of these lines require a long adjustment period between initiation of the primary culture and the first successful subculture. The extent of this adjustment is also reflected in the slower growth rate of cells in the early subpassages than in the later passages. The cell types which survive are only a fraction of those originally present and, of course, are of unknown origin. In addition, it has been known for a long time that the composition of insect hemolymph changes, often quite markedly, as the insect advances from the embryonic to the adult stage, doubtless reflecting the changing requirements of the cells (Florkin and Jeuniaux, 1974). Yet all but a few of the continuous mosquito cell lines have been initiated from the embryonic or neonatal stage. Such cells even *in situ* may not be fully able to support development of the parasites. The supportive capabilities of the descendants of these cells, substantially altered both biochemically and physiologically by the long adjustment period *in vitro,* may be even further reduced. Another factor, yet to be investigated, is the possible influence of the hormonal balance of the intact insect on the development of the parasite.

The partial successes of Ball and Chao (1971) and Rosales-Ronquillo *et al.* (1974) in using such substrates as a moth cell line and fathead minnow cells to support growth of the oocyst and ookinete stages of *P. relictum* and *P. berghei,* respectively, suggest that unidentified growth factors may be equally as important, if not more so, than the specific origin of the cells themselves. This possibility, unfortunately, has been only briefly addressed (Rosales-Sharp and Silverman, 1976).

If cells from continuous lines no longer show sufficient affinity to those of the intact mosquito vector in supporting parasite development, a logical assumption is that primary cultures would provide a more adequate substrate. This approach has been tried by a few investigators (Schneider, 1972; Rosales-Ronquillo and Silverman, 1974; Speer *et al.,* 1975) but with only modest success. However, valid comparisons between the two types of culture systems are not yet possible because of pronounced differences in the growth rates of the respective cells. Adequate evaluations of the effectiveness of organ cultures are equally difficult to make, as whole organs rarely remain healthy *in vitro* for any length of time or, if they do, tend to enter a state of "suspended animation" (Schneider, 1967), a decidedly unpromising environment for actively growing parasites.

Reducing the interval of adjustment for primary cell cultures and/or developing truly adequate conditions for insect organ cultures might well lead to additional development of the malaria parasites. Since most media for mosquito cell or organ cultures have been designed as a result of empirical observations, one obvious starting point is to formulate a medium based on adult hemolymph analysis, followed if possible by an assessment of the value of the individual components in the medium. As seen in the following section, some progress has been made in this direction.

IV. ADULT ANOPHELINE HEMOLYMPH ANALYSIS
AND THE DESIGN OF CULTURE MEDIA

The environment of the mosquito hemocoel is important not only as a source of nutrients for parasite growth but also presumably in furnishing environmental stimuli that regulate parasite differentiation. The malaria parasite is known to possess a complete genome at all stages of its development. Thus, the strikingly different stages of preerythrocytic schizogony, erythrocytic schizogony, gametogony, and sporogony the parasite passes through may be reflections of the different environmental stimuli it encounters within its hosts. Different milieus may control different phenotypic expressions of the parasite. A better understanding of the mosquito environment may lead to better control over the differentiation of the parasite stages occurring within the mosquito.

There are three main approaches that may be followed in the design of a suitable *in vitro* medium for cell culture: the *imitative approach* that seeks to duplicate the normal *in vivo* environment of the cell, the *empirical approach* that attempts to determine by trial and error which additive, and in what concentration, gives the best results of growth and differentiation of the cells being cultured, and the *depletive approach* that attempts to measure which nutrients are removed from the culture medium by the growing cells. There is a considerable amount of evidence indicating that the nutrition of the developing *Plasmodium* oocyst is mediated through the hemolymph rather than through the interface between the oocyst and its attachment to the midgut (Vanderberg *et al.*, 1977). Thus, the composition of this hemolymph should be taken into consideration in formulating a culture medium designed to support oocyst differentiation *in vitro*. At first consideration, cells *in vitro* should be expected to grow best in a culture medium that is an exact duplication of their normal *in vivo* milieu. However, this rarely works out in practice. For instance, early workers in vertebrate cell culture found that attempts to grow cells in 100% serum were unsuccessful. Thus, the imitative approach to designing culture media has its limitations. There are a number of reasons why this may be so.

1. Almost immediately after metabolizing cells are placed in culture, the composition of the medium changes. Nutrients are removed from the medium, and metabolic products of the cell pass into it. Under normal *in vivo* conditions, the environment around the cell remains in better homeostasis because of the replenishment of nutrients and removal of toxic products. Thus, in the design of culture medium, some nutrients may have to be included in higher than normal *in vivo* concentrations to allow for these losses to the cell.

2. Chemical analyses of *in vivo* fluids are always imperfect. Because of the small quantities of hemolymph that can be collected from mosquitoes, only estimates of the concentrations of the different components can be made. Many

components such as hormones and various growth factors may be totally undetectable.

3. Even if an accurate analysis of hemolymph could be made, it should be kept in mind that this composition changes at different times during the adult life of the mosquito. Hemolymph composition is likely to be quite different, for instance, shortly after a blood meal versus immediately after egg deposition. Thus, the concept of a single normal *in vivo* environment is not a valid one.

4. At a given time in the life of a mosquito, there may be differences in hemolymph composition at different points throughout the body because of the relatively inefficient circulation within the mosquito. Hemolymph within the thorax, where the large flight muscles are concentrated, is likely to be different in composition from the hemolymph adjacent to the ovaries and midgut, located within the abdomen. An analysis of hemolymph collected from whole mosquitoes reflects an average of the hemolymph components found throughout the hemocoel, which might be quite different from the concentrations of these components within the microenvironment surrounding the oocysts.

5. As will be discussed subsequently, an analysis of the chemical components found within the hemolymph may include some constituents that are normally bound or chelated to macromolecules *in vivo*. Thus, the total amounts determined by analysis and the amounts actually free and available to the oocyst may differ considerably.

In spite of all these theoretical shortcomings an analysis of the normal *in vivo* milieu is an important starting point in the rational design of a suitable culture medium. Subsequent empirical culture studies can then be done to change and improve the culture medium. Relatively little has been done, however, on the analysis of mosquito hemolymph. A number of studies have attempted to determine the chemical constituents of the whole mosquito by the analysis of homogenates prepared from batches of whole mosquitoes (citations in Vanderberg *et al.*, 1977). Most of these studies were done with culicine rather than anopheline mosquitoes. This is unfortunate, since most current interest in malaria parasite cultivation centers on mammalian malaria, with the prospect of ultimate application to *P. falciparum*.

In an attempt to resolve this problem, recent studies were undertaken on an analysis of the hemolymph of *A. stephensi,* an efficient vector of both rodent and human malaria (Mack and Vanderberg, 1978a; Mack *et al.*, 1979a,b). Hemolymph was collected from adult female mosquitoes by two different procedures: centrifugation of whole mosquitoes whose body wall had been incised to permit escape of the hemolymph, and perfusion of the mosquito hemocoel by introducing fluid into the hemocoel with a fine pipet and collecting the perfusate that flowed out of the incised body wall. Quantitative determinations were made of the physical characteristics of the hemolymph (Mack and Vanderberg, 1978a), and of the free amino acids (Mack *et al.*, 1979a) and carbohydrates present (Mack *et al.*, 1979b).

In discussing the design of a suitable culture medium, the following factors are considered separately: osmolarity, inorganic components, free amino acids, sugars, and macromolecules. By assessing some of the theoretical considerations involved, by summarizing the results of the hemolymph analyses thus far conducted, and by evaluating the successes and failures of the empirical approaches that have so far been taken, a better understanding of how to approach the problem in the future may be obtained.

A. Osmolarity

In general, animal cell lines, including those from insects, can withstand a wide range of osmolarities *in vitro*, but within definite high and low limits. This range bears a relationship to the osmolarity of the normal body fluid of the animal from which the culture is initiated. For instance, Kurtti *et al.*, (1974) found that a cell line of lepidopteran origin showed excellent *in vitro* growth rates within a range of osmolalities between 290 and 360 mOsmoles. The hemolymph of the insect from which the cell line originated was 318 mOsmoles (Adams and Wilcox, 1973). The osmolality of the blood of vertebrates is known to vary within relatively narrow limits (generally at levels between 290 and 305 mOsmoles), while that of insect hemolymph may vary considerably under different physiological conditions even within the same species.

The range of osmolalities tolerated by the oocysts of the malaria parasite, or by mosquito tissues in culture, is yet to be determined. The newly emerged adult female *A. stephensi* contains hemolymph with an osmolality of 412 mOsmoles. By 11 days after the mosquito has ingested a blood meal infected with *P. berghei* the hemolymph osmolality has reached 490 mOsmoles, and even higher (550 mOsmoles) after a noninfected blood meal (Mack and Vanderberg, 1978a). Interestingly, these levels are considerably higher than levels (325–390 mOsmoles) found in the media currently used to culture mosquito tissues (Stone and Hink, 1973). Schneider's (1969) modification of Grace's medium, employed in the only reported study on cultivation of the oocysts of a mammalian malaria parasite, has an osmotic pressure of 325 mOsmoles. In view of the rather high findings with *A. stephensi* hemolymph, it would be of interest to raise the osmotic pressure of culture media used for malaria parasites to levels approximating these estimated *in vivo* values.

B. Inorganic Constituents

Lockwood (1961) has pointed out that a satisfactory physiological saline solution for the *in vitro* maintenance of tissues may not necessarily be an exact duplicate of the normal *in vivo* fluid. One of the reasons for this is that some of the inorganic constituents may be bound to other components and thus are not freely available within the solution. Willis and Sunderman (1952) have found that about 50% of the divalent cations (Ca^{2+} and Mg^{2+}) are not freely ionized, being bound instead to organic components. Thus, if one were to use the inorganic elemental analysis of serum or hemolymph as a guide in preparing an imitative culture medium, the high degree of ionization might result in a medium with much higher concentrations of ions than are actually present *in vivo*. Such high concentrations may be toxic to tissues. Hoyle (1957) has shown that a saline with the measured magnesium concentration found in locust hemolymph sends the muscles of the insect into fibrillation. Therefore, an appropriate analysis of the inorganic constituents of mosquito hemolymph should include not only a quantitative elemental analysis but also a determination of the degree of ionization of these constituents.

No such analysis is yet available for mosquito hemolymph. Some analyses of homogenized mosquito organs (Bradford and Ramsey, 1949) or whole mosquitoes (Clark and Ball, 1954) are suspect because they include concentrations of both intracellular and extracellular components. The Na^+/K^+ ratio, for instance, is normally quite different intracellularly and extracellularly. Determination of the ratio for the insect as a whole gives no helpful information about the ratio of these ions in the extracellular fluid. The classic studies of Ringer (1883) with vertebrate tissues demonstrated that the ratios of the constituent inorganic ions to one another may be more important than their actual concentrations. These ratios may be of considerable importance in insect physiology, in view of Kroeger and Müller's (1973) findings which suggest that changes in these ratios may be involved in gene activation in dipteran polytene chromosomes. On the other hand, data on the cultivation of a wide variety of cells indicate that many cells *in vitro* can withstand a considerable range of Na^+/K^+ ratios but may be sensitive to the actual amounts of K^+ present (Kurtti *et al.*, 1975; Fish *et al.*, 1973). Other ratios that may be of importance *in vivo* or *in vitro* are Mg^{2+}/Ca^{2+} and the ratio of the monovalent cations (Na^+ plus K^+) to the divalent cations (Mg^{2+} plus Ca^{2+}).

C. Sugars and Organic Acids

Glucose and trehalose are known to be the chief sugars in insects and have been shown to be the most abundant sugars in the hemolymph of *A. stephensi* (Mack *et al.*, 1979b). These sugars have also been identified in whole-body homogenates of adult *Culex* mosquitoes (Lakshmi and Subrahmanyan, 1975). After the discovery by Wyatt and Kalf (1957) that trehalose, a nonreducing disaccharide, was a major sugar in insect hemolymph, many workers in insect tissue culture added this sugar to their media in an attempt to obtain better cell growth. However, no one has yet been able to demonstrate that trehalose has any special virtue over glucose in supporting growth of insect cell lines. Media containing only glucose as an energy source seems to be quite adequate for the growth of insect cell lines (Vaughn, 1971; Stone and Hink, 1973). However, it is conceivable that the sporogonic stages of *Plasmodium* may have special requirements for trehalose. Mack and Vanderberg (1978b) report that this sugar, as well as glucose, can be used directly by sporozoites for energy metabolism. These authors have also presented evidence that the reduced levels of hemolymph sugar found in malaria-infected mosquitoes may be due to direct utilization of sugar by the growing parasites. Until it can be demonstrated that the mosquito stages of the malaria parasite have no special requirement for trehalose, it seems prudent to include it together with glucose in the medium. Total sugar levels found in *A. stephensi* hemolymph were found to be on the order of 1–4 mg/ml at different stages of adult life. These are well within the levels generally reported for the hemolymph of other insects. However, insect cell lines are able to withstand considerably higher levels of sugars. Grace (1962) used total carbohydrate levels of over 25 mg/ml in his medium, which has been widely used for the culture of insect tissues.

In addition to the use of sugars in energy metabolism, they are also utilized as precursors in lipid synthesis by the mosquito (Van Handel, 1965; Lakshmi and Subrahmanyam, 1975). Sugars may likewise be the source of some of the lipids required by the parasite, either directly by synthesis of lipids within the parasite or by transport of these synthesized lipids from the hemolymph to the parasite.

Large quantities of organic acids are also found in insect hemolymph, chiefly tricarboxylic acid (TCA) cycle intermediates such as citrate, α-ketoglutarate, succinate, fumarate, malate, and oxaloacetate. At physiological pH values these acids tend to be in their salt form and accordingly may account for a considerable proportion of the anionic components of the hemolymph. Thus, by binding cations, these organic acids may affect the ion ratios, the osmotic pressure, and the buffering capacity of hemolymph (Florkin and Jeuniaux, 1974). The only TCA cycle intermediate found in *A. stephensi* hemolymph was malate, though other organic acids and esters were also found including glucuronate, glycerophosphate, lactate, and phosphoethanolamine (Mack *et al.*, 1979b).

D. Amino Acids

Insect hemolymph is uniquely characterized by relatively high levels of free amino acids which may contribute as much as 40% of the total osmotic pressure of the hemolymph (Vaughn, 1971). Mack *et al.* (1979a) were able to identify 24 free amino acids or their derivatives in the hemolymph of *A. stephensi* females at various stages of their adult life. Total free amino acid levels of approximately 1.4 mg/ml of hemolymph were found after mosquitoes had taken a blood meal, the major amino acids being alanine, glutamic acid, histidine, lysine, methionine, proline, and valine. Mosquitoes infected with the rodent malaria parasite *P. berghei* had levels of total free amino acids that were about one-third of the levels found in noninfected ones. The chief differences that occurred with individual free amino acids were that infected mosquitoes had greater increases in arginine, greater decreases in valine and histidine, and a total loss of detectable methionine. It is known that free amino acids can be directly utilized by the sporogonic stages of the malaria parasite. The studies of Ball and Chao (1976) have suggested that *P. relictum* oocysts remove free amino acids from the medium in which they are growing, and other studies have demonstrated the incorporation of tritiated leucine *in vivo* into oocysts of *P. gallinaceum* (Vanderberg *et al.*, 1967) and *in vitro* into ookinetes of *P. berghei* (Weiss and Vanderberg, 1976). In addition, *P. berghei* sporozoites appear to be capable of utilizing amino acids as substrates for energy metabolism (Mack and Vanderberg, 1978b).

The depletion of an essential amino acid *in vivo* or *in vitro* by the parasite may serve as a factor limiting further growth of the parasite. It is thus important that all amino acids, especially those heavily used by the parasite, be in adequate supply. One can establish the general principle that the parasite itself is best able to establish its own nutritional needs. If an excess of a mixture of amino acids is included in a medium, the parasite should be able to select those that it needs for its growth and development. However, some amino acids may have a toxic effect. Mitsuhashi (1976) has shown that β-alanine may have detrimental effects on the growth of cell cultures from butterfly pupal ovaries, and on these grounds Wyatt and Wyatt (1976) have suggested that this amino acid should be omitted from insect tissue culture media. One must also be cautious about interactions between amino acids and other components of the medium. Histidine, for instance, is an effective chelator for divalent cations. Its presence in large amounts may thus distort ionic ratios within the media. If histidine becomes depleted from the medium, however, the increased availability of the divalent cations could cause precipitation of the relatively insoluble phosphates of calcium and magnesium (Wyatt and Wyatt, 1976).

E. Proteins and Other Macromolecules

Many of the early workers in insect tissue culture found a need to supplement their media with hemolymph collected from the species of insect being cultured (Vaughn, 1971). Though adequate quantities of hemolymph can be collected from large insects such as lepidopterans and orthopterans, it obviously becomes an impossibility with smaller insects approaching the size of a mosquito. Fortunately, it is possible to replace insect hemolymph with vertebrate serum as a supplement to the medium for maintaining the growth, if perhaps not all of the specialized functions, of mosquito cells. A number of different lines of mosquito cells have now been grown in media containing bovine sera without the addition of insect hemolymph (reviewed in Hink, 1976). Based on this, *Plasmodium* oocysts cocultured with insect cell lines have been grown in media supplemented with only small quantities of insect hemolymph or none at all. Schneider (1972) cultured *P. cynomolgi* oocysts in the presence of *A. stephensi* cells in a medium that included 15% fetal bovine serum. Ball and Chao (1971) cultured *P. relictum* oocysts together with mosquito or lepidopteran cells in a medium supplemented with 10% fetal bovine serum and a low concentration (0.5%) of hemolymph from the moth *Samia cynthia*. Whether complete sporogonic development can be supported *in vitro* without the presence of mosquito hemolymph remains to be determined. Perhaps essential growth factors normally obtained from mosquito hemolymph can eventually be supplied by cocultivation with mosquito cells or organs.

Nothing is known, of course, about which components of hemolymph are required by mosquito cells or malaria parasites *in vitro*, while studies on the components of serum specifically utilized by mosquito cells in culture have barely begun (Kuno *et al.*, 1971). Insect hemolymph generally contains considerably lower quantities of protein than vertebrate serum. *Anopheles stephensi* hemolymph has a protein content on the order of only 0.1% (S. R. Mack and J. P. Vanderberg, unpublished results). This content presumably fluctuates considerably, being highest during vitellogenesis when large quantities of yolk protein are being transferred through the hemolymph from the fat body to the ovaries. *In vitro* duplication of normal *in vivo* protein concentrations is clearly not essential (and may even be harmful), since vertebrate and invertebrate cell lines are quite successfully grown in media typically supplemented with only about 10–20% serum. Aside from the specific role that some proteins may play in tissue maintenance *in vitro*, the overall protein content may significantly affect other attributes of the medium. These proteins not only exert osmotic effects themselves but may also bind ions and small molecules, including water. This could have a subsequent effect on the overall osmotic pressure of the medium (since osmolality depends upon the number of osmotically active particles available), as well as on the relative ratios of the different ions in solution.

Serum supplements may also supply other essential requirements for cell growth, including vitamins, lipids, and nucleotides. Virtually nothing is known about either the presence of these components in mosquito hemolymph, or the requirement for them by the malaria parasite. There is probably, however, a requirement for purines by the developing sporogonic stages. These stages, like the erythrocytic stages of the parasite, may rely on *de novo* synthesis of pyrimidines but may require exogenous sources of purines during development (Weiss and Vanderberg, 1976). Any of the essential nutrients, if known, can be supplied in defined form. Otherwise, they may be supplied in undefined additives such as serum, hemolymph, embryo extracts, or hydrolysates of yeast or animal tissues. The appropriate addition of these can be made only by the empirical approach. Some of the principles that should be considered in the addition of these supplements have been discussed by Vaughn (1971, 1973) and Wyatt and Wyatt (1976).

V. CONCLUDING REMARKS

Until recently, the culture of the sporogonic stages of malaria parasites has been, by default, a rather exclusive field of endeavor. The number of individuals who attempted to culture these stages in the 30 years between 1946 and 1976 was few and rarely were they contemporaries of one another. Not surprisingly, the extent of progress was very limited. This situation, fortunately, has been somewhat rectified during the past few years.

One of the most recent and significant advances has been the demonstration of ookinete formation *in vitro* from gametocyte-containing blood. Given the difficulty of obtaining mature gametocytes in continuous cultures of the erythrocytic stages, the use of ookinetes for assessing the factors required to support further sporogonous development *in vitro* is a very attractive alternative. Additional refinements in obtaining the ookinetes are needed, however, since present techniques are not sufficiently rigorous to exclude large numbers of parasitized red blood cells.

Thus far, it has not been possible to culture any of the sporogonous stages *in vitro* for more than a limited amount of time, usually 5 days or less. More substantial results may be forthcoming once culture media are designed to reflect more adequately the *in vivo* milieus of the vector mosquitoes. Such media, at least for anopheline species, should now be more readily formulated using information gained from recent analyses of adult hemolymph. Quite possibly, such media might also encourage a more rapid growth rate in primary cultures of mosquito cells and a shorter interval of adaptation for continuous cell lines. These cultures, in turn, might prove more supportive for parasite growth and development than is presently the case.

If the momentum of the past few years continues and all stages of the parasite are equally scrutinized, many current unknowns of this phase will undoubtedly be revealed quite readily. However, the ultimate goal of culturing the complete sporogonous phase *in vitro* still appears to be a good many years in the future.

REFERENCES

Adams, J. R., and Wilcox, T. A. (1973). Determination of osmolalities of insect hemolymph from several species. *Ann. Entomol. Soc. Am.* **66,** 575–577.

Akov, S. (1962). A qualitative and quantitative study of the nutritional requirements of *Aedes aegypti* L. larvae. *J. Insect Physiol.* **8,** 319–335.

Alger, N. E. (1968). *In vitro* development of *Plasmodium berghei* ookinetes. *Nature (London)* **218**, 774.

Ball, G. H. (1947). Attempts to cultivate the mosquito phase of *Plasmodium relictum*. *Am. J. Trop. Med.* **27**, 301–307.

Ball, G. H. (1948). Extended persistence of *Plasmodium relictum* in culture. *Am. J. Trop. Med.* **28**, 533–536.

Ball, G. H. (1954). Prolonged contraction of mosquito digestive tract *in vitro* with partial development of oocysts of *Plasmodium relictum*. *Exp. Parasitol.* **3**, 358–367.

Ball, G. H. (1964). *In vitro* culture of the mosquito phase of avian malaria. *J. Parasitol.* **50**, 3–10.

Ball, G. H. (1972). Use of invertebrate tissue culture for the study of plasmodia. *In* "Invertebrate Tissue Culture" (C. Vago, ed.), Vol. 2, pp. 321–342. Academic Press, New York.

Ball, G. H., and Chao, J. (1957). Development *in vitro* of isolated oocysts of *Plasmodium relictum*. *J. Parasitol.* **43**, 409–412.

Ball, G. H., and Chao, J. (1960). *In vitro* development of the mosquito phase of *Plasmodium relictum*. *Exp. Parasitol.* **9**, 47–55.

Ball, G. H., and Chao, J. (1961). Infectivity to canaries of sporozoites of *Plasmodium relictum* developing *in vitro*. *J. Parasitol.* **47**, 787–790.

Ball, G. H., and Chao, J. (1963a). Contributions of *in vitro* culture towards understanding the relationships between avian malaria and the invertebrate host. *Ann. N. Y. Acad. Sci.* **113**, 322–331.

Ball, G. H., and Chao, J. (1963b). The relationship of the mosquito stomach and other organs to malaria parasites as indicated by *in vitro* culture. *Ann. Epiphyt.* **14**, 205–210.

Ball, G. H., and Chao, J. (1964). Temperature stresses on the mosquito phase of *Plasmodium relictum*. *J. Parasitol.* **50**, 748–752.

Ball, G. H., and Chao, J. (1971). The cultivation of *Plasmodium relictum* in mosquito cell lines. *J. Parasitol.* **57**, 391–395.

Ball, G. H., and Chao, J. (1976). The use of amino acids by *Plasmodium relictum* oocysts *in vitro*. *Exp. Parasitol.* **39**, 115–118.

Bates, M. (1949). "The Natural History of Mosquitoes." Macmillan, New York.

Bishop, A., and McConnachie, E. W. (1956). A study of factors affecting the emergence of the gametocytes of *Plasmodium gallinaceum* from the erythrocytes and the exflagellation of the male gametocytes. *Parasitology* **46**, 192–215.

Bishop, A., and McConnachie, E. W. (1960). Further observations on the *in vitro* development of the gametocytes of *Plasmodium gallinaceum*. *Parasitology* **50**, 431–448.

Boorman, J. (1967). Aseptic rearing of *Aedes aegypti* Linn. *Nature (London)* **213**, 197–198.

Boyd, M. F., Christophers, R., and Coggeshall, L. T. (1949). Laboratory diagnosis of malaria infections. *In* "Malariology" (M. F. Boyd, ed.), Vol. 1, pp. 155–204. Saunders, Philadelphia, Pennsylvania.

Bradford, S., and Ramsey, R. W. (1949). Analysis of mosquito tissues for sodium and potassium and development of a physiological salt solution. *Fed. Proc., Fed. Am. Soc. Exp. Biol.* **8**, 15–16.

Brooks, M. A., and Kurtti, T. J. (1971). Insect cell and tissue culture. *Annu. Rev. Entomol.* **16**, 27–52.

Canning, E., and Sinden, R. E. (1973). The organization of the ookinete and observations on nuclear division in oocysts of *Plasmodium berghei*. *Parasitology* **67**, 29–40.

Carter, R., and Beach, R. F. (1977). Gametogenesis in culture by gametocytes of *Plasmodium falciparum*. *Nature (London)* **270**, 240–241.

Carter, R., and Chen, D. H. (1976). Malaria transmission blocked by immunization with gametes of the malaria parasite. *Nature (London)* **263**, 57–60.

Carter, R., and Miller, L. H. (1979). A method for the study of gametocytogenesis by *Plasmodium falciparum* in culture: Evidence for environmental modulation of gametocytogenesis. *Bull. W.H.O.* (in press).

Carter, R., and Nijhout, M. M. (1977). Control of gamete formation (exflagellation) in malaria parasites. *Science* **195**, 407–409.

Carter, R., Gwadz, R. W., and Green, I. (1979). *Plasmodium gallinaceum:* Transmission blocking immunity in chickens. II. The effects of antigamete antibodies *in vitro* and *in vivo* and their elaboration during infection. *Exp. Parasitol.* **47**, 202–216.

Chao, J., and Ball, G. H. (1964). Cultivation of the insect cycle of plasmodia. *Am. J. Trop. Med. Hyg.* **13**, 181–192.

Chen, D. H., Seeley, D., and Good, W. C. (1977). *In vitro Plasmodium berghei* (malaria) ookinete formation. *Abstract Int. Congr. Protozool., 5th, 1977* No. 21.

Chorine, V. (1933). Conditions que régissent la fécondation de *Plasmodium praecox. Arch. Inst. Pasteur Alger.* **11**, 1–8.

Clark, E. W., and Ball, G. H. (1952). The free amino acids in the whole bodies of culicid mosquitoes. *Exp. Parasitol.* **1**, 339–346.

Clark, E. W., and Ball, G. H. (1954). The major inorganic constituents of whole bodies of adult *Culex tarsalis* and *C. stigmatosoma. Physiol. Zool.* **27**, 334–341.

Clark, E. W., and Ball, G. H. (1956). Preliminary microelectrophoretic studies of insect proteins. *Physiol. Zool.* **29**, 206–212.

Clyde, D. F., Most, H., McCarthy, V. C., and Vanderberg, J. P. (1973). Immunization of man against sporozoite-induced falciparum malaria. *Am. J. Med. Sci.* **266**, 169–177.

Clyde, D. F., McCarthy, V. C., Miller, R. M., and Woodward, W. E. (1975). Immunization of man against falciparum and vivax malaria by use of attenuated sporozoites. *Am. J. Trop. Med. Hyg.* **24**, 397–401.

Davies, E. E. (1974). Ultrastructural studies on the early ookinete stage of *Plasmodium berghei nigeriensis* and its transformation into an oocyst. *Ann. Trop. Med. Parasitol.* **68**, 283–290.

Federoff, S. (1967). Proposed usage of animal tissue culture terms. *Exp. Cell Res.* **46**, 642–648.

Field, J. W., and Shute, P. G. (1956). ''The Microscopic Diagnosis of Human Malaria. II. A. Morphological Study of the Erythrocytic Parasites.'' Government Press, Kuala Lumpur.

Fish, D. C., Dobbs, J. P., and Elliott, J. M. (1973). Effect of osmotic pressure, Na^+/K^+ ratio and medium concentration on the enzyme activity and growth of L cells in suspension culture. *In Vitro* **9**, 108–113.

Florkin, M., and Jeuniaux, C. (1974). Hemolymph: Composition. *In* ''The Physiology of Insecta''. (M. Rockstein, ed.), 2nd ed., Vol. 5, pp. 255–307. Academic Press, New York.

Garnham, P. C. C., Bird, R. G., Baker, J. R., Desser, S. S., and El-Nahal, H. M. S. (1969). Electron microscope studies on motile stages of malaria parasites. VI. The ookinete of *Plasmodium berghei yoelii* and its transformation into the early oocyst. *Trans. R. Soc. Trop. Med. Hyg.* **63**, 187–194.

Gavrilov, W., and Cowez, S. (1941). Essai de culture *in vitro* de tissus de moustiques et d'intestins de lapins adultes infectes. *Ann. Parasitol.* **18**, 180–186.

Grace, T. D. C. (1962) Establishment of four strains of cells from insect tissues grown *in vitro. Nature (London)* **195**, 788–789.

Grace, T. D. C. (1966). Establishment of a line of mosquito (*Aedes aegypti* L.) cells grown *in vitro. Nature (London)* **211**, 366–367.

Greene, A. E., and Charney, J. (1971). Characterization and identification of insect cell cultures. *Curr. Top. Microbiol. Immunol.* **55**, 54–64.

Gubler, D. J. (1968). A method for the *in vitro* cultivation of ovarian and midgut cells from the adult mosquito. *Am. J. Epidemiol.* **87**, 502–508.

Gwadz, R. W. (1976). Malaria: Successful immunization against the sexual stages of *Plasmodium gallinaceum. Science* **193**, 1150–1151.

Hagedorn, H. H., and Judson, C. L. (1972). Purification and site of synthesis of *Aedes aegypti* yolk proteins. *J. Exp. Zool.* **182**, 367–378.

Hawking, F., Wilson, M. E., and Gammage, K. (1971). Evidence for cyclic development and short-lived maturity in the gametocytes of *Plasmodium falciparum. Trans. R. Soc. Trop. Med. Hyg.* **65,** 549–559.

Haynes, J. D., Diggs, C. L., Hines, F. A., and Desjardins, R. E. (1976). Culture of human malaria parasites *Plasmodium falciparum. Nature* (*London*) **263,** 767–769.

Hink, W. F. (1976). A compilation of invertebrate cell lines and culture media. *In* "Invertebrate Tissue Culture: Research Applications" (K. Maramorosch, ed.), pp. 319–369. Academic Press, New York.

Hoyle, G. (1957). "Comparative Physiology of the Nervous Control of Muscular Contraction." Cambridge Univ. Press, London and New York.

Hsu, S. H., Mao, W. H., and Cross, J. H. (1970). Establishment of a line of cells derived from ovarian tissue of *Culex quinquefasciatus* Say. *J. Med. Entomol.* **7,** 703–707.

Hsu, S. H., Li, S. Y., and Cross, J. H. (1972). A cell line derived from ovarian tissue of *Culex tritaeniorhynchus summorousus* Dyar. *J. Med. Entomol.* **9,** 86–91.

James, S. P. (1934). The Shute method of making preparations of exflagellating gametocytes and ookinetes of malarial parasites. *Trans. R. Soc. Trop. Med. Hyg.* **28,** 104–105.

Jeffrey, G. M. (1960). Infectivity to mosquitoes of *Plasmodium vivax* and *Plasmodium falciparum* under various conditions. *Am. J. Trop. Med. Hyg.* **9,** 315–320.

Jensen, J. B. (1979). Observations on gametocytogenesis in *Plasmodium falciparum* from continuous culture. *J. Protozool.* **26,** 129–132.

Jones, J. C. (1970). Hemocytopoiesis in insects. *In* "Regulation of Hemopoiesis" (A. S. Gordon, ed.), Vol. 1, pp. 7–65. Appleton, New York.

Kitamura, S. (1970). Establishment of a cell line from *Culex* mosquito. *Kobe J. Med. Sci.* **16,** 41–50.

Kitchen, S. F., and Putnam, P. (1942). Observations on the mechanism of the parasite cycle in falciparum malaria. *Am. J. Trop. Med.* **22,** 361–386.

Kroeger, H., and Müller, G. (1973). Control of puffing activity in three chromosomal segments of explanted salivary gland cells of *Chironomous thummi* by variation in extracellular Na^+, K^+, and Mg^{++}. *Exp. Cell Res.* **82,** 89–94.

Kuno, G., Hink, W. F., and Briggs, J. D. (1971). Growth promoting serum proteins for *Aedes aegypti* cells cultured *in vitro. J. Insect Physiol.* **17,** 1865–1879.

Kurtti, T. J., Chaudhary, S. P. S., and Brooks, M. A. (1974). Influence of physical factors on the growth of insect cells *in vitro*. I. Effect of osmotic pressure on growth rates of a moth line. *In Vitro* **10,** 149–156.

Kurtti, T. J., Chaudhary, S. P. S., and Brroks, M. A. (1975). Influence of physical factors on the growth of insect cells *in vitro*. II. Sodium and potassium as osmotic pressure regulators of moth cell growth. *In Vitro* **11,** 274–285.

Lakshmi, M. B., and Subrahmanyam, D. (1975). Trehalose of *Culex pipiens fatigans. Experientia* **31,** 898–899.

Laveran, A. (1880). Note sur un nouveau parasite trouvé dans le sang de plusieurs malades atteints de fièvre palustre. *Bull. Acad. Med., Paris* **9,** 1235–1236.

Lockwood, A. M. (1961). "Ringer" solutions and some notes on the physiological basis of their ionic composition. *Comp. Biochem. Physiol.* **2,** 241–289.

MacCallum, W. G. (1897). On the flagellated form of the malaria parasite. *Lancet* **2,** 1240–1241.

MacCallum, W. G. (1898). On the haematozoan infections of birds. *J. Exp. Med.* **3,** 117–136.

Mack, S. R., and Vanderberg, J. P. (1978a). Hemolymph of *Anopheles stephensi* from noninfected and *Plasmodium berghei*-infected mosquitoes. I. Collection procedure and physical characteristics. *J. Parasitol.* **64,** 918–923.

Mack, S. R., and Vanderberg, J. P. (1978b). *Plasmodium berghei:* Energy metabolism of sporozoites. *Exp. Parasitol.* **46,** 317–322.

Mack, S. R., Samuels, S., and Vanderberg, J. P. (1979a). Hemolymph of *Anopheles stephensi* from noninfected and *Plasmodium berghei*-infected mosquitoes. 2. Free amino acids. *J. Parasitol.* **65**, 130-136.

Mack, S. R., Samuels, S., and Vanderberg, J. P. (1979b). Hemolymph of *Anopheles stephensi* from noninfected and *Plasmodium berghei*-infected mosquitoes. 3. Carbohydrates. *J. Parasitol.* **65** 217-221.

Marchoux, E., and Chorine, V. (1932). La fecondation des gametes d'hematozoaires. *Ann. Inst. Pasteur, Paris* **49**, 75-102.

Marhoul, Z., and Pudney, M. (1972). A mosquito cell line (Mos. 55) from *Anopheles gambiae* larvae. *Trans. R. Soc. Trop. Med. Hyg.* **66**, 183-184.

Martin, S. K., Miller, L. H., Nijout, M. M. and Carter, R. (1978). *Plasmodium gallinaceum:* Induction of male gametocyte exflagellation by phosphodiesterase inhibitors. *Exp. Parasitol.* **44**, 239-242.

Micks, D. W., and Ferguson, M. J. (1961). Microorganisms associated with mosquitoes. III. Effect of reduction in the microbial flora of *Culex fatigans* Wiedermann on the susceptibility of *Plasmodium relictum* Grassi and Feletti. *J. Insect Pathol.* **3**, 244-248.

Micks, D. W., DeCaires, P. F., and Franco, L. B. (1948). The relationship of exflagellation in avian plasmodia to pH and immunity in the mosquito. *Am. J. Hyg.* **48**, 182-190.

Mitchell, G. H., Butcher, G. A., and Cohen, S. (1976). A note on the rapid development of *Plasmodium falciparum* gametocytes *in vitro. Trans. R. Soc. Trop. Med. Hyg.* **70**, 12-13.

Mitsuhashi, J. (1976). Insect cell line: Amino acid utilization and requirements. *In* "Invertebrate Tissue Culture: Applications in Medicine, Biology and Agriculture" (E. Kurstak and K. Maramorosch, eds.), pp. 257-262. Academic Press, New York.

Nijhout, M. M. (1977). Gamete development in malaria parasites stimulated by a specific mosquito factor. *Abstr., Int. Congr. Protozool., 5th, 1977* Abstract No. 207.

Nijhout, M. M., and Carter, R. (1978). Gamete development in malaria parasites: Bicarbonate-dependent stimulation by pH *in vitro. Parasitology* **76**, 39-53.

Nussenzweig, R. S., and Chen, D. (1974). The antibody response to sporozoites of simian and human malaria parasites: Its stage and species specificity and strain cross-reactivity. *Bull. W.H.O.* **50**, 293-297.

Nussenzweig, R. S., Vanderberg, J., Most, H., and Orton, C. (1967). Protective immunity produced by injection of x-irradiated sporozoites of *Plasmodium berghei. Nature (London)* **222**, 488-489.

Nussenzweig, R. S., Vanderberg, J., Spitalny, G. L., Rivera, C. I. O., Orton, C., and Most, H. (1972). Sporozoite-induced immunity in mammalian malaria: A review. *Am. J. Trop. Med. Hyg.* **21**, 722-728.

Phillips, R. S., Wilson, R. J. M., and Pasvol, G. (1976). Differentiation of gametocytes of *Plasmodium falciparum in vitro. Trans. R. Soc. Trop. Med. Hyg.* **70**, 286.

Phillips, R. S., Wilson, J. M., and Pasvol, G. (1978). Differentiation of gametocytes in microcultures of human blood infected with *Plasmodium falciparum. J. Protozool.* **25**, 394-398.

Puck, T. T., and Marcus, P. I. (1955). A rapid method for viable cell titration and clone production with HeLa cells in tissue culture. *Proc. Natl. Acad. Sci. U.S.A.* **41**, 432-437.

Pudney, M., and Varma, M. G. R. (1971). *Anopheles stephensi* var. *mysorensis:* Establishment of a larval cell line (Mos. 43). *Exp. Parasitol.* **29**, 7-12.

Ragab, H. A. (1949). Observations on the isolated gut of the mosquito. *Trans. R. Soc. Trop. Med. Hyg.* **43**, 225-230.

Rieckmann, K., Carson, P., Beaudoin, R., Cassels, J., and Sell, K. (1974). Sporozoite-induced immunity in man against an Ethiopian strain of *Plasmodium falciparum* (Letter). *Trans. R. Soc. Trop. Med. Hyg.* **68**, 258-259.

Rinaldini, L. M. (1954). A quantitative method for growing animal cells *in vitro. Nature (London)* **173**, 1134-1135.

Ringer, S. (1883). A further contribution regarding the influence of the different constituents of the blood on the contraction of the heart. *J. Physiol. (London)* **4**, 29–42.

Rosales-Ronquillo, M. C., and Silverman, P. H. (1974). *In vitro* ookinete development of the rodent malaria parasite, *Plasmodium berghei*. *J. Parasitol.* **60**, 819–824.

Rosales-Ronquillo, M. C., Simons, R. W., and Silverman, P. H. (1972). Long-term primary culture of cells of the mosquito *Anopheles stephensi*. *Ann. Entomol. Soc. Am.* **65**, 721–729.

Rosales-Ronquillo, M. C., Simons, R. W., and Silverman, P. H. (1973). Aseptic rearing of *Anopheles stephensi* (Diptera: Culicidae). *Ann. Entomol. Soc. Am.* **66**, 949–954.

Rosales-Ronquillo, M. C., Nienaber, G., and Silverman, P. H. (1974). *Plasmodium berghei* ookinete formation in a nonvector cell line. *J. Parasitol.* **60**, 1039–1040.

Rosales-Sharp, M. C., and Silverman, P. H. (1976). Application of tissue culture to problems in malariology. *In* "Invertebrate Tissue Culture: Applications in Medicine, Biology and Agriculture" (E. Kurstak and K. Maramorosch, eds.), pp. 77–86. Academic Press, New York.

Ross, R. (1897). Observations on a condition necessary to the transformation of the malaria crescent. *Br. Med. J.* **1**, 251–255.

Row, R. (1929). On some observations on the malarial parasite grown aerobically in simple cultures with special reference to the evolution and degeneration of the crescents. *Indian J. Med. Res.* **16**, 1120–1125.

Schneider, I. (1967). Insect tissue culture. *In* "Methods in Developmental Biology" (F. H. Wilt and N. K. Wessells, eds.), pp. 543–554. Crowell-Collier, New York.

Schneider, I. (1968a). Cultivation *in vitro* of *Plasmodium gallinaceum* oocysts. *Exp. Parasitol.* **22**, 178–186.

Schneider, I. (1968b). Cultivation of *Plasmodium gallinaceum* oocysts in Grace's cell strain of *Aedes aegypti* (L.). *Proc. Int. Colloq. Invertebr. Tissue Cult., 2nd, 1967* pp. 247–253.

Schneider, I. (1969). Establishment of three diploid cell lines of *Anopheles stephensi* (Diptera: Culicidae). *J. Cell Biol.* **42**, 603–606.

Schneider, I. (1972). A comparative study of the development of the mosquito cycle of *Plasmodium cynomolgi* in primary cultures versus an established cell line of *Anopheles stephensi*. *Proc. Helminthol. Soc. Wash.* **39**, 438–444.

Schneider, I. (1973). Preparation of primary cultures: Dipteran embryos and larvae (diploid lines). *In* "Tissue Culture: Methods and Applications" (P. F. Krause, Jr. and M. K. Patterson, Jr. eds.), pp. 150–153. Academic Press, New York.

Schneider, I., and Blumenthal, A. B. (1978). *Drosophila* cell and tissue culture. *In* "The Genetics and Biology of Drosophila" (M. Ashburner and T. R. F. Wright, eds.), Vol. 2a, pp. 266–316. Academic Press, New York.

Shapiro, M., Espinal-Tejada, C., and Nussenzweig, R. S. (1975). Evaluation of a method for *in vitro* ookinete development of the rodent malarial parasite, *Plasmodium berghei*. *J. Parasitol.* **61**, 1105–1106.

Shute, P. G., and Maryon, M. (1951). A study of gametocytes in a West African strain of *Plasmodium falciparum*. *Trans. R. Soc. Trop. Med. Hyg.* **44**, 421–438.

Shute, P. G., and Maryon, M. (1966). "Laboratory Technique for the Study of Malaria," 2nd ed. Churchill, London.

Sinden, R. E., and Croll, N. A. (1975). Cytology and kinetics of microgametogenesis and fertilization in *Plasmodium yoelii nigeriensis*. *Parasitology* **70**, 53–65.

Sinden, R. E., and Garnham, P. C. C. (1973). A comparative study on the ultrastructure of *Plasmodium* sporozoites within the oocyst and salivary glands, with particular reference to the incidence of the microscope. *Trans. R. Soc. Trop. Med. Hyg.* **67**, 631–637.

Sinden, R. E., and Smalley, M. E. (1976). Gametocytes of *Plasmodium falciparum*: Phagocytosis by leucocytes *in vivo* and *in vitro*. *Trans. R. Soc. Trop. Med. Hyg.* **70**, 344–345.

Singh, K. R. P. (1967). Cell cultures derived from larvae of *Aedes albopictus* (Skuse) and *Aedes aegypti* (L.). *Curr. Sci.* **36**, 506–508.

Singh, K. R. P., and Bhat, U. K. M. (1969). Primary cell cultures derived from embryos of *Anopheles stephensi* Liston. *Indian J. Med. Res.* **57**, 52–55.

Smalley, M. E. (1976). *Plasmodium falciparum* gametocytogenesis *in vitro*. *Nature (London)* **264**, 271–272.

Smith, D. S. (1968). "Insect Cells, Their Structure and Function." Oliver & Boyd, Edinburgh.

Speer, C. A., Rosales-Ronquillo, M. C., and Silverman, P. H. (1975). Motility of *Plasmodium berghei* ookinetes *in vitro*. *J. Invertebr. Pathol.* **25**, 73–78.

Sterling, C. R., Aikawa, M., and Vanderberg, J. P. (1973). The passage of *Plasmodium berghei* sporozoites through the salivary glands of *Anopheles stephensi:* An electron microscope study. *J. Parasitol.* **59**, 593–605.

Stone, R. P., and Hink, W. F. (1973). *In vitro* culture of cells and tissues from the mosquito *Anopheles quadrimaculatus* Say. *In Vitro* **8**, 362–367.

Terzakis, J. A. (1971). Transformation of the *Plasmodium cynomolgi* oocyst. *J. Protozool.* **18**, 62–73.

Terzakis, J. A., Sprinz, H., and Ward, R. A. (1966). Sporoblast and sporozoite formation in *Plasmodium gallinaceum* infection of *Aedes aegypti*. *Mil. Med.* **131**, 984–992.

Trager, W. (1941). Studies on conditions affecting the survival *in vitro* of a malarial parasite (*Plasmodium lophurae*). *J. Exp. Med.* **74**, 441–462.

Trager, W. (1943). Further studies on the survival and development *in vitro* of a malarial parasite. *J. Exp. Med.* **77**, 411–420.

Trager, W. (1971). A new method for intraerythrocytic cultivation of malaria parasites (*Plasmodium coatneyi* and *P. falciparum*). *J. Protozool.* **18**, 239–242.

Trager, W., and Jensen, J. P. (1976). Human malaria parasites in continuous culture. *Science* **193**, 673–675.

Vanderberg, J. P. (1974). Studies on the motility of *Plasmodium* sporozoites. *J. Protozool.* **21**, 527–537.

Vanderberg, J. P. (1975). Development of infectivity by the *Plasmodium berghei* sporozoite. *J. Parasitol.* **61**, 43–50.

Vanderberg, J. P., and Rhodin, J. (1967). Differentiation of nuclear and cytoplasmic fine structure during the sporogonic development of *Plasmodium berghei*. *J. Cell Biol.* **32**, C7–C10.

Vanderberg, J. P., Rhodin, J., and Yoeli, M. (1967). Electron microscopic and histochemical studies of sporozoite formation in *Plasmodium berghei*. *J. Protozool.* **14**, 82–103.

Vanderberg, J. P., Nussenzweig, R. S., and Most, H. (1969). Protective immunity produced by the injection of x-irradiated sporozoites of *Plasmodium berghei*. V. *In vitro* effects of immune serum on sporozoites. *Mil. Med.* **134**, Suppl. 1183–1190.

Vanderberg, J. P., Nussenzweig, R. S., Sanabria, Y., Nawrot, R., and Most, H. (1972). Stage specificity of antisporozoite antibodies in rodent malaria and its relationship to protective immunity. *Proc. Helminthol. Soc. Wash.* **39**, 514–525.

Vanderberg, J. P., Weiss, M. M., and Mack, S. R. (1977). *In vitro* cultivation of the sporogonic stages of *Plasmodium:* A review. *Bull. W.H.O.* **55**, 377–392.

Van Handel, E. (1965). The obese mosquito. *J. Insect Physiol.* **11**, 478–486.

Vaughn, J. L. (1971). Cell culture media and methods. *In* "Invertebrate Tissue Culture", (C. Vago, ed.), Vol. 1, pp. 4–40. Academic Press, New York.

Vaughn, J. L. (1973). Insect cell nutrition: Emphasis on sterols and fatty acids. *In Vitro* **9**, 122–128.

Walliker, D., and Robertson, E. (1970). Cultivation *in vitro* of sporozoites of *Plasmodium berghei*. *Trans. R. Soc. Trop. Med. Hyg.* **64**, 5.

Wallis, R. C., and Lite, S. W. (1970). Axenic rearing of *Culex salinarius*. *Mosq. News* **30**, 427–429.

Weathersby, A. B. (1952). The role of the stomach wall in the exogenous development of *Plasmodium gallinaceum* as studied by means of haemocoel injections of susceptible and refractory mosquitoes. *J. Infect. Dis.* **91**, 198–205.

Weiss, M. M., and Vanderberg, J. P. (1976). Studies on *Plasmodium* ookinetes. 1. Isolation and concentration from mosquito midguts. *J. Protozool.* **23,** 547–551.

Weiss, M. M., and Vanderberg, J. P. (1977). Studies on *Plasmodium* ookinetes. 2. *In vitro* development. *J. Parasitol.* **63,** 932–934.

Willis, M. J., and Sunderman, F. W. (1952). Studies in serum electrolytes. XIX. Nomograms for calculating Mg ions and ultrafiltrates. *J. Biol. Chem.* **197,** 343–345.

Wyatt, G. R., and Kalf, G. F. (1957). The chemistry of insect hemolymph. II. Trehalose and other carbohydrates. *J. Gen. Physiol.* **40,** 833–847.

Wyatt, G. R., and Wyatt, S. S. (1976). The development of an insect tissue culture medium. *In* ''Invertebrate Tissue Culture: Applications in Medicine, Biology and Agriculture'' (E. Kurstak and K. Maramorosch, eds.), pp. 249–255. Academic Press, New York.

Yoeli, M., and Upmanis, R. S. (1968). *Plasmodium berghei* ookinete formation *in vitro. Exp. Parasitol.* **22,** 122–128.

Cultivation of Erythrocytic and Exoerythrocytic Stages of Plasmodia

William Trager and James B. Jensen

I. INTRODUCTION

Propagation of a parasite *in vitro* is both an end in itself and a means to many other ends. A successful culture method inevitably supplies information about the developmental requirements of the parasite. At the same time it opens the way to studies difficult or impossible to do with parasites maintained in their host animals. This is especially true of such parasites as the protozoa of human malaria, for which there are few suitable experimental animal hosts.

In approaching the cultivation of forms with complex life cycles, each separate phase of multiplication and differentiation must be considered separately. With malaria parasites the sporogonic cycle occurring in the mosquito host is largely extracellular. It begins with a union of gametes and ends with the formation of sporozoites, forms incapable of further development in the mosquito and specifically adapted for initiation of the preerythrocytic cycle in a suitable vertebrate host. Studies on the duplication of this self-limiting sporogonic cycle *in vitro* are

Malaria, Vol. 2
Copyright © 1980 by Academic Press, Inc.
All rights of reproduction in any form reserved.
ISBN 0-12-426102-7

considered in this volume, Chapter 5. Here we will deal with cultivation of the two cycles of development that occur in the vertebrate host and that are largely intracellular.

The first, the preerythrocytic or exoerythrocytic cycle, is initiated by the sporozoites. In avian plasmodia it occurs in reticuloendothelial cells and soon gives rise to merozoites infective to erythrocytes; these begin the erythrocytic cycle. It also gives rise, however, to other merozoites that continue the exoeryhrocytic cycle. Thus in birds this cycle is capable of indefinite propagation; accordingly it lends itself to methods for continuous *in vitro* culture (see Section IV). In mammalian plasmodia, however, the preerythrocytic cycle occurs in hepatic cells and typically involves one cycle of development that produces only merozoites infective to erythrocytes (see Section IV for further details).

With both avian and mammalian plasmodia the erythrocytic cycle is capable of indefinite asexual propagation as long as the parasites have available to them living erythrocytes of appropriate type maintained under appropriate conditions. All development occurs intracellularly. Only the merozoites, products of schizogony especially equipped for entry into a red cell, are able to survive briefly extracellularly (Dennis *et al.*, 1975; McAlister, 1977). Under natural conditions the interval between the liberation of the merozoites at the time of rupture of the host cell in which they have been formed and their subsequent entry into new cells must be very short.

The erythrocytic cycle also gives rise, under conditions not now understood, to a small proportion of gametocytes, forms which do not develop further in the vertebrate host but produce male and female gametes. These initiate the sporogonic cycle if they are ingested by a suitable mosquito. Here again growth and differentiation of the gametocytes occur intracellularly, but the mature gametes can live extracellularly.

Since erythrocytes are cells of limited metabolic capability (for example, mature red cells no longer have a protein-synthesizing system), it seemed possible that one might be able to grow the erythrocytic cycle of malaria extracellularly in a nonliving medium. In this way one might be able to dissect the host cell–parasite relationship and learn what essential roles the living host cell plays for obligate intracellular protozoan parasites. Some partially successfuly attempts at extracellular cultivation of erythrocytic parasites will be considered in Section III. But intracellular cultures in erythrocytes maintained *in vitro,* comparable to tissue cultures of viruses, can provide answers to many kinds of questions, especially now that some species can be grown continuously *in vitro* (Trager and Jensen, 1976; Trager and Jensen, 1978).

II. CULTURE OF ERYTHROCYTIC STAGES WITHIN THEIR HOST CELLS

A. Short-Term Culture

1. Methods Used and Typical Results

Bass and Johns (1912) were the first to report *in vitro* development of malaria parasites. They added glucose to whole defibrinated blood from patients with malaria and incubated small amounts of the mixture in upright vials at 37°C. They observed that rings of both *Plasmodium falciparum* and *P. vivax* matured *in vitro* and sometimes gave rise to another generation and rarely even to one or two additional cycles. These results caused a considerable flurry of excitement among malariologists, but in the hands of most other workers only the initial maturation could be obtained. The method was, therefore, largely abandoned. It should be noted, however, that even this brief period of *in vitro* development can be used for experiments with chemotherapeutic agents (Black, 1946) and that it is the basis of the *in vitro* test for chloroquine resistance developed by Rieckmann (Rieckmann and Lopez Antunano, 1971).

When the subject was again attacked about 20 years later, short-term cultures were obtained with several species of malaria of birds and primates (see World Health Organization, 1975). The best results were those with *P. lophurae* in chicken or duck erythrocytes (Trager, 1947a; McGhee and Trager, 1950) and with *P. knowlesi* in rhesus monkey erythrocytes (Ball *et al.*, 1945; Geiman *et al.*, 1946). Both of these species show initial development with reinvasion and small increases in number under the following conditions. Blood from an infected animal is mixed with uninfected blood (duck or chicken for *P. lophurae*, rhesus monkey for *P. knowlesi*) to give an initial parasite count of about 1%. The washed cells are suspended in a culture medium [the Harvard medium or its modifications (Siddiqui and Schnell, 1972)] and placed in vessels (erlenmeyer flasks or ''boats'') so as to have a relatively large surface exposed (e.g., 6 ml of suspension in a 50-ml erlemeyer flask). The flasks (or other vessels) are equipped with tubes for delivery of a slow current of 5% carbon dioxide in air and are rocked gently on a rocking table (16 cycles/min) held in an incubator at 37°C (*P. knowlesi*) or at 40°C (*P. lophurae*). For both species of parasites the best results were obtained if the starting parasite number was made relatively low, e.g., 50,000 parasites to 1,000,000 red cells per cubic millimeter of the final suspension for *P. lophurae* (Trager, 1947a) and 16,000–25,000 parasites to 1,000,000 cells per cubic millimeter for *P. knowlesi* (Geiman *et al.*, 1946). Typical early results are shown in Tables I and II.

2. Information Gained from Short-Term Cultures

Nutritional Requirements and Mode of Action of Drugs. The earliest *in vitro* experiments with both *P. lophurae* and *P. knowlesi* had already revealed

TABLE I

Growth of *Plasmodium lophurae* in Duck Erythrocytes *in Vitro*[a]

| | | | | Extent of multiplication[c] between days | | | | |
| | | | | Original culture | | Subculture | | |
Experiment	Flask	Medium[b]	Initial parasites per 10,000 red cells	0–1	1–2	2–3	3–4	0–4
1	1	RCE	410	2.9	1.4	4.2	1.2	21.0
	2	BGM	580	3.3	1.0	2.9	1.0	9.6
2	1	RCE	565	1.7	1.2	2.5	1.3	6.7
	2	BGM	540	1.9	1.6	2.5	1.7	13.0
3	1	BGM	670	2.7	1.5	2.5	1.7	17.2
4	1	BGM	587	1.4	1.7	2.5	1.4	8.2
	2	BGM	660	1.2	1.8	2.1	1.8	8.2

[a] The cultures were held at 40°C in erlenmeyer flasks gassed with 5% carbon dioxide in air and rocked at 16 cycles/min. From Trager (1947a).

[b] RCE, A medium with high potassium and a duck erythrocyte extract; BGM, modified Harvard medium (Geiman *et al.*, 1946).

[c] Ratio of count on later day to count on earlier day.

specific nutritional requirements. Most striking was the demonstration of the requirement by *P. lophurae* for calcium pantothenate (Trager, 1943) and by *P. knowlesi* for *p*-aminobenzoic acid (PABA) (Fig. 1). A requirement for PABA by malaria parasites had already been indicated by the finding by Maier and Riley (1942) that the antimalarial effect of sulfonamides against *P. lophurae* infection

TABLE II

Multiplication of *Plasmodium knowlesi* during a 20- to 24-Hour Period with Different Culture Methods[a]

| | | No. of experiments with the amount of multiplication | | | | | | | | |
Culture method	Total no. of experiments	2×	3×	4×	5×	6×	7×	8×	9–11×	Average multiplication
Rocker–dilution	131	28	41	19	14	11	8	6	4	4.1
Perfusion, type 1	51	7	15	12	8	3	5	1		4.1
Perfusion, type 2[b]	53	12	17	12	7	4	1			3.6
Total, all types	235	47	73	43	29	18 (19)	14	7	4	3.9

[a] From Geiman *et al.* (1946).

[b] This method of cultivation makes use of the continuous flow of nutrient medium through the blood being cultivated.

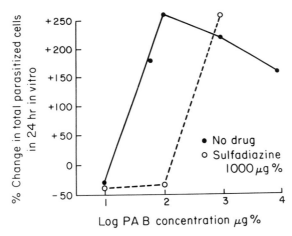

FIG. 1. Sulfadiazine-*P*-aminobenzoic acid antagonism as observed on the second generation of *P. knowlesi* grown in culture (from Ball, 1946.)

in ducklings was antagonized by PABA. This work has had far-reaching ramifications in the use of long-acting sulfa drugs as antimalarials, in Hawking's finding that a milk diet (essentially lacking PABA) protects mice against otherwise lethal *P. berghei* infections, and in present understanding of the folate metabolism of malaria parasites (Ferone, 1977).

The discovery of the requirement for pantothenate led to demonstration of the antimalarial effect of antimetabolites of this vitamin (Table III). These compounds unfortunately were not sufficiently effective to become of practical use,

TABLE III

Effects of Antipantothenates on *Plasmodium falciparum* in *Aotus* monkey Erythrocytes after 2 Days *in vitro*[a]

Flask	Anti-pantothenate	Concentration (μg/ml)	Parasites per 10,000 erythrocytes	
			Normal	Abnormal
1	None	0	25	2
2	None	0	23	5
3	SN 14622	150	5	8
4	SN 14622	150	2	12
5	WR 54036	75	1	8
6	WR 54036	75	1	8
7	WR 54036	50	2	6
8	WR 54036	50	0	10

[a] From Trager (1971a); see this paper for details.

possibly because they act on the parasite not directly but rather via an effect on the host cell (see Section III).

Other specific requirements demonstrated by short-term cultures include a requirement for biotin, methionine, and purines (see Trager, 1977). In 1-day experiments with *P. knowlesi* (which has a 24-hour cycle of schizogonic development) serum was successfully replaced with stearate (Siddiqui *et al.*, 1969). Whereas human plasma fractions rich in albumin or γ-globulin had no effect on the growth of *P. lophurae* in chick erythrocytes, a fraction containing α-globulin and rich in lipoproteins inhibited growth (Trager, 1947a). This seemed to be in keeping with the *in vivo* inhibitory effects observed with duck and chicken plasmas high in a bound, fat-soluble factor measured by its biotin-like growth-promoting activity (Trager, 1947b; Trager and McGhee, 1950). In light of the recent finding that high-density lipoprotein disappears from the plasma of individuals undergoing an attack of *P. vivax* malaria (Lambrecht *et al.*, 1978) this subject deserves much more attention.

Short-term cultures of *P. knowlesi* and *P. lophurae,* as well as similar cultures of *P. gallinaceum* of chickens, *P. coatneyi* of rhesus monkeys, and even *P. falciparum* of humans, have been used to study certain aspects of metabolism of the parasites (see Polet and Conrad, 1969) and the mode of action of antimalarial drugs (Ryley, 1953; McCormick *et al.*, 1971; Siddiqui *et al.*, 1972).

B. Prolonged Cultivation

1. Early Attempts with Experimental Malarias

Viable male gametocytes of *P. lophurae* were present after up to 16 days of incubation *in vitro* (Trager, 1943). Asexual parasites were also present, but in decreased numbers. By preparing subcultures every second day, *P. lophurae* was regularly sustained for 4-day periods with parasite increases ranging up to 20-fold, and in one series for 8 days with a 170-fold increase in the parasitemia (about 3.5 times for each cycle of 48 hours). At each subculture, however, it was necessary to add such a quantity of new red cells that the rate of multiplication of the parasites did not keep up with the dilution, resulting in progressively lower overall parasitemia.

The same kind of result was obatained with *P. knowles* (Geiman *et al.*, 1946), sustained for 6 days despite its shorter (24 hour) cycle of reproduction. Trigg and Shakespeare (1976) later documented that there was progressivley less multiplication of *P. knowlesi* with each successive cycle of development *in vitro*.

One result indicating the possibility of continuous cultivation was reported by Anderson (1953) with *P. gallinaceum*. He used a medium consisting of chicken erythrocyte extract prepared in chicken serum and found that, after 10 days, with a dilution with fresh red cells every second day, the parasitemia was the same as it had been initially, showing that extensive multiplication had occurred. Attempts to repeat this result with *P. gallinaceum* or other species were, however, not successful, suggesting that some subtle unknown factor was not being duplicated. That small, subtle changes in environmental conditions can markedly affect prolonged *in vitro* development has been repeatedly noted now that methods for continuous culture are available (see below).

It seemed evident that the rocker flask method had failed to lead to continuous culture. Several perfusion methods (see Bertagna *et al.*, 1972) proved to be more cumbersome without giving significantly better results. Trager (1971b) then reasoned that, at least for species such as *P. coatneyi* and *P. falciparum,* which spend two-thirds of each 48-hour cycle sequestered in deep organs and attached to capillary walls, it might be desirable to have a stationary settled layer of red cells with a slow flow of medium over them. This led to development of the so-called flow vial. With the modified Harvard medium in this setup both *P. coatneyi* and *P. falciparum* showed a second cycle of reinvasion but no overall increase in parasite number. Experiments with a number of different tissue culture media, using *P. coatneyi* in rocker dilution flasks, then revealed the great superiority of medium RPMI-1640 supplemented with 25 mM N-2-hydroxyethylpiperazine-N'-2-ethanesulfonic acid (HEPES) buffer (Trager, 1976). RPMI 1640 is a medium originally prepared by George Moore and his associates (1967) for the culture of human leukocytes. When this medium with 25 mM HEPES and 15% rhesus monkey serum was used with *P. coatneyi* in flow vials, the parasites continued to cycle for over a week and persisted for 2 weeks with decreased numbers.

2. Continuous Culture of Plasmodium falciparum (Trager and Jensen, 1976)

Application of what had been learned from the work with *P. coatneyi* to experiments with *P. falciparum* then gave in two flow vials the first continuous cultures of this, or any, species of malarial parasite (Table IV). It was soon found that the parasites could also be propagated in simple petri dishes held in a candle jar with the medium changed manually once a day (Jensen and Trager, 1977). These methods are applicable to the cultivation of most strains of *P. falciparum* (Jensen and Trager, 1978; personal communications from others). We will now describe the methods in detail not from a historical point of view but as they are best understood at the present time. We will also consider the advantages and limitations of the several methods now in use, what they have already revealed concerning growth requirements of the parasites, and their potentialities for future work.

a. The Medium. This is prepared from powdered RPMI-1640 with glutamine but without bicarbonate (Table V). The amount required for 1 liter (10.4 g) is dissolved in 900 ml of glass-redistilled water, and to this is added 5.94

TABLE IV

Establishment of the First Continuous Culture Line (FCR-1/FVO) of *Plasmodium falciparum*[a]

		Parasites per 10,000 red cells[b]			
Days *in vitro*	Total dilution	R	T	S	Total
0	1	32	0	0	32
2	1	6	23	24	53
4	1	18	5	7	30
4	3	1	1	4	6
6	3	27	7	4	38
11	36	5	2	2	9
13	36	19	13	6	38
14	36	40	9	1	50
22	1,728	9	2	1	12
24	1,728	30	20	9	59
25	1,728	29	32	21	82
28	18,000	11	3	0	14
31	18,000	34	25	7	66
46	10.8×10^6	3	1	0	4
48	10.8×10^6	22	5	4	31

[a] Representative counts during the first weeks in culture in a flow vial are shown. At 0 time erythrocytes from an *A. trivirgatus* monkey infected with the Vietnam–Oak Knolls strain were diluted 10-fold with a human erythrocyte suspension to give 32 parasites per 10,000 red cells. Dilutions with fresh human erythrocytes were performed at 3- or 4-day intervals and usually a 4-fold dilution was effected. From Trager and Jensen (1976).

[b] R, Rings; T, trophozoites (one nucleus); S, schizonts (two or more nuclei).

g of HEPES. The solution is diluted to 960 ml and sterilized by filtration through a Millipore filter of 0.45-μm porosity. This solution may be stored up to 1 month at 4°C. The medium is completed by the addition of sterile 5% sodium bicarbonate (sterilized by filtration through a 0.45-μm Millipore filter) at the rate of 4 ml to 96 ml of the RPMI-1640–HEPES solution. This medium without serum is designated RP. It can be stored up to a week in the refrigerator in screw-capped bottles. It is used for washing cells. Complete medium is prepared from it by the addition of serum.

No useful modification of the medium has yet been found. Medium 199, which closely resembles RPMI-1640 but has several additional ingredients, has been used by several workers (Haynes *et al.*, 1976) and might be equally suitable for long-term culture, but this has never been demonstrated. There is no advantage to its use.

b. Serum. The best results have been obtained with human serum at 15 or 10% (v/v). The serum should be obtained from a unit of blood freshly collected

TABLE V

Composition of RPMI-1640[a]

Component	Amount (mg/liter)
Inorganic salts	
$Ca(NO_3)_2 \cdot 4\,H_2O$	100.0
KCl	400.0
$MgSO_4$	48.84
NaCl	6000.0
$NaHCO_3$	2000.0[b]
Na_2HPO_4	800.0
Other	
Glucose	2000.0
Glutathione (reduced)	1.0
Phenol red	5.0
Amino acids	
L-Arginine (free base)	200.0
L-Asparagine	50.0
L-Aspartic acid	20.0
L-Cystine	65.0 (2 HCl)
L-Glutamic acid	20.0
L-Glutamine	300.0
Glycine	10.0
L-Histidine (free base)	15.0
L-Hydroxyproline	20.0
L-Isoleucine (allo-free)	50.0
L-Leucine (methionine-free)	50.0
L-Lysine–HCl	40.0
L-Methionine	15.0
L-Phenylalanine	15.0
L-Proline (hydroxy-L-proline-free)	20.0
L-Serine	30.0
L-Threonine (allo-free)	20.0
L-Tryptophan	5.0
L-Tyrosine	28.94 (Sodium salt)
L-Valine	20.0
Vitamins	
Biotin	0.20
D-Calcium pantothenate	0.25
Choline chloride	3.00
Folic acid	1.00
Isoinositol	35.00
Nicotinamide	1.00
p-Aminobenzoic acid	1.00
Pyridoxine–HCl	1.00
Riboflavin	0.20
Thiamine–HCl	1.00
Vitamin B_{12}	0.005

[a] From Gibco catalogue.
[b] Added before use.

without anticoagulant and kept overnight in a refrigerator to permit shrinkage of the clot. The serum, with some cells, is run into centrifuge tubes by a plasma transfer tube, centrifuged to remove the cells, and placed in sterile tubes or flasks in suitable amounts. It is stored frozen at $-20°C$. Old serum or serum from outdated cells cannot be used. However, plasma from blood freshly collected in citrate [acid–citrate–dextrose (ACD) or citrate–phosphate–dextrose (CPD)] can be used once the clotting elements have been removed by the addition of calcium chloride (1.0 ml of a 10% solution per 100 ml plasma) while gently stirring with a magnetic stirrer.

The ABO type of the blood used for serum depends on the cells to be used and the particular experimental purpose. When new cultures are to be started with infected cells either from human patients or from *Aotus trivirgatus* monkeys, type AB^+ serum should be used. This is compatible with any type of human cell and with *Aotus* erythrocytes. For the maintenance of established culture lines and for large-scale propagation, type A^+ serum (with A^+ or O^+ red cells) is used, since it is the most readily obtainable.

The complete medium with serum (designated RP-S) is best prepared fresh by aseptic addition of sterile serum to sterile RP. If necessary, however, the medium may be mixed with nonsterile serum and the final mixture sterilized through an appropriate filter. RP-S can be safely stored up to a week at refrigerator temperature.

Individual human sera appear to vary somewhat in the extent of growth they support. No correlation has been observed with suitability and time after a meal (hence with abundance or scarcity of lipid). An adequate concentration is 10%; 5% is not dependable. For starting new lines and for reactivating cultures from the frozen state (see below) 15% appears desirable.

Commercially obtained sera are not suitable (Table VI). Neither is freshly collected fetal calf serum (Jensen, 1978b). However, fresh rabbit serum can replace human serum (K. H. Rieckmann, personal communication). It is clear that much more attention must be given both to attempts to replace human serum partially or completely and to determine the nature of the factors it contains that are essential to development of erythrocytic stages of *P. falciparum*.

In malarious countries it will be important to avoid two possible sources of unsuitable serum: (1) serum from individuals with a high degree of immunity to falciparum malaria, and (2) serum from individuals who have recently taken any drug with an antimalarial effect. Unpublished results from several laboratories already show that both of the above kinds of serum have inhibitory effects.

c. Erythrocytes. Since *P. falciparum* in nature is exclusively a parasite of humans, since human erythrocytes have a longer *in vivo* lifetime that those of *A. trivirgatus* (the only suitable experimental host), since more is known about human erythrocytes than about any other cell, and since in any case human red

TABLE VI

Comparison of the Growth of a *Plasmodium falciparum* Culture Supplemented with Fresh Human Type A+ Serum and Commercially Available Animal and Human Sera[a]

Serum	Percentage growth in comparison to control	Comments
Control[b]	100	The $\bar{m}$ parasitemia at 96 hours for controls in all experiments was 6.8%, representing an average increase of 60–70 times
Freshly collected fetal bovine	35[c]	The first few cycles were encouraging, but growth declined with each subculture
Adult bovine	7.2	
Newborn bovine	1.0	
Horse	19.0	
Sheep	2.3	
Swine	14.0	After 48 hours cultures RBC showed some agglutination of RBCs; at 96 hours a considerable amount of hemolysis
Human frozen[d]	27.0	
Human lyophilized (Miles)	4.4	Hemolysis began after 72 hours *in vitro*; became extensive at 96 hours
Human lyophilized[e] (Difco)	17.6	Hemolysis began after 48 hours *in vitro*; became extensive at 96 hours
Human lyophilized in laboratory	100	Stored at 23°C for 6 weeks before reconstituting by the addition of distilled water

[a] All sera, except controls, were heat-inactivated 30 minutes at 56°C. Petri dish cultures were placed in a candle jar.
[b] Fresh human serum obtained from freshly clotted blood supplied by New York Blood Center.
[c] The average of all samples tested for the first 96 hours *in vitro*.
[d] Commercially pooled fresh frozen human serum from Miles Laboratories, Inc.
[e] Reconstituted and added to culture medium at an equivalent of 20% serum.

cells are the easiest to obtain in quantity, they are the host cell of choice for *in vitro* cultivation of *P. falciparum*.

The cells are obtained as a unit of blood collected either in ACD (per liter: 8 g citric acid, 22 g sodium citrate, 24.5 g glucose; for each 100 ml whole blood add 15 ml ACD) or in CPD (per liter: 3.27 g citric acid, 26.3 g sodium citrate, 25.5 g glucose, 2.22 g sodium monobasic phosphate; for each 100 ml whole blood add 14 ml CPD). It is convenient to transfer the blood, after thorough mixing, to flasks in amounts of 50–100 ml. Cells may be used immediately after collection and after up to 4 weeks of storage at 4°C. Hence cells outdated for transfusion purposes can still be used for another week for cultivation. Usually cells stored for a week after collection support better growth than freshly collected cells, perhaps because the leukocytes have died by that time. Certainly individual bloods vary somewhat in the extent of growth they support, and it will be of great interest to try to correlate this with certain biochemical properties of erythrocytes.

The ABO type of cell to be used depends on the particular experiment and the type of serum. With AB$^+$ serum any type of cell can be used. For routine maintenance and large-scale cultivation, A$^+$ cells with A$^+$ serum are used.

Red cells are prepared as follows: An appropriate volume (e.g., 20 ml) of stored blood is transferred aseptically to a conical, graduated 50-ml centrifuge tube and centrifuged 10 minutes at 2000 rpm (650 g). The supernatant, the buffy coat, and the upper layer of red cells are removed. The cells are then resuspended in 10 ml RP (complete medium but without serum) and recentrifuged. This constitutes the first wash. The procedure is repeated for a second wash. The final supernatant and upper layer of red cells are again removed. There usually then remain, from 20 ml blood, 4–5 ml of packed cells. These are resuspended in an equal volume of RP-S (complete medium with 10% serum) to make a 50% suspension.

d. Culture Systems—Their Preparation and Maintenance

i. Petri Dish Cultures (Jensen and Trager, 1977). If 3.5-cm plastic dishes are used, each is provided with 1.5 ml of an 8% red cell suspension containing infected cells to give an initial parasitemia of about 0.1%. Since the surface area of such a dish is about 900 mm^2, the 1.5 ml gives an initial depth of less than 2 mm, but this is increased on subsequent days with the change in medium (see below). In actual practice, an infected erythrocyte suspension is prepared from a previous culture, from a patient's blood, or from an infected *Aotus* monkey. The parasitemia of this material should be determined by a count on a stained film. If either a previous culture in human cells or a patient's blood is used, the material is centrifuged [8–10 minutes at 1500 rpm (500 g)], the supernatant is removed (including the buffy coat for a patient's blood), and the cells are resuspended in an equal volume of complete medium with serum. If the inoculum is heparinized blood from an infected *Aotus*, it should be similarly treated except that the final 50% suspension should in addition receive $^1/_{10}$ its volume of a solution of heparin (30 mg heparin in 100 ml 0.85% sodium chloride solution, sterilized by autoclaving). An appropriate volume of infected cell suspension is added to the 50% suspension of uninfected erythrocytes (see Section II, B, 2, c). For example, if the starting material is from a culture or a patient with 2% parasitemia, one adds infected cell suspension at the rate of 1 part to 20 parts of uninfected cells to give a calculated starting parasitemia of 0.1%. In any case, a "0-time" smear is prepared from this mixture and used to determine the actual starting parasitemia.

The 50% cell suspension made by mixing infected and uninfected cells is diluted with enough complete RP-S medium to make an 8% cell suspension, and this is then placed in the petri dishes. For larger dishes, appropriately larger volumes of suspensions are used.

The dishes are placed in a glass desiccator with a candle. The candle is lit, and the cover put on (sealed with silicone grease) with the stopcock open. When the candle flame goes out, the stopcock is closed and the desiccator is set in an incubator at 37°C. Once a day (or more often with high parasitemias—see below) the dishes are removed from the desiccator and provided with fresh medium. This is done by gently tipping the dish and aspirating off the clear medium overlying the settled red cell layer. Normally 1–1.2 ml can be removed; 1.5 ml fresh RP-S medium is added, the cells are resuspended by swirling, and the cultures are returned to the candle jar and the incubator. Blood films are ordinarily made at 48 and 96 hours. This is best done immediately after the removal of old medium by taking up a small droplet of the concentrated cell suspension from the bottom of the dish.

The extent of growth depends on a number of factors: strain, time of culture, suitability of red cells, and serum. With an established strain a 0-time parasitemia of 0.1% usually gives 2–5% after 96 hours. This is an increase of 20-to-50-fold in two cycles, or a maximal increase of 7-fold per cycle. The cells are then ready for subculture. When higher parasitemias are desired in dish cultures, it is necessary to provide fresh medium at 12- or 8-hour intervals. Cultures can be started at 1–2% and brought in 2 days to 10–20% or even higher with special handling and with a reduction in the percentage of red cells. If a 5% cell suspension is used, 30% parasitemia gives the same actual number of parasites as 20% parasitemia in an 8% red cell suspension.

This simple petri dish–candle jar method is ideal for many kinds of work and lends itself especially well to screening for new antimalarial agents (Trager *et al.*, 1978) and to experiments on drug resistance (Nguyen-Dinh and Trager, 1978). It can readily be modified for particular purposes. Thus the gas phase in a candle jar usually has 2–3% carbon dioxide and 14–17% oxygen. If one wishes a different gas phase, it can be introduced into the desiccator (see Friedman, 1978; and especially Scheibel, et al. 1979).

ii. Flask Cultures. W. A. Siddiqui (personal communication) uses the following modification of the dish method. The cultures are held in 125-ml erlenmeyer flasks containing 10 ml of a 5% erythrocyte suspension in RP-S medium. The flasks are equipped with delivery tubes for flow of a gas mixture of 8% carbon dioxide, 2% oxygen, and the balance nitrogen delivered by amber latex tubing. The medium is changed by removing the overlying medium carefully with a pasteur pipet and adding fresh medium. The following weekly schedule has been used for the Uganda–Palo Alto strain. Day 0, Friday: Preparation of culture with parasitemia of 1–2%. Day 1, Saturday: No treatment. Day 2, Sunday: Change of medium. Day 3, Monday: Change of medium. Day 4, Tuesday: Subculture; erythrocytes are resuspended, the total volume is measured, and a sample is removed for a red cell and parasite count (now 10–20%); the bulk of the suspension is harvested, and fresh, washed cells are then added to reduce the parasite count back to the 0-time condition with 1–2%. Day 1 of subculture, Wednesday: No treatment. Day 2 of subculture, Thursday: Change medium. Day 3 of subculture, Friday: Harvest parasites and dilute as on Tuesday. Typical results for weeks 9–11 of culture are given in Table VII (W. A. Siddiqui, personal communication). This is clearly a satisfactory system. In view of recent work on the effects of the gas phase (Scheibel et al. 1979) and in view of the permeability of latex tubing to gases, it would be of interest to determine the proportions of carbon dioxide and oxygen actually going through the flasks.

Yet another modification, by J. D. Haynes (personal communication), uses tissue culture flasks gassed and then stoppered after each manual change of medium.

iii. Continuous-Flow Methods. The type of flow vial originally used has been superseded and will not be described here. It is worth noting that, for one

TABLE VII

Growth of *Plasmodium falciparum* (Uganda–Palo Alto Strain, Line FUP/5-77) in Type A+ Human Erythrocytes[a]

Week in culture	Day of week	Parasites per 100 red cells	Red cells/ml culture $\times 10^6$	Parasites/ml culture $\times 10^6$	Total yield of parasites per culture[b] flask $\times 10^6$
9	0	1.7	510	8.7	
	4	17.4	425	73.9	776
	0	2.0	490	9.8	
	3	13.9	410	53.3	533
10	0	0.9	500	4.5	
	4	14.9	370	55.1	606
	0	1.0	540	5.4	
	3	15.3	405	62.0	620
11	0	1.9	450	8.5	
	4	19.5	290	56.5	650
	0	1.8	520	9.4	
	3	18.2	430	78.0	820

[a] Data from W.A. Siddiqui, personal communication.
[b] Volume in flask, 10–11 ml. Total weekly yield about 1.2×10^9 parasites.

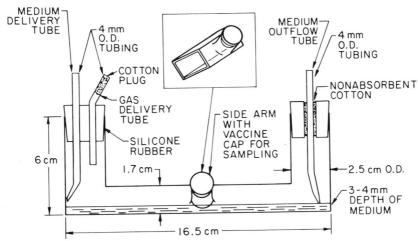

FIG. 2. The flow vessel is made from rectangular 17 × 25 mm tubing with two vertical cylindrical necks of 25-mm diameter and a side arm about 25 mm long and of 11 mm diameter attached at an angle so as to permit access to the bottom by means of a syringe and needle. For sterilization the side arm is capped with aluminum foil, and each vertical neck is plugged with cotton and the whole wrapped in paper. For use, the aluminum foil is removed and a sterile vaccine stopper is inserted in the side arm. An infected blood suspension (12 ml of a 10 or 8% red cell suspension with appropriate, usually 1%, parasitemia) is introduced aseptically through the right-hand vertical neck. This cotton plug is then replaced with a no. 4 silicone rubber stopper bearing the outflow tube. The left-hand cotton plug is similarly replaced with a no.4 silicone stopper bearing the inflow tube and the gas inlet tube. Both stoppers are individually wrapped and autoclaved separately. Both the inflow and outflow tubes are capped with aluminum foil to protect their sterility until they are connected (from Trager, 1979).

South American strain of *P. falciparum* with evidently a rather low growth potential, a culture was established by the flow vial method but not by the petri dish method (Jensen and Trager, 1978).

The culture vessel (Trager, 1979) that has been used for long-term maintenance of two different lines of *P. falciparum* at parasitemias reaching 10–15% 3 days each weeks is illustrated in Fig. 2. It is aseptically connected at its inflow end to tubing from a reservoir flask of medium (400 ml RP-S). The outflow is connected to a sterile receiving flask (ordinarily a 500-ml erlenmeyer flask). Both inflow and outflow are controlled by peristaltic pumps. The rate of inflow is about 50–60 ml/day. The outflow is adjusted to a faster rate, so that the level of medium in the vessel is controlled by the height to which the tip of the outflow tube is adjusted.

To set up a new culture system a 500-ml flask holding 350 ml of sterile RPMI-1640 with HEPES but without bicarbonate is provided with 14.7 ml sterile 5% sodium bicarbonate solution and 40 ml sterile serum. The flask is then equipped with a separately sterilized rubber stopper bearing a cotton-plugged air inlet tube and a glass delivery tube reaching to the bottom of the flask. The outer end of this tube is capped with aluminum foil. The flask is set in a small refrigerator with holes through which sterile tubing capped with aluminum foil has been introduced. By quick removal of the aluminum caps this tubing is connected to the delivery tube from the flask. The tubing after leaving the refrigerator passes through a peristaltic pump and into an adjacent incubator. This tubing may be of silicone rubber or of Tygon, or it may be Teflon-lined. With the last-mentioned type, which is quite hard, it is necessary to have a section of silicone rubber in the peristaltic pump and at each end for ease of connection to glass tubing. The end of the tubing passing into the incubator is capped with aluminum foil.

The outflow assembly consists of a 500-ml flask bearing a silicone rubber stopper with a cotton-plugged outlet to the air and with a glass delivery tube running to the bottom of the flask. This carries a length of silicone rubber tubing capped at its far end with aluminum foil. This tubing goes through the peristaltic pump into the incubator.

After the reservoir and outflow assemblies are in place the culture vessel is prepared (see legend for Fig. 2). This is attached in the incubator in a horizontal position. It is connected to the inflow and outflow tubes by removing the aluminum foil caps from the glass tubes of the culture vessel and the corresponding silicone rubber tubes and rapidly making aseptic connections. The gas delivery tube from a tank holding 7% carbon dioxide, 5% oxygen, and the balance nitrogen is then connected. The gas bubbles first through a large bottle of distilled water and then through a small flask at about 1 bubble/second before entering the incubator. The silicone rubber tubing used to deliver the gas is permeable, resulting in an actual gas phase in the culture vessel of 2% carbon dioxide and 10% oxygen. The gas escapes through the cotton packing around the outflow tube at the right of the vessel, and this tube is adjusted so that its tip just makes contact with the surface of the medium in the culture vessel.

After an hour, when the red cells are well settled, the flow is begun by setting the inflow pump at a high speed until the tubing is full and the medium just begins to enter the culture vessel. The pump is then reset to the desired speed, and the outflow pump is turned on.

Such a culture setup theoretically could be kept in continuous operation indefinitely as long as fresh red cells are provided at appropriate intervals, the reservoir flask is replaced once a week, and the outflow flask is replaced when it is full. In practice, however, it has been found advisable to replace the complete setup after about 2 months. A new setup is begun with an infected cell suspension from an old one. When such a new preparation is started, the first reservoir flask suffices for only 6 days, rather than a week, since a portion of medium must be used to fill the tubing.

For continuous production of parasites we harvest and add fresh red cells every

Monday, Wednesday, and Friday. With the flows shut off the vessels are rocked gently to resuspend the cells, and a sample is taken by a syringe and needle inserted aseptically through the vaccine cap. This sample is used to prepare a Giemsa-stained film for counting the parasites. In the meantime an appropriate amount of washed 8% red cell suspension is prepared (see Section II, C), e.g., 12 ml per culture vessel. Depending on the parasite count (usually about 10%), 10 ml (or more) of the suspension in the culture vessel is removed aseptically by a syringe and needle inserted through the vaccine stopper. This constitutes the harvest of infected red cell suspension. The same volume of fresh red cell suspension is then introduced with a separate 10-ml syringe and no. 20 needle. These are left in place while the contents of the vessel are thoroughly mixed. A small sample is then drawn into the syringe and used to make a stained film for determining the parasite count just after dilution with fresh cells.

Typical results with this method are shown in Table VIII, and the parasites are illustrated in Fig. 3. Note that the extent of multiplication in 2-day intervals averaged 10-fold, a higher rate of increase than that seen with any of the manual methods. At each harvest one vessel yields $0.6-1.0 \times 10^9$ parasites, a weekly yield of $2-3 \times 10^9$.

It is easy to conceive modifications of this method, and one has already been described (Brackett and Green, personal communication). In our laboratory we now use a single pump for both inflow and outflow. By using larger tubing for the outflow, the same pump gives a more rapid rate of outflow than the delivery of the medium.

iv. "Tipping Vessel" Automated Medium Changer.   This apparatus (Jensen *et al.,* 1979), based in part on a medium changer used with extracellular cultures of *P. lophurae,* was designed to automatically perform the same operation done manually in changing media in petri dish cultures.

The vessel (Figs. 4–6) consists of upper and lower chambers connected by a U-shaped side arm. The upper chamber contains a small recess at one end. The U-shaped side arm originates above this recess and connects the upper chamber with the lower one. Both chambers have vertical, round chimneys fitted with silicone rubber stoppers containing two glass tubes each and a serum-stoppered side port (D in Fig. 4). During use, the upper chamber contains a settled layer of infected erythrocytes and a covering layer of RP-S. To change the culture medium the vessel is slowly tipped forward, allowing the exhausted medium to flow into the U-shaped side arm and the erythrocytes into the anterior recess (Fig. 5). As the vessel is then tipped in reverse, the exhausted medium flows into position below the chimney of the lower chamber and the erythrocytes into a similar position in the upper chamber (Fig. 6). At this time, the infected cells can be removed, and freshly washed, uninfected cells can be added by hypodermic needle via the serum-stoppered side port. Also, while in the reverse position, the

TABLE VIII

Growth of *Plasmodium falciparum* (Line FCR-3/FMG) in Two
Continuous-flow Vessels[a]

| | Percentage Parasitemia[b] | | | |
| | Vessel A | | Vessel B | |
Date (1978)	Before	After	Before	After
Sept. 18	19	2	15	1.6
Sept. 20	13	1.4	11	1.2
Sept. 22	14	1.2	8	0.8
Sept. 25	17	0.7	20	1.5
Sept. 27	8	1.6	11	0.7
Sept. 29	14	1.6	6	0.9
Oct. 2	19	1	15	0.9
Oct. 4	9	0.8	11	1.3
Oct. 6	13	0.4	13	0.9
Oct. 9	14	1.5	17	1.2
Oct. 11	13	0.9	14	1.5
Oct. 13	12	1.2	13	1.1
Oct. 16	21	1.2	15	1.2
Oct. 18	12		17	

[a] This culture line was begun in August 1976 in petri dishes (see Jensen and Trager, 1978) and grown continuously *in vitro* until June 30, 1978. The culture was then frozen and stored until Sept. 4, 1978, when it was reactivated in petri dishes and returned to flow vessels on Sept. 8, 1978.

[b] The figures give the number of parasites per 100 red cells just before and just after the addition of a fresh 8% red cell suspension, done every Monday, Wednesday, and Friday. The ratio between the count just after dilution on one date and just before dilution on the next date (2 or 3 days later) gives the extent of multiplication. For the 3-day intervals this ranged from 12- to 35-fold, with an average of 20 for one vessel and 15 for the other. For the 2-day intervals the extent of multiplication ranged from 6 to 16, with an average of 10 for both vessels.

FIG. 4. Culture vessel consisting of an upper chamber (A) connected by a U-shaped side arm to a lower chamber (B), Upper and lower chambers have chimneys fitted with silicone rubber stoppers containing glass tubes (E–H). The upper chamber contains a settled layer of infected erythrocytes with a covering layer of culture medium. Cells can be added or removed through the side port (D).

FIG. 5. Forward tipping of vessel permits exhausted medium to spill into the side arm (C), while erythrocytes flow into small anterior recess.

FIG. 6. When vessel is reversed from forward position, the exhausted medium flows to a position below the lower-chamber chimney where it can be removed through tube E. Fresh culture medium can be added through tube H, stirring the cells as it enters.

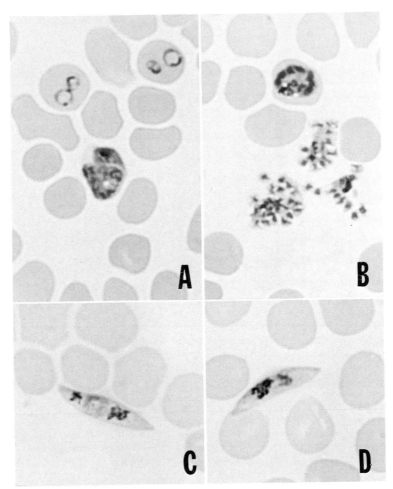

FIG. 3. Erythrocytic stages of *P. falciparum* from continuous *in vitro* cultures. The cultures do not show the characteristic synchrony found *in vivo*, thus all stages of the asexual cycle can be readily seen together, such as the ring stages and trophozoites in (A) (×1600) and schizonts and merozoites in (B) (× 1600). Sexual stages, such as the macrogametocyte and the microgametocyte (C and D, respectively) (× 2000) are commonly seen in newly isolated cultures but are rarely seen after a few months *in vitro* (from Trager and Jensen, 1978).

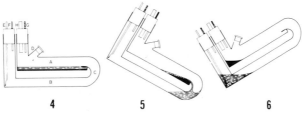

4   5   6

FIGS. 4–6. Schematic drawings of culture vessels in their different operational positions.

TABLE IX

The Growth Rate of *Plasmodium falciparum* (FCR3/FMG Strain) in a Tipping Apparatus[a]

Group	No. of hours in culture	Parasites per 10,000 erythrocytes[f]					Increase in parasitemia
		R	T	2N	>2N	Total	
A	0[b]	25	16	1	7	49	
	48[c]	353	157	18	70	598	12×
	96[d]	636	356	60	468	1520	31×
B	0[b]	58	38	7	18	121	
	48[c]	423	442	68	114	1047	8.7×
C	0[b]	92	103	16	24	235	
	48[c]	832	555	53	183	1623	7×
	0[b]	150	59	10	42	261	
	48[c]	575	541	71	117	1304	5×
D	0[b]	77	21	1	12	111	
	72[e]	697	352	35	282	1366	12.3×
	0[b]	158	56	6	21	241	
	72[e]	1084	603	33	370	2090	8.7×

[a] The growth rate depends upon the relative parasitemias after the addition of fresh cells and the length of culture time. Group A represents typical parasite growth rates when initial parasitemias were approximately 0.5%, group B when approximately 1–1.5%, and group C when 2–2.5%. Group D represents typical growth rates seen over the 3-day, Friday–Monday period when initial parasitemias were approximately 1 and 2.5%, respectively.

[b] Represents parasitemia after the addition of fresh erythrocytes.

[c] Represents parasitemia 48 hours after the addition of fresh cells.

[d] Represents parasitemia 96 hours after the addition of fresh cells.

[e] Represents parasitemia 72 hours (from Friday to Monday) after the addition of fresh cells.

[f] R, rings; T, trophozoites; 2N, binucleated stage; >2N, schizonts.

exhausted medium can be removed from the lower chamber through tube E (Fig. 4) and fresh medium added to the cells in the upper chamber through tube H (Fig. 4). Humidified gas (3% carbon dioxide, 10% oxygen, and 87% nitrogen) flows continuously through the vessel from tube F to tube G, (Fig. 4), both of which are cotton-plugged to maintain sterility.

A tipping platform, with places for eight culture vessels, has its position controlled by an electrically driven cam. The medium is fed into the vessels from a glass manifold filled with RP-S medium from a small refrigerator by a peristaltic pump. The tipping platform and filling manifold all fit into an incubator held at 37°C. Parasite multiplication with this apparatus is comparable to the continuous-flow method, with parasitemias ranging between 1–2% and 10–16% per 48-hour cycle (Table IX).

3. Large-Scale Production and Concentration of Parasite Material

Any of the methods considered above can be scaled up for the production of large amounts of parasites.

In addition we have used a large, flat-bottomed vessel (Fig. 7) patterned somewhat after the flow vessel but designed for manual intermittent change of medium without the use of peristaltic pumps. This holds 75 ml of red cell suspension (5 ml packed cells) to give 20% parasitemia (10×10^9 parasites).

Large parasites (trophozoites through segmenters) can be readily separated from uninfected red cells, and those with rings by the use of gelatin solutions, e.g., the plasma expander Physiogel (Pasvol *et al.*, 1978a; Reese *et al.*, 1978a) or gelatin (Jensen, 1978a). A suspension of infected cells is mixed with the gelatin solution and allowed to stand at 37°C for ½ hour. Cells with a normal biconcave shape (this includes cells with ring forms) aggregate in rouleaux and sediment rapidly, whereas deformed cells (this includes all those with trophozoites or later stages) remain suspended in the supernatant. By such treatment a 7% parasite suspension can yield a supernatant containing 70% parasites. The sedimented material with rings can be placed back in culture. This method is effective only for culture lines that still produce knobs on the surface of the host erythrocyte (see Langreth *et al.*, 1979).

If a culture is first made relatively synchronous, e.g., by treatment with 5% sorbitol (Vanderberg, personal communication), and then cultured to the late schizont stage, a fairly homogeneous concentrate of late segmenters can then be obtained by treatment with gelatin.

4. Cryopreservation of Cultures

We have modified a cryopreservation method originally reported by Rowe *et al.* (1968) that is simple and gives consistently repeatable results. The cryoprotectant is prepared by adding 70 ml glycerol to 180 ml 4.2% sorbitol in 0.9% sodium chloride and sterilizing through a 0.45-μm Millipore filter. Infected erythrocytes are centrifuged, the supernatant fluid is discarded, and the erythrocytes are resuspended in an equal volume of the cryoprotectant. After a 5-minute equilibration time the cells are distributed in 0.5-ml amounts to small screw-cap vials and frozen quickly by immersion in a dry ice–alcohol mixture or liquid nitrogen. Frozen vials are stored in a liquid nitrogen refrigerator. To reclaim cultures they are quickly thawed in a 37°C water bath, transferred to a sterile centrifuge tube, and spun at 500 *g* for 10 minutes. The glycerol supernatant is discarded and replaced with an equal volume of 3.5% sodium chloride. The cells are recovered by centrifugation, and the saline supernatant is discarded and replaced by an equal volume of RP-S containing 15% serum. This wash is

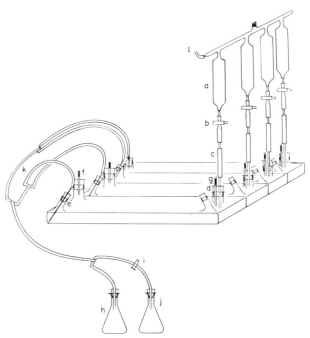

FIG. 7. Culture vessels for large-scale laboratory cultivation of *P. falciparum*. This apparatus allows large-scale production of parasites for immunological or biochemical purposes. Although it requires a daily manual change of culture medium, this operation takes only about 15–20 minutes, does not require peristaltic pumps, and can be accomplished without exposing the cultures to possible microbial contamination. The culture vessels, made from rectangular glass tubing (22 × 75 × 400 mm), with a cylindrical chimney (d) and a serum stoppered side port (e) at each end, are connected by glass and silicone tubing (c) to a four-place manifold whose arms (a) contain the premeasured, prewarmed culture medium. To renew the culture medium it is allowed to flow (by siphon) via the hypodermic needle inserted through the serum stoppered side port (c) into a flask (h) below. All the medium can be thus removed with few, if any, erythrocytes being lost. Fresh medium is delivered to the vessels from the manifold (a) through tubing (c) by opening the clamp (b). After the fresh medium is added, the erythrocytes are evenly suspended by gently rocking the vessels. Usually 2 hours before the medium is changed, the manifold is filled (by siphon) with chilled culture medium through tubing (1) from a reservoir held in a small refrigerator above the incubator. To harvest the parasitized erythrocytes, the medium is first removed, as above, the clamp (i) is shifted from flask j to flask h, and the vessels are tilted to a 45° angle which allows the cells to flow into flask j. Subcultures can be made by leaving sufficient infected erythrocytes in the vessels to seed new erythrocytes added through the serum stoppered side port located at the manifold end of the vessel. A gas mixture of 2% carbon dioxide, 3% oxygen, and 95% nitrogen flows continuously through the vessels from the cotton-plugged tube (f to g).

repeated once, and then the infected erythrocytes are mixed with a 5–10× volume of uninfected erythrocytes, diluted to an 8% cell suspension with RP-S (15%), distributed at 1.5 ml each into 35-mm petri dishes, and placed in a candle jar at 37°C (see above for details).

5. Information from Continuous Cultures

a. Gametocyte Formation. In infections produced by the inoculation of single erythrocytic parasites of *P. gallinaceum* into chicks (Downs, 1947) or *P. berghei* into mice (Walliker, 1976) gametocytes of both sexes appear. This shows that the asexual erythrocytic forms carry the information for gametocyte formation. What determines its expression is completely unknown. Continuous cultures provide an opportunity for attack on this problem.

So far it has been observed that recently isolated culture lines are more likely to produce gametocytes (Jensen, 1979), though immature gametocytes have also been occasionally seen after a year or more *in vitro* (Trager, 1979). Gametocytes capable of exflagellation have been produced in culture (Carter and Beach, 1977), but mosquitoes have not yet been infected from culture material. Such infections would be of practical importance in any attempt to develop a sporozoite vaccine.

b. Effect on Parasite Growth of the Genetic Character of Host Erythrocytes. The geographic distribution of a number of human red cell polymorphisms is highly correlated with the presence of hyperendemic malaria (Allison, 1961). It has been postulated that this is so because polymorphisms confer a measure of resistance to malaria, especially to *P. falciparum*, a parasite which causes an infection highly lethal to young children. Good statistical evidence supporting this hypothesis exists for only one of these polymorphisms—sickle hemoglobin (HbS). The heterozygote trait carriers of HbS on the average show lower parasitemia with *P. falciparum* than individuals with HbA. This must be an effect sufficient to permit relatively higher survival of the trait carriers, in this way supporting the continued presence of the gene for HbS even though in the homozygous state it is highly deleterious and usually results in death before reproductive age is reached.

How HbS acts to reduce the parasitemia has only recently been clarified. Friedman (1978) used an African strain of *P. falciparum* growing in continuous culture. He exposed cells from both homozygous (SS) and heterozygous (SA) individuals to infections *in vitro* and found that both types of cells supported as good growth of the parasites as normal AA cells if they were in an atmosphere with 17–18% oxygen. If, however, they were transferred to an atmosphere with 5% oxygen or less, the results were very different (Fig. 8). In the SS cells the parasite number went down sharply during the first day. Electron microscope

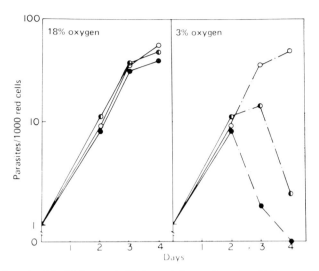

FIG. 8. Growth of *P. falciparum* in HbS-containing erythrocytes. Cultures were grown under an atmosphere of 18% oxygen–3% carbon dioxide for 2 days and then either maintained in this gas mixture (left) or shifted to 3% oxygen–3% carbon dioxide (right). Data shown are typical of growth in AA (○), SA (◐), and SS (●) red cells (from Friedman, 1978).

(EM) study of such parasites showed them to be damaged by the paracrystalline formation of the HbS (which is responsible for the sickling that occurs at low oxygen). Most interesting was the effect in the SA cells. Here during the first day there was a small increase in parasite number, indicating that maturation of late segmenters and reinvasion were not affected. By the second day parasites had decreased, and EM examination revealed a fine structure characteristic of degenerating trophozoites. It is possible that the partial paracrystalline formation of the HbS (which in SA cells may constitute up to 40% of the total hemoglobin) interferes with the phagocytic feeding of the parasite (Rudzinska and Trager, 1959). Other effects probably also play a role. Thus SA cells at low oxygen lose potassium, and M. J. Friedman (personal communication) has shown that prevention of this loss permits normal parasite development. Since the growing trophozoite stage of *P. falciparum* is ordinarily attached to capillary endothelium and sequestered in deep organs, it will be exposed to low oxygen tension, about 5%, so that the unfavorable conditions produced experimentally *in vitro* occur naturally *in vivo*. Independent confirmation of these results using short-term cultures and rather different methods has been reported by Pasvol *et al.* (1978b). Thus the relative resistance of sickle trait carriers to *P. falciparum* is accounted for at the cellular level.

The culture method now permits similar studies to be done with HbC, HbE, thalassemia, and the several glucose-6-phosphate dehydrogenase deficiencies, as well as with genetic membrane abnormalities such as ovalocytosis.

   c. **Chemotherapy and Drug Resistance.**   Petri dish cultures provide a simple, straightforward method for testing drugs directly for their effect on *P. falciparum* developing in human erythrocytes (Table X) (see Trager *et al.,* 1978). There is no need for an animal screen for compounds effective against the erythrocytic stage of this species. It is true that the culture method will not reveal drugs activated (or inactivated) by host metabolic reactions, but since these reactions often differ in mice and humans, the animal screen is not entirely reliable in this respect either. Compounds active *in vitro* will of course have to be studied in animals for their pharmacological properties. Those that appear safe will still have to be tested in humans, especially for the determination of blood levels, since these can be correlated with effective concentrations *in vitro*.

   Drug resistance shows up readily *in vitro* (Siddiqui *et al.,* 1972), and indeed this provided the basis for the very useful Rieckmann test (Rieckmann and Lopez-Antunano, 1971) for chloroquine resistance. The original method as developed by Rieckmann required a blood sample of at least 10 ml. This had to be taken by venipuncture, which severely limited the applicability of the method for field surveys, especially with children. Recently, however, Rieckmann has modified the continuous-culture method and developed a microtest for drug resistance that can be carried out with 20 μl of blood obtained by fingerprick (Rieckmann *et al.,* 1978; and personal communication).

   The continuous-culture method was used to produce *in vitro* a chloroquine-resistant line of an African strain of *P. falciparum* (Nguyen-Dinh and Trager, 1978) (Fig. 9). This indicated that there was no special genetic constraint in African *P. falciparum* against the development of chloroquine resistance. Drug-resistant lines produced *in vitro* from sensitive lines will provide material for direct biochemical comparison and perhaps for determination of the basis of drug resistance.

   d. **Nutrition and Metabolism.**   The continuous-culture method on the one hand permits study of the organisms under conditions optimal for their development. This should lead to determination of the exogenous nutrients required by the parasite host–cell complex and of metabolic products. The culture method also provides a means of producing large amounts of parasite material for the preparation of free parasites and for subcellular fractionation of the parasites. Work along both these two main lines is only beginning. It will be based on earlier work with experimental malarial infections, especially those caused by *P. lophurae* and *P. knowlesi*. These have been used for nutritional studies in short-term cultures (see Section II, I) and for free parasite preparations and subcellular

TABLE X

Antimalarial Effect *in Vitro* of Deaza-S-isobutyladenosine[a] on Culture Line FCR-3 of *Plasmodium falciparum*[b]

Dish	Concentration of drug (mM)	Parasite counts at 2 days per 10,000 red cells					Average normal parasites per 100 red cells
		Rings	Trophozoites	Schizonts	Total normal	Abnormal	
1	0	246	138	148	532	0	5
2	0	208	200	120	528	0	5
3	0	258	124	168	548	0	5
4	0.1	218	124	74	416	0	4
5	0.1	164	142	100	406	0	4
6	0.1	178	136	102	418	0	4
7	0.2	30	12	4	46	124	0.4
8	0.2	8	28	4	40	78	0.4
9	0.2	10	18	4	32	136	0.4
10	0.3	8	6	0	14	66	0.1
11	0.3	10	6	4	20	90	0.1
12	0.3	0	0	0	0	76	0.1

[a] A sample of this inhibitor of adenosyl homocysteine hydrolase was kindly supplied by P. K. Chiang and G. L. Cantoni, National Institute of Mental Health, Bethesda, Maryland.

[b] An 8% red cell suspension with a parasitemia of 1% was incubated for 2 days in petri dishes in a candle jar without and with drug.

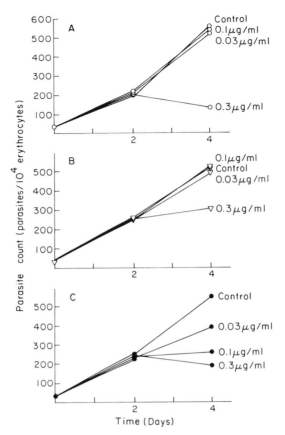

FIG. 9. Response to chloroquine of the Vietnamese (FCR-1), African (FCR-3), and adapted (R-FCR-3) strains with the petri dish test. Parasites from the three strains were grown for 2 days in normal medium under identical conditions and then exposed for 2 days to media containing no chloroquine or 0.3, 0.1, or 0.03 μg of chloroquine base per milliliter of medium. Each point represents the average of duplicate dishes. (A) Vietnamese (FCR-1) strain. (B) Adapted (R-FCR-3) strain. (C) Original African (FCR-3) strain (from Nguyen-Dinh and Trager, 1978).

fractionation (for example, see Sherman, 1977; Kilejian, 1974, 1975; Scheibel and Pflaum, 1970).

   e. Immunology (see Chapters 2, 3, 4, 5, 6, 7, Vol. 3).   Parasites after a year in continuous culture have been used to immunize *A. trivirgatus* monkeys (Reese *et al.,* 1978b), thus extending the earlier work on immunization with parasites produced by a 1-day incubation of infected *Aotus* blood (Siddiqui, 1977) or human blood (Mitchell *et al.,* 1977). The cultures will be of special use in providing merozoite material free of contaminating erythrocyte membranes.

They may also lead to the preparation of specific antigens involved in protective immunity.

Combined cultures of parasites with lymphocytes from immune and nonimmune hosts, using serum from immune and nonimmune hosts, are already being used to investigate in detail the nature of the immune reaction.

f. Changes Apparent after Long-Term Culture. After up to a year and a half of continuous culture, the parasites retained their original fine structure (Langreth *et al.*, 1978). All culture lines grown continuously for longer periods show progressive loss of the knobs on the surface of the infected erythrocytes (Langreth *et al.*, 1979). The knobs contain an antigen produced by the parasite (Kilejian *et al.*, 1977). Presumably, under culture conditions there occurs either a phenotypic change or selection in favor of a mutant that does not produce the knob protein (Kilejian, 1979). Although mostly "knobby" or "knobless" culture lines are available, choice between the alternative explanations will require establishment of clones (see Chapter 5, Vol. 3 for further details).

III. EXTRACELLULAR CULTURE OF ERYTHROCYTIC STAGES

A. *Plasmodium lophurae*

The avian malaria parasite *P. lophurae* is the only obligate intracellular protozoon that has been kept alive and developing extracellularly *in vitro* (Trager, 1957, 1958, 1971c). For this purpose the parasites were freed from their host erythrocytes by immune lysis and cultured in a nutrient medium containing an extract of duck red cells supplemented with certain essential cofactors. Electron microscopy (Fig. 10) (Trager *et al.*, 1972; Langreth and Trager, 1973) has shown that the parasites used as inoculum are completely freed from the plasma membrane of their host erythrocytes. They have, however, two membranes, their own parasite plasma membrane and a closely apposed outer parasitophorous membrane. The latter is derived by invagination of the erythrocyte plasma membrane at the time the merozoite invades, but quickly becomes modified (McLaren *et al.*, 1977; Langreth, 1977). This membrane grows with the parasite, extracellularly *in vitro* as well as in the normal intracellular situation (Fig. 11). When merozoites are formed during extracellular development *in vitro*, they separate from the parasitophorous membrane just as they do normally *in vivo*. It has not been possible to determine with certainty whether merozoites formed under these conditions *in vitro* are capable of further development. If medium is changed twice daily, many parasites of normal appearance are present up to the fourth day. On the third day young trophozoites of normal ultrastructure are seen without a parasitophorous membrane. They could have developed from

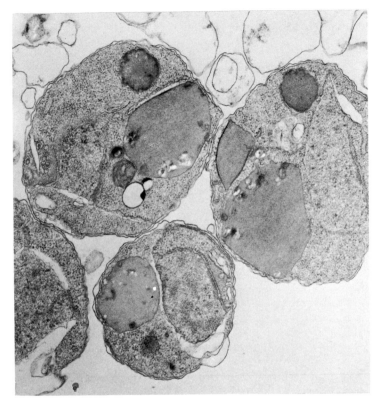

FIG. 10. Parasites of *P. lophurae* freshly isolated from their host erythrocytes by immune lysis. The parasites are bounded by two membranes, the outermost, the parasitophorous vacuole membrane, is derived from the erythrocyte plasmalemma. ×21,000 (from Langreth and Trager, 1973).

merozoites formed *in vitro,* or they could represent surviving forms that have lost the parasitophorous membrane. After the second day the cultures become too asynchronous to permit detailed assessment.

For this reason the cultures are most useful for short-term studies. In these studies the parasites are put in culture when they are young, uninucleate trophozoites. One day later their growth and development are assessed by morphological criteria (proportions of multinucleate and degenerate parasites) and by their activity in incorporating various ^{14}C-labeled precursors, e.g., amino acids, into trichloracetic acid (TCA)-precipitable material. Such short-term experiments, as well as those involving longer maintenance, have shown the importance of the red cell extract and the requirement of the parasites for exogenous sources of ATP and CoA (Trager, 1950, 1971c).

The requirement for CoA (Table XI) seems to rest on a major biosynthetic

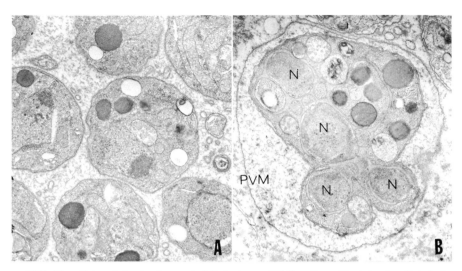

FIG. 11. Extracellular development of *P. lophurae*. (A) Parasites cultivated extracellularly *in vitro* for 1 day. The fine structure of these trophozoites suggests healthy normal cells. ×20,000. (B) A schizont after 2 days of extracellular development. Note the four nuclei (N), as well as the greatly expanded parasitophorous vacuole membrane (PVM). ×20,000 (from Langreth and Trager, 1973).

defect of the parasite. It has not so far been possible to demonstrate in *P. lophurae* any of the enzymes of the pathway from pantothenic acid to CoA. All these enzymes are easily demonstrated in the host duck erythrocyte (Trager and Brohn, 1975; Brohn and Trager, 1975). Similar studies with other species of malaria would be of great interest.

The ATP requirement probably has a rather different basis, for *P. lophurae* has its own glycolytic enzymes able to form ATP (Trager, 1967). The requirement itself is a striking one (Table XII). Bongkrekic acid, an inhibitor of mitochondrial ATP translocase, as well as of ATPase and cation transport, was found to inhibit extracellular development of *P. lophurae* (Table XIII) at concentrations down to 2 μg/ml, and this inhibition was partly reversed by high concentrations of ATP (Trager, 1973). These results suggest that the requirement for exogenous ATP may be related to transport across the parasitophorous membrane, a membrane that has ATPase demonstrable at its inner surface (Langreth, 1977).

The erythrocyte extract surely contributes hemoglobin, a principal source of amino acids, and probably also other essential materials (Trager, 1958). It is clear that only a small beginning has been made toward dissection of the intimate physiological relationships between an intracellular parasite and its host cell. As already emphasized in another connection (Trager, 1978), this should become a

TABLE XI

Effect of CoA on the Extracellular Development of *Plasmodium lophurae* and Its Partial Replacement by Phosphopantetheine (PPS) but Not by Phosphopantothenoylcysteine (PPC) or Phosphopantothenic acid (PPA)[a]

Experiment	Flasks	Supplement	Concentration (mM)	Average percentage of parasites after 1 day[b]		Incorporation (cpm/100 × 10⁶ parasites per hour of exposure)
				>1 Nucleus	Degenerate	
1	1–3	None	0	16	9	398
	4–6	PPA	0.06	15	7	414
	7–9	CoA	0.05	21	4	665
2	1–3	None	0	12	16	207
	4–6	PPA	0.06	16	22	266
	7–9	CoA	0.05	16	7	356
3	1–3	CoA	0.05	30	11	646
	4–6	PPC	0.05	16	16	473
	7–9	PPS	0.05	21	13	602
	10–12	None	0	15	16	347

[a] The medium was one-third strength erythrocyte extract with all supplements except CoA as indicated. At 16 hours each flask received, in experiments 1 and 2, 2.5 μCi of L-[*methyl*-¹⁴C]methionine, and in experiment 3, 2.5 μCi of L-[U-¹⁴C]isoleucine. Samples were taken 3–4 hours later. From Trager and Brohn (1975).

[b] At 0 time the percentages with >1 nucleus were 6, 4, and 9 for experiments 1–3, respectively.

TABLE XII

Incorporation of L-[U-¹⁴C]Proline by Extracellular *Plasmodium lophurae*[a]

Flasks	Medium	Average percentage of parasites[b]			Average cpm per culture per hour of exposure
		>1N	>2N	Degenerate	
1–3	0.3 RCE in A, no ATP pyruvate	5	1	21	167
4–6	0.3 RCE in A, complete	18	4	5	253
7–9	0.3 RCE in B, no ATP pyruvate	7	2	24	150
10–12	0.3 RCE in B, complete	19	4	3	256

[a] Effect of ATP and pyruvate omission in 0.3 red cell extract (RCE) made with two different diluents: (A) Standard diluent containing adenine sulfate, guanine, xanthine, and uracil each at 0.5 mg/liter and cytidylic acid at 0.2 mg/liter. (B) Modified diluent with these materials replaced by adenosine at 10 mg/liter and orotic acid at 4 mg/liter. Each flask received 50 × 10⁶ parasites. Tracer (2.5 μCi per flask, specific activity 260 mCi/mmole) was added after 16 hours, and samples taken 3–4 hours later. Data from Trager, 1971c.

[b] At 0 time there were 2% with >1 nucleus (>1N) and 0.5% with >2 nuclei (>2N).

TABLE XIII

Effects of Bongkrekic Acid (BK), Oligomycin (O), and Atractyloside (A) on *Plasmodium lophurae* **Developing Extracellularly** *in Vitro*[a]

Experiment	Flasks	Inhibitor (μg/ml)	With >1 nucleus	With >2 nuclei	Degenerate	Average cpm per 100×10^6 parasites per hour of exposure
			Average percentage of parasites after 20 hours[b]			
A	1–3	None	35	9	1.0	348
	4–6	BK, 1.4	20	3	0.5	217
	7–9	BK, 2.8	16	3	0.5	204
	10–12	BK, 14.0	24	5	1.0	177
B	1–3	None	32	10	3	420
	4–6	BK, 50	26	6	0.5	206
	7–9	O,[c] 5	31	9	2	350
	10–12	A, 100	31	10	4	354
C	1–3	None	30	10	3	344
	4–6	O,[c] 30	8	1	11	104
	7–9	BK, 15	15	3	4	212
	10–12	BK, 38	23	4	2	200
D	1–3	None	46	17	2	545
	4–6	EtOH, 2500	36	18	3	460

[a] The medium was a 0.3 strength red cell extract with all supplements. After a 15- to 16-hour incubation at 40°C, each flask received 2.5 μCi [U-^{14}C]proline. Sampling was done 3–4 hours later. From Trager (1973).

[b] At 0 time there were the following percentages of parasites with >1 and >2 nuclei, respectively: experiment A,6 and 0.5; B,5 and 0; C,6 and 3; D,12 and 3.

[c] Oligomycin (Sigma, 15% oligomycin A, 85% B) added as an ethanol (95%) solution to give a final ethanol concentration of 0.27%, which itself had a small inhibitory effect (experiment D).

major field of study and should include other kinds of intracellular parasitic protozoa.

1. Methods for Extracellular Cultivation of Plasmodium lophurae

Only those used for *P. lophurae* will be treated, since the work with *P. falciparum* is at too premature a stage.

a. Medium. This is an extract of duck erythrocytes in a complex nutrient mixture (Table XIV). It is prepared aseptically from defibrinated blood taken from ducks not over 3 months old. The blood is centrifuged in 25-ml amounts, and the serum and most of the buffy coat are removed. The approximately 10 ml of cells in each tube is frozen in a dry ice–ethanol bath and stored overnight in a dry ice chest. The cells are thawed by immersion of the tube in ice water, suspended in 13.3 ml of diluent A-1 (Table XIV), and centrifuged 50 minutes at 1800 g at 20°C. A low temperature cannot be used, since the diluent contains gelatin. Each such tube yields 8–9 ml of a deep-red supernatant designated full strength (1×) extract. This contains about 14% hemoglobin, or roughly one-half the concentration of hemoglobin present in the erythrocytes. The pH of the extract is adjusted to 6.9 with sterile 0.1 M hydrochloric acid.

For many types of work it is convenient to use more dilute red cell extracts. A one-quarter strength (0.25×) extract is prepared by mixing 1 part 1× extract (before pH adjustment) with 3 parts diluent A-1. The pH of this mixture is brought to 6.9 with sterile 0.1 M potassium hydroxide. The final extracts then receive, at the rate of 0.2 ml/10 ml medium, a solution containing (at pH 6.0) L-malic acid, yeast adenylic acid (2′ and 3′ mixed isomers), and nicotinamide adenine dinucleotide to give final concentrations of 6.0, 1.4, and 0.15 mM, respectively. To complete the medium ATP, pyruvate, CoA, and folinic acid are added as small volumes of concentrated solutions to give final concentrations of 2, 5, 0.05, and 0.01 mM, respectively.

b. Preparation of Free Parasites.   The inoculum of free parasites is prepared by immune lysis from the blood of infected young Pekin ducklings on the fourth day after inoculation, showing a fairly synchronous parasitemia of close to 100%, with 90% or more of the parasites in the uninucleate trophozoite stage (see Trager, 1950). An appropriate amount of blood is drawn aseptically, using as anticoagulant a solution with 30 mg heparin/100 ml of 0.85% sodium chloride at the rate of 0.1 ml/ml blood. The blood is centrifuged, the plasma removed, and the cells suspended in 1× red cell extract to make a 20% suspension. To 6.3 ml of such a suspension in a 50-ml erlenmeyer flask with a silicone rubber stopper are added 0.13 ml sterile guinea pig serum (as a complement source) and 0.7 ml of a potent rabbit anti-duck erythrocyte serum (hemolytic titer of 1:10,000). The mixture is incubated ½ hour at 40°C on a rocker, with shaking at 15 minutes, and is then transferred to a conical centrifuge tube and centrifuged 1 minute to a speed of 500 rpm. Red cells that are hemolyzed but that still have their plasma membranes are agglutinated, hence sedimented, by this very brief centrifugation. Free parasites (and small numbers of free red cell nuclei) remain in the supernatant which is used to inoculate experimental flasks.

c. Preparation of the Cultures and Assessment of Growth.   Erlenmeyer flasks (50 ml) are equipped with a sterile silicone rubber stopper bearing a cotton-plugged gas inlet and an outlet tube. Each flask receives 0.25 ml of sterile duck plasma obtained by carefully bleeding a duckling without an anticoagulant and centrifuging the blood. To this is added 0.2 ml of chick embryo extract. The flask is then rotated in such a way that as the plasma clots it forms a layer lining

TABLE XIV

Composition of Solution A-1 Used to Make the Erythrocyte Extract[a]

		Stock solution	For 100 ml of final medium	
No.	Ingredient	Concentration (mg/100 ml)	Volume stock solution (ml)	Final concentration (mg/100 ml)
1	NaCl	6,600	5.0	330.0
	KCl	8,800		440.0
2	$NaH_2PO_4 \cdot H_2O$	550	2.5	13.8
	K_2HPO_4	6,270		156.8
3	$NaHCO_3$	5,000	1.8	90.0
4	$CaCl_2$	260	1.5	3.9
5	$MnSO_4 \cdot H_2O$	170	2.0	3.4
6	Sodium acetate	1,500	1.0	15.0
	Glycerol	2,500		25.0
7	Dextrose	5,000	4.3	215.0
8	Hexose diphosphate (magnesium salt)	5,000	1.4	70.0
9	Glutathione (reduced)	2,000	5.0	100.0
	L-Ascorbic acid	20		1.0
	Nicotinamide	8,000		400.0
115	Lactalbumin hydrolysate	1,500	52.0	750
	Bovine plasma fraction V	1,200		600
12-2	Gelatin (Wilson PF)	36,000	20.0	7,200
13 h	Riboflavin	5	1.0	0.05
	Thioctic acid	1		0.01
	Thiamine–HCl	5		0.05
	Pyridoxine–HCl	5		0.05
	Pyridoxamine–2HCl	2		0.02
	Pyridoxal–HCl	2		0.02
	Vitamin B_{12}	1		0.01
	Inositol	10		0.10
	Nicotinamide	50		0.50
	Choline chloride	50		0.50
13 b	Calcium pantothenate	200	0.5	1.0
13 d	p-Aminobenzoic acid	100	0.1	0.1
14 B	Biotin	5	0.01	0.0005
14 F	Folic acid	5	0.02	0.001
15 c	Adenosine	100	1.0	1.0
	Orotic acid	40		0.4

[a] All solutions were prepared in water redistilled in a Pyrex glass still. Stock solutions 1, 2, 4, 5, 7, 13 b, 13 d, 14 B, and 14 F were placed in tubes and sterilized by autoclaving. Solution 12-2 was placed in tubes and sterilized by steaming 20 minutes on each of three successive days. Solutions 3, 6, 8, 13 h, and 15 c were sterilized by filtration (porcelain Selas 03 filter) and aseptically placed in tubes. Solution 115 was similarly sterilized and placed, in 52-ml amounts, in 250-ml erlenmeyer flasks. The final mixture was prepared by addition aseptically to such a flask of the designated amount of each solution in the order 1, 2, 3, 7, 8, 12-2, 4, 5, 6, 13 h, 13 b, 13 d, 14 B, 14 F, and 15 c. Finally freshly prepared and sterilized (through a glass ultrafine filter) solution 9 was added, followed by 15 ml of duck serum (from defibrinated blood of ducks not over 3 months old). The stock solutions were stored up to 3 months in a refrigerator, except for 13 h, which was kept frozen at $-20°C$, and solution 9, which was always freshly prepared. The final mixture was used on the day of preparation. From Trager and Brohn (1975).

the lower portion of the wall of the flask. The flask then receives 3 ml of red cell extract medium, the appropriate supplements (ATP, pyruvate, CoA, and folinic acid for a complete medium), and finally the inoculum of free parasites, ordinarily $50-150 \times 10^6$/flask. The flasks are set on a rocking table (at 16 cycles/min) and receive a slow current of air with 5% carbon dioxide. After overnight incubation about one-half of the free parasites form a visible "scum" sticking to the plasma clot lining the wall of the flask. Bits of this scum can be conveniently removed with capillary-tip pipets for the preparation of slides or for electron microscopy. Giemsa-stained films are used to count the proportions of degenerate parasites and of parasites with two or more nuclei. The starting material contains 90–95% uninucleate forms and essentially no degenerate parasites. Under optimal conditions after 1 day there will be very few degenerating parasites and up to 50% with two or more nuclei (Fig. 12).

If incorporation of radioactive tracers is to be followed, they are added usually after 16 hours of incubation, and the cultures are incubated for an additional 4 hours. The fluid portion is then removed to a centrifuge tube while 10% TCA is added to the flask. The material in the centrifuge tube is centrifuged 10 minutes at 3000 rpm (1800 g) to sediment those parasites that have not adhered in the scum. The supernatant is removed, and the small pellet is fixed with cold 10%

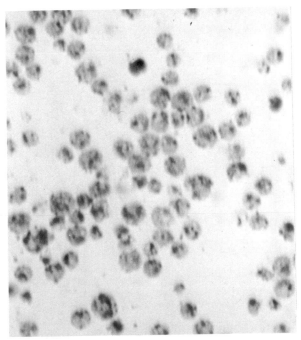

FIG. 12. Light micrograph of a thin film of trophozoites and young schizonts of *P. lophurae* grown extracellularly for 1 day. Note numerous parasites with two or more nuclei. ×3000.

TCA. This and the material in the flask are combined for further treatment and scintillation counting to determine the radioactivity incorporated by the parasites during their last 4 hours of incubation (see Trager, 1971c).

d. Prolonged Cultures. This is possible only with a full-strength red cell extract. The old medium is removed, and fresh medium is added after 1 day (18–20 hours) and thereafter at 12-hour intervals. This means that parasites suspended in the medium and not adherent in the scum are removed with the first change of medium. Under these conditions free parasites showed excellent survival for 2 days, but by the end of the third day about 10% appeared degenerate (Langreth and Trager, 1973). When the inoculum after hemolysis was not subjected to differential centrifugation, so that it included parasites still within the plasma membrane of hemolyzed cells, a majority of the free parasites appeared morphologically normal even after 4 days, and infectivity could be demonstrated (Trager, 1957) through the fifth day. Results from such preparations, however, are not readily interpretable.

If the parasitophorous membrane is essential for the parasites' development, then continuous extracellular cultivation would require either that merozoites be provided with such membranes or that the functions of the membrane be somehow performed by other constituents of the medium. Attempts to maintain merozoites extracellularly might lead to important results in this connection. Such attempts should be made with exoerythrocytic as well as erythrocytic merozoites of *P. lophurae* and with the erythrocytic merozoites of *P. falciparum* derived from continuous cultures.

B. *Plasmodium falciparum*

Preliminary experiments with *P. falciparum* rings from infected *Aotus* monkeys freed by immune lysis and placed in a human erythrocyte extract suggest that this parasite also is capable of limited extracellular development (Trager, 1974). Now that *P. falciparum* can be grown *in vitro* in human erythrocytes, it should be possible to start cultures with uninucleate trophozoites freed from their host cells and in this way to duplicate more closely the experiments with *P. lophurae*. That *P. falciparum* might have a requirement for exogenous ATP has already been indicated by its better development in hosts whose erythrocytes have a relatively higher ATP level (Brewer and Powell, 1965).

IV. EXOERYTHROCYTIC STAGES IN CULTURE

A. Avian Exoerythrocytic Parasites

The exoerythrocytic stages of plasmodia, as the term implies, are the developmental stages occurring in vertebrate host cells other than erythrocytes or their immediate precursors, reticulocytes and erythroblasts. In avian species of *Plasmodium* these stages may be preerythrocytic, developing from sporozoites with cryptozoic (primary) and metacryptozoic (secondary) schizogony producing cryptozoites and metacryptozoites, respectively; or they may be initiated from erythrocytic forms that invade tissue cells to become phanerozoites (Huff and Coulston, 1944). These terms, "cryptozoite," "metacryptozoite," and "phanerozoite," are used to denote exoerythrocytic zoites according to their origin, but these stages are essentially indistinguishable otherwise (Huff, 1969). In avian species the exoerythrocytic stages occur in cells of the reticuloendothelial system, whereas in mammalian species they develop in hepatic parenchymal cells.

The exoerythrocytic stages of avian plasmodia have been grown routinely in tissue culture for over 30 years. Detailed reviews of early work have been published by Porter (1948), Hawking (1951), Pipkin and Jensen (1956), and Huff (1964), thus only a brief historical account will be given here. The first attempts at exoerythrocytic parasite cultivation by Huff and Bloom (1935) consisted of cultures of bone marrow cells from canaries infected with *P. elongatum*. Although these investigators saw no parasites in their cultures, the material remained infective when injected into susceptible canaries after 48 hours *in vitro*. Gavrilov *et al.* (1938) cultured exoerythrocytic stages of *P. gallinaceum* in bone marrow explants from infected chicks maintained by plasma clot or hanging-drop techniques, which remained infective after 10 days in culture. It is not clear whether these meager results reflect unsatisfactory methods or the use of poor sources of exoerythrocytic parasites. Their cultures were made from tissues of birds in the early stages of infections which had been initiated by the inoculation of infected blood. Any exoerythrocytic schizonts would certainly be rare in the course of such infections. These investigators tried to infect cultures of normal tissues with blood from infected birds and failed consistently.

The work of Hawking (1944, 1945) demonstrated that cultures started from a rich source of exoerythrocytic parasites and maintained in a susceptible cell line could be grown abundantly *in vitro* for long periods of time. His starting material was either splenic or peripheral blood macrophages obtained from chicks infected by sporozoites of *P. gallinaceum*. His cultures remained viable and infective to young chicks for 89 days. This work was confirmed by Zuckerman (1946) who, in addition, made the significant observation that chick embryonic spleen was a far richer source of exoerythrocytic stages than hatched chicks. The first long-term cultures were those of Meyer and Musacchio (1959) who grew the exoerythrocytic stages of *P. gallinaceum* for 4 years in explants of chick embryonic myocardial cells using alternately the plasma clot and hanging-drop techniques. Concurrent with the work of culturing exoerythrocytic parasites in tissue explants was the development of serial passages of these parasites in embryonated chicken, duck, and turkey eggs (see review of techniques by Pipkin and Jensen, 1956). The most successful techniques involved suprachorioallantoic implantation of infected tissue from other embryos. Today numerous strains of avian plasmodia are routinely maintained by regular passage from embryo to embryo by chorioallantoic grafting. Tissues from infected embryos were an excellent source of seed material for initiating cultures in monolayers of avian cells and led to the development by Huff and his co-workers of the techniques used today for long-term cultures (Huff *et al.*, 1960; Huff, 1964).

Cultures of avian exoerythrocytic parasites are generally started from tissues of infected birds or embryonated eggs but may also be initiated from sporozoites, and perhaps also from erythrocytic stages. Meyer (1947) demonstrated exoerythrocytic stages in embryonic chick brain cells after adding erythrocytic stages to them. Later she repeated this work (Meyer, 1949) but suggested that her experiments did not prove that erythrocytic stages could give rise to exoerythrocytic forms in culture, because some exoerythrocytic merozoites may have been present. The first successful cultures started from sporozoites were those of Dubin *et al.* (1949, 1950) who grew the preerythrocytic parasites of *P. gallinaceum* by adding sporozoites of this parasite to cultures of chick tissues. This method has not been generally successful, however, because of the difficulty of obtaining sporozoites free of the bacterial and fungal contaminants that are part of the normal flora of the mosquitoes that produce the sporozoites.

TABLE XV

Components and Stock Solutions Needed for the Culture Medium Used in Exoerythrocytic Stage Cultures of *Plasmodium fallax* and *Plasmodium lophurae*[a,b]

Components[c]	Amount	Stock	Supplier[d]
Medium 199 with Earle's salts	9.87 g	Powdered base	Gibco
BME with Earle's salts	9.00 g	Powdered base	Gibco
BME, vitamin mixture	10.0 ml	Commercial stock, 100×	MBA
Folinic acid, calcium salt	2.0 ml	6 mg/100 ml H_2O	Gibco
MEM, nonessential amino acids	10.0 ml	Commercial stock, 100×	MBA
L-Glutamine	0.292 g		Sigma
Sodium bicarbonate	2.45 g		Sigma
Penicillin–streptomycin	20.0 ml	Stock: 5000 units plus 5000 μg/ml	
Fetal bovine serum, heat-inactivated	10.0 ml		Gibco
Glass-redistilled water	Sufficient to total 2000 ml		

[a] Adjust final pH to 7.4 with 1.0 N Sodium hydroxide.
[b] Filter final solution through 0.45-μm Millipore apparatus.
[c] Basal medium (Eagle's); MEM, minimal essential medium.
[d] Gibco, Grand Island Biological Company, Grand Island, New York; MBA, Microbiological Associates, Bethesda, Maryland, Sigma, Sigma Chemical Company, St. Louis, Missouri.

1. Method for Cultivation

Details of procedures for the long-term culture of avian exoerythrocytic forms were given by Davis *et al.* (1966) and recently modified by Beaudoin (1977). Cultures are initiated from embryonic turkey brain tissue infected with *P. fallax* or *P. lophurae* maintained by weekly serial passage from embryo to embryo, or from cryopreserved stabilates of infected embryonic turkey brain cells. A third species, *P. gallinaceum*, has been grown in cultured chicken brain cells with only limited success. The constituents of the culture medium are listed in Table XV. The embryonic turkey brains (infected on days 7–11 and harvested 6 days later) are excised, minced, trypsinized, and distributed in the culture medium into T-30 culture flasks. Once these primary cultures form a confluent monolayer, they are subcultured by standard procedures, i.e., trypsinization to break up the cell sheet, dilution, and distribution into two or three new culture flasks. Routinely, the generation time of the parasites is shorter than that of the brain cells to the extent that the cultures usually become overparasitized by the fourth subculture. When the cultures become overparasitized, new cultures are started either by diluting at the time of subculture with uninfected embryonic turkey brain cells, or by using the medium from highly parasitized cultures, which contains many parasitized cells sloughed from the monolayer, to seed new cultures of turkey brain cells.

2. Uses of Cultured Exoerythrocytic Parasites

The first obvious advantages of cultures of exoerythrocytic stages over *in vivo* studies was the opportunity for detailed observation of the morphology and development of these stages (Figs. 13 and 14). The first direct observations of these forms *in vitro* were made by Hegner and Wolfson (1939) who examined stages of *P. cathemerium* from canary lung in a hanging-drop culture. A thorough study of the morphology and behavior of living exoerythrocytic stages of *P. gallinaceum* and *P. fallax* was reported by Huff *et al.* (1960) using phase-contrast microscopy and time-lapse photography. The first fine-structural studies on cultured exoerythrocytic parasites, those of Meyer and de Oliveira-Musacchio (1960, 1965), were lacking in precise detail. However, a complete study with excellent detail was reported by Hepler *et al.* (1966). Since most studies on the fine structure of exoerythrocytic parasites were made on material grown in tissue culture, a comparative study was done with material fixed *in vivo* by Aikawa *et al.* (1968) on exoerythrocytic stages of *P. gallinaceum* in chick embryo liver.

In vitro cultures of exoerythrocytic forms allow the testing of chemotherapeutic agents on these stages. The first attempts to study the direct action of drugs upon exoerythrocytic stages were reported by Tonkin (1946). She tested the effects of different drugs at various concentrations using primary cultures of

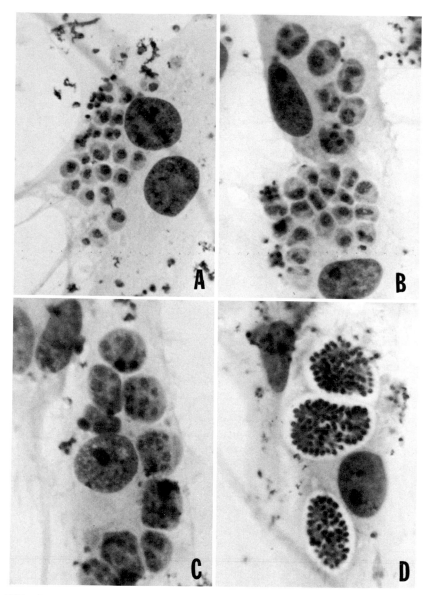

FIG. 13. Developmental stages of *P. fallax* in embryonic turkey brain cells. (A) Binucleate host cell with young trophozoites. (B) Two parasitized turkey brain cells, one with several trophozoites (bottom) and the other with young schizonts. (C) Host cell with multinucleate schizonts. (D) Host cell with three mature schizonts containing exoerythrocytic merozoites. All micrographs are ×3000. (Micrographs kindly provided by Richard Beaudoin, Naval Medical Research Institute, Bethesda, Maryland.)

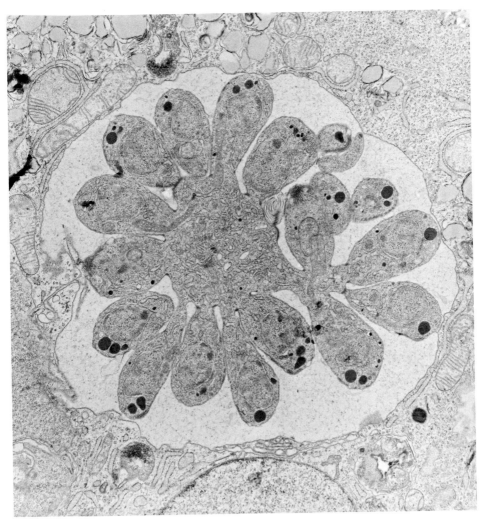

FIG. 14. Electron micrograph of a *P. lophurae* schizont showing numerous merozoite anlagen forming within the cultured embryonic turkey brain cell. ×21,000. (Micrograph kindly provided by Richard Beaudoin, Naval Medical Research Institute, Bethesda, Maryland.)

chick tissue infected with *P. gallinaceum*. Antiparasitic effects were observed when sulfathiazole, sulfadiazine, *m*-aminobenzenesulfonamidopyrimidine, and α-anisylguanidine nitrate were used. Streptothricin and streptomycin also caused some inhibition of parasitic growth. Quinine sulfate was slightly effective at concentrations that were toxic to the cells. Little or no activity was observed for mepacrine, pamaquine, stilbamidine, chlorguanide, and sontoquine. Although these earlier studies by Tonkin (1946), and also by Coulston and Huff (1948), using the light microscope, indicated that the drugs effected some damage to the parasites, they showed little more than that. Later, using refined culture techniques and ultrastructural studies, Beaudoin and Aikawa (1968) reported on the action of primaquine on the exoerythrocytic stages of *P. fallax* in embryonic turkey brain cells. Their study revealed that the site of drug action was apparently the parasite mitochondria which, unlike those of the host cell, were greatly swollen in cultures containing the drug. In another study, Beaudoin *et al.* (1967) showed that a strain of *P. gallinaceum* could retain its ability to transmit resistance to pyrimethamine through several subcultures of exoerythrocytic stages in the absence of an erythrocytic cycle. With this demonstration they supplied the last link in the life cycle of the parasite through which drug resistance had been transmitted.

Another field of study utilizing *in vitro* cultures of the exoerythrocytic stages of plasmodia is the immunology of malarial infections. Evidence of immunity to exoerythrocytic stages was demonstrated in experiments reported by Graham *et al.* (1973) where turkey poults, inoculated with serum from birds recovering from *P. fallax* infections, were later challenged with exoerythrocytic stages produced in cell cultures. Birds that received serum showed 90% fewer exoerythrocytic forms than the controls. Later, Holbrook *et al.* (1974) extended the study by immunizing birds with exoerythrocytic merozoites harvested from cultured turkey fibroblasts. Strong protective immunity was demonstrated in the vaccinated birds, 90% of which survived challenge versus 30% in the controls. Immunization with exoerythrocytic merozoites failed to protect against challenge with erythrocytic forms.

Experiments by Holbrook *et al.* (1976) showed that merozoites harvested from cell cultures of *P. fallax,* when used to immunize mice, offered some protection when challenged with sporozoites of *P. berghei,* a mammalian *Plasmodium.* In their conclusions the authors suggested that the immunity may have been nonspecific but did not rule out the possibility that some cross-immunization had occurred.

B. Mammalian Exoerythrocytic Parasites

The exoerythrocytic stages of mammalian plasmodia occur in hepatic parenchymal cells and, unlike those of avian species, develop principally from sporozoites. They are then preerythrocytic, having no phanerozoites, and it is becoming generally accepted that most mammalian species have only one, or at most, only a few exoerythrocytic schizogonous cycles (Garnham, 1977). Early attempts to culture exoerythrocytic forms in various tissue explants from monkeys infected with *P. cynomolgi* (Hawking *et al.,* 1948) and human bone marrow explants from patients infected by sporozoites of *P. vivax* and *P. fal-*

ciparum (Dubin, 1947, 1948) were uniformly unsuccessful. Recently, however, Foley *et al.* (1978) were successful in culturing rat liver cells infected with exoerythrocytic forms of *P. berghei* for up to 44 hours and found the cultures to be infective when inoculated into recipient rodents. They were able to rule out the presence of erythrocytic stages or sporozoites in their cultures by showing that the blood from the donor rats was not infective when injected into susceptible rodents and by immunizing the recipient rats against *P. berghei* sporozoites. They concluded therefore that the primary liver cultures contained viable exoerythrocytic schizonts that had been maintained *in vitro* for 44 hours. This report is reminiscent of that by Huff and Bloom (1938) who cultured bone marrow explants of canaries infected with *P. elongatum* for 48 hours and found them to be still infective to susceptible birds.

Dubin *et al.* (1950) reported that attempts to infect human liver and bone marrow cultures with sporozoites of *P. vivax* were unsuccessful. Their liver tissue cultures, however, contained only fibroblasts and Kupffer cells. They suggested that the lack of parenchymatous liver cells might account for their failure. Recently, Doby and Barker (1976) reported finding intracellular bodies in human liver cell cultures into which sporozoites of *P. vivax* had been introduced. They concluded that these bodies were the preerythrocytic stages of this parasite but offered no further evidence as to their parasitological nature. Unfortunately their material was lost soon after the original observations, thus no further examination was possible.

Recent investigations by Beaudoin and co-workers (1974) greatly undermined the hypothesis of parasite–host cell specificity by successful cultivation of the avian plasmodia *P. fallax* and *P. lophurae* in embryonic mouse liver parenchymal cells. They were able to grow these exoerythrocytic stages in mouse liver cells through several subcultures until the cultures became overparasitized. These findings illustrate that cultures of mammalian liver parenchymal cells can support avian malaria parasites and that the presumed host specificity does not necessarily hold true for *in vitro* systems. Their laboratory has recently followed up these remarkable findings with a preliminary report on the successful cultivation of exoerythrocytic stages of *P. berghei* (Strome *et al.,* 1979). They used sporozoites of *P. berghei* to infect monolayers of embryonic turkey brain cells and observed development from sporozoite through cryptozoic schizogony to merozoites. Reinvasion or initiation of a second exoerythroyctic cycle was not observed.

REFERENCES

Aikawa, M., Huff, C. G., and Sprinz, H. (1968). Electron microscope observation of the exoerythrocytic stages of *Plasmodium gallinaceum* in chick embryo liver. *Am. J. Trop. Med. Hyg.* **17**, 156–169.

Allison, A. C. (1961). Genetic factors in resistance to malaria. *Ann. N. Y. Acad. Sci.* **91,** 710–729.

Anderson, C. R. (1953). Continuous propagation of *Plasmodium gallinaceum* in chicken erythrocytes. *Am. J. Trop. Med. Hyg.* **2,** 234–242.

Ball, E. G. (1946). Chemical and nutritional observations on malarial parasites grown *in vitro. Fed. Proc., Fed. Am. Soc. Exp. Biol.* **5,** 397–399.

Ball, E. G., Anfinsen, C. B., Geiman, Q. M., McKee, R. W., and Ormsbee, R. A. (1945). *In vitro* growth and multiplication of the malaria parasite, *Plasmodium knowlesi. Science* **101,** 542–544.

Bass, C. C., and Johns, F. M. (1912). The cultivation of malarial plasmodia (*Plasmodium vivax* and *Plasmodium falciparum*) *in vitro. J. Exp. Med.* **16,** 567–579.

Beaudoin, R. L. (1977). Should cultivated exoerythrocytic parasites be considered as a source of antigen for a malaria vaccine? *Bull. W. H. O.* **55,** 373–376.

Beaudoin, R. L., and Aikawa, M. (1968). Primaquine-induced changes in morphology of exoerythrocytic stages of malaria. *Science* **160,** 1233–1234.

Beaudoin, R. L., Strome, C. P. A., and Huff, C. G. (1967). Persistance of pyrimethamine resistance in exoerythrocytic stages of *Plasmodium gallinaceum. Exp. Parasitol.* **20,** 156–159.

Beaudoin, R. L., Strome, C. P. A., and Clutter, W. G. (1974). Cultivation of avian malaria parasites in mammalian liver cells. *Exp. Parasitol.* **36,** 355–359.

Bertagna, P., Cohen, S., Geiman, Q. M., Haworth, J., Königk, E., Richards, W. H. G., and Trigg, P. I. (1972). Cultivation of malaria parasites. *Bull. W.H.O.* **47,** 357–373.

Black, R. H. (1946). The effect of antimalarial drugs on *Plasmodium falciparum* (New Guinea strains) developing *in vitro. Trans. R. Soc. Trop. Med. Hyg.* **40,** 163–170.

Brewer, G. J., and Powell, R. D. (1965). A study of the relationship between the content of adenosine triphosphate in human red cells and the course of falciparum malaria: A new system that may confer protection against malaria. *Proc. Natl. Acad. Sci. U.S.A.* **54,** 741–745.

Brohn, F. H., and Trager, W. (1975). Coenzyme A requirement of malaria parasites: Enzymes of coenzyme A biosynthesis in normal duck erythrocytes and erythrocytes infected with *Plasmodium lophurae. Proc. Natl. Acad. Sci, U.S.A.* **72,** 2456–2458.

Carter, R., and Beach, R. F. (1977). Gametogenesis in culture by gametocytes of *Plasmodium falciparum. Nature (London)* **270,** 240–241.

Coulston, F., and Huff, C. G. (1948). Symposium on exoerythrocytic forms of malarial parasites. IV. The chemotherapy and immunology of pre-erythrocytic stages in avian malaria. *J. Parasitol.* **34,** 290–299.

Davis, A. G., Huff, C. G., and Palmer, T. T. (1966). Procedures for maximum production of exoerythrocytic stages of *Plasmodium fallax* in tissue culture. *Exp. Parasitol.* **19,** 1–8.

Dennis, E. G., Mitchell, G. H., Butcher, G. A., and Cohen, S. (1975). *In vitro* isolation of *Plasmodium knowlesi* merozoites using polycarbonate sieves. *Parasitology* **71,** 475–481.

Doby, J. M., and Barker, R. (1976). Essais d'obtention *in vitro* des formes préerythrocytaires de *Plasmodium vivax* en cultures de cellules hepatiques humaines inoculées par sporozoites. *C. R. Seances Soc. Biol. Rennes* **170,** 661–665.

Downs, W. G. (1947). Infection of chicks with single parasites of *Plasmodium gallinaceum* Brumpt. *Am. J. Hyg.* **46,** 41–44.

Dubin, I. N. (1947). Bodies suggesting exoerythrocytic forms of *Plasmodium vivax* in tissue culture. *Proc. Soc. Exp. Biol. Med.* **65,** 154–156.

Dubin, I. N. (1948). A search for exoerythrocytic forms in human malaria by means of tissue cultures of bone marrow. *J. Natl. Malar. Soc.* **7,** 330–332.

Dubin, I. N., Laird, R. L., and Drinnon, V. P. (1949). The development of sporozoites of *Plasmodium gallinaceum* into cryptozoites in tissue cultures. *J. Natl. Malar. Soc.* **8,** 175–180.

Dubin, I. N., Laird, R. L., and Drinnon, V. P. (1950). Further observations on the development of sporozoites of *Plasmodium gallinaceum* into cryptozoites in tissue cultures. *J. Natl. Malar. Soc.* **9,** 119–131.

Ferone, R. (1977). Folate metabolism in malaria. *Bull. W.H.O.* **55**, 291–298.

Foley, D. A., Kennard, J., and Vanderberg, J. P. (1978). *Plasmodium berghei:* Infective exoerythrocytic schizonts in primary monalayer cultures of rat liver cells. *Exp. Parsitol.* **46**, 179–188.

Friedman, M. J. (1978). Erythrocytic mechanism of sickle cell resistance to malaria. *Proc. Natl. Acad. Sci. U.S.A.* **75**, 1994–1997.

Garnham, P. C. C. (1977). The continuing mystery of relapses in malaria. *Commonw. Inst. Helminthol., Protozool. Abstr.* **1**, 1–12.

Gavrilov, W., Bobkoff, G., and Laurencin, S. (1938). Essai de culture en tissus de *Plasmodium gallinaceum. Ann. Soc. Belge Med. Trop.* **18**, 429–438.

Geiman, Q. M., Anfinsen, C. B., McKee, R. W., Ormsbee, R. A., and Ball, E. G. (1946). Studies on malarial parasites. VII. Methods and techniques for cultivation. *J. Exp. Med.* **84**, 583–606.

Graham, H. A., Palczuk, N. C., and Stauber, L. A. (1973). Immunity to exoerythrocytic forms of malaria. II. Passive transfer of immunity to exoerythrocytic form. *Exp. Parasitol.* **34**, 372–381.

Hawking, F. (1944). Tissue culture of malaria parasites (*Plasmodium gallinaceum*). *Lancet* **1**, 693–694.

Hawking, F., (1945). Growth of protozoa in tissue culture. I. *Plasmodium gallinaceum,* exoerythrocytic forms. *Trans. R. Soc. Trop. Med. Hyg.* **39**, 245–263.

Hawking, F. (1951). Tissue culture of plasmodia. *Br. Med. Bull.* **8**, 16–21.

Hawking, F., Perry, W. L. M., and Thurston, J. P. (1948). Tissue forms of a malaria parasite, *Plasmodium cynomolgi. Lancet* **1**, 783–789.

Haynes, J. D., Diggs, C. L., Hines, F. A., and Desjardins, R. E. (1976). Culture of human malaria parasites (*Plasmodium falciparum*). *Nature (London)* **263**, 767–769.

Hegner, R., and Wolfson, F. (1939). Tissue culture studies of parasites in reticuloendothelial cells in birds infected with *Plasmodium. Am. J. Hyg.* **29**, 83–85.

Hepler, P. K., Huff, C. G., and Sprinz, H. (1966). The fine structure of the exoerythrocytic stages of *Plasmodium fallax. J. Cell Biol.* **30**, 333–358.

Holbrook, T. W., Palczuk, N. C., and Stauber, L. A. (1974). Immunity to exoerythrocytic forms of malaria. III. Stage specific immunization of turkeys against exoerythrocytic forms of *Plasmodium fallax. J. Parasitol.* **60**, 348–354.

Holbrook, T. W., Spitalny, G. L., and Palczuk, N. C. (1976). Stimulation of resistance in mice to sporozoite-induced *Plasmodium berghei* malaria by injections of avian exoerythrocytic forms. *J. Parasitol.* **62**, 670–675.

Huff, C. G. (1964). Cultivation of the exoerythrocytic stages of malarial parasites. *Am. J. Trop. Med. Hyg.* **13**, 171–177.

Huff, C. G. (1969). Exoerythrocytic stages of avian and reptilian malarial parasites. *Exp. Parasitol.* **24**, 383–421.

Huff, C. G., and Bloom, W. (1935). A malarial parasite infecting all blood and blood-forming cells of birds. *J. Infect. Dis.* **57**, 315–336.

Huff, C. G., and Coulston, F. (1944). The development of *Plasmodium gallinaceum* from sporozoite to erythrocytic trophozoites. *J. Infect. Dis.* **75**, 231–249.

Huff, C. G., Pipkin, A. C., Weathersby, A. B., and Jensen, D. V. (1960). The morphology and behavior of living exoerythrocytic stages of *Plasmodium gallinaceum* and *P. fallax* and their host cells. *J. Biophys. Biochem. Cytol.* **7**, 93–102.

Jensen, J. B. (1978a). Concentration from continuous culture of erythrocytes infected with trophozoites and schizonts of *Plasmodium falciparum. Am. J. Trop. Med. Hyg.* **27**, 1274–1276.

Jensen, J. B. (1979). Some aspects of serum requirements for continuous cultivation of *Plasmodium falciparum. Bull. W.H.O.* **57**(Suppl. 1), 27–31.

Jensen, J. B. (1979). Observations on gametocytogenesis in *Plasmodium falciparum* from continuous culture. *J. Protozool.* **26**, 129–132.

Jensen, J. B., and Trager, W. (1977). *Plasmodium falciparum* in culture: Use of outdated erythrocytes and description of the candle jar method. *J. Parasitol.* **63,** 883–886.

Jensen, J. B., and Trager, W. (1978). *Plasmodium falciparum* in cultures: Establishment of additional strains. *Am. J. Trop. Med. Hyg.* **27,** 743–746.

Jensen, J. B., Trager, W., and Doherty, J. (1979). *Plasmodium falciparum:* Continuous cultivation in a semi-automated apparatus. *Exp. Parasitol.* **48,** 36–41.

Kilejian, A. K. (1974). A unique histidine-rich polypeptide from the malaria parasite *Plasmodium lophurae. J. Biol. Chem.* **249,** 4650–4655.

Kilejian, A. (1975). Circular mitochondrial DNA from the avian malarial parasite *Plasmodium lophurae. Biochem. Biophys. Acta* **390,** 276–284.

Kilejian, A. (1979). Characterization of a protein correlated with the production of knob-like protrusions on membranes of erythrocytes infected with *Plasmodium falciparum. Proc. Natl. Acad. Sci.* USA **76,** 4650–4653.

Kilejian, A., Abati, A., and Trager, W. (1977). *Plasmodium falciparum* and *Plasmodium coatneyi:* immunogenicity of "knob-like protrusions" on infected erythrocyte membranes. *Exp. Parasitol.* **42,** 157–164.

Lambrecht, A. J., Snoeck, J., and Timmermans, U. (1978). Transient an-alpha-lipoproteinemia in man during infection by *Plasmodium vivax. Lancet* **1,** 1206.

Langreth, S. G. (1977). Electron microscope cytochemistry of host-parasite membrane interactions in malaria. *Bull. W.H.O.* **55,** 171–178.

Langreth, S. G., Jensen, J. B., Reese, R. T., and Trager, W. (1978). Fine structure of human malaria. *J. Protozool.* **25,** 443–452.

Langreth, S. G., Reese, R. T., Motyl, M. R., and Trager, W. (1979). *Plasmodium falciparum:* Loss of knobs on the infected erythrocyte surface after long-term cultivation. *Exp. Parasitol.* **48,** 213–219.

Langreth, S. G., and Trager, W. (1973). Fine structure of the malaria parasite *Plasmodium lophurae* developing extracellularly *in vitro. J. Protozool.* **20,** 606–613.

McAlister, R. O. (1977). Time-dependent loss of invasive ability of *Plasmodium berghei* merozoites *in vitro. J. Parasitol.* **63,** 455–463.

McCormick, G. J., Canfield, C. J., and Willet, G. P. (1971). *Plasmodium knowlesi: In vitro* evaluation of antimalarial activity of folic acid inhibitors. *Exp. Parasitol.* **30,** 88–93.

McGhee, R. B., and Trager, W. (1950). The cultivation of *Plasmodium lophurae in vitro* in chicken erythrocyte suspensions and the effects of some constituents of the culture medium upon its growth and multiplication. *J. Parasitol.* **36,** 123–127.

McLaren, D. J., Bannister, L. H., Trigg, P. I., and Butcher, G. A. (1977). A freeze-fracture study on the parasite-erythrocyte interrelationship in *Plasmodium knowlesi* infections. *Bull. W.H.O.* **55,** 199–204.

Maier, J., and Riley, E. (1942). Inhibition of antimalarial action of sulfonamides by *p*-aminobenzoic acid. *Proc. Soc. Exp. Biol. Med.* **50,** 152–154.

Masouredis, S. D. (1977). Preservation and clinical use of blood and blood components. *In* "Hematology" (W. J. Williams, E. Beutler, A. J. Erslev, and R. W. Rundles, eds.), 2nd ed., pp. 1530–1546. McGraw-Hill, New York.

Meyer, H. (1947). Cultivation of the exoerythrocytic form of *Plasmodium gallinaceum* in tissue culture of embryonic chicken brain. *Nature (London)* **160,** 155–156.

Meyer, H. (1949). Cultivo de "*Plasmodium gallinaceum*" en culturas de tecido a partir de sangre fectado. II. *Riv. Brasil. Biol.* **9,** 211–216.

Meyer, H., and Musacchio, M. O. (1959). *Plasmodium gallinaceum* in tissue cultures: Results obtained during 4 years of uninterrupted cultivation of the parasite *in vitro. Proc. Int. Congr. Trop. Med Malaria, 6th, 1958* Vol. 7, pp. 10–13.

Meyer, H., and de Oliverira Musacchio, M. (1960). Estudo electron microscopio da forma exo-eritrocitaria do *Plasmodium gallinaceum* en culturas de tecido. *An. Acad. Bras. Cienc.* **32,** 91–94.

Meyer, H., and de Oliveira Musacchio, M. (1965). An electron microscopic study of the final and initial forms of *Plasmodium gallinaceum* in thin sections of infected tissue cultures. *J. Protozool.* **12**, 193–202.

Mitchell, G. H., Richards, W. H. G., Butcher, G. A., and Cohen, S. (1977). Merozoite vaccination of douroucouli monkeys against falciparum malaria. *Lancet* **1**, 1335–1338.

Moore, G. E., Gerner, R. E., and Franklin, H. A. (1967). Culture of normal human leukocytes. *J. Am. Med. Assoc.* **199**, 519–524.

Nguyen-Dinh, P., and Trager, W. (1978). Chloroquine resistance produced *in vitro* in an African strain of human malaria. *Science* **200**, 1397–1398.

Pasvol, G., Wilson, R. J. M., Smalley, M. E., and Brown, J. (1978a). Separation of viable schizont-infected red cells of *Plasmodium falciparum* from human blood. *Ann. Trop. Med. Parasitol.* **72**, 87–88.

Pasvol, G., Weatherall, D. J., and Wilson, R. J. M. (1978b). Cellular mechanism for the protective effect of haemoglobin S against *P. falciparum* malaria. *Nature (London)* **274**, 701–703.

Pipkin, A. C., and Jensen, D. V. (1956). Avian embryos and tissue culture in the study of parasitic protozoa. I. Malarial parasites. *Exp. Parasitol.* **7**, 491–530.

Polet, H., and Conrad, M. E. (1969). The influence of three analogs of isoleucine on *in vitro* growth and protein synthesis of erythrocytic forms of *Plasmodium knowlesi*. *Proc. Soc. Exp. Biol. Med.* **130**, 581–586.

Porter, R. J. (1948). Studies in tissue culture of exoerythrocytic schizogony in avian malarial parasites: Symposium on exoerythrocytic forms of malarial parasites. *J. Parasitol.* **34**, 300–305.

Reese, R. T., Trager, W., Jensen, J. B., Miller, D. A., and Tantravahi, R. (1978). Immunization against malaria with antigen from *Plasmodium falciparum* cultivated *in vitro*. *Proc. Natl. Acad. Sci. U.S.A.* **75**, 5665–5668.

Reese, R. T., Langreth, S. G., and Trager, W. (1979a). Isolation of stages of the human parasite *Plasmodium falciparum* from culture and from animal blood. *Bull. W.H.O.* **57**(Suppl. 1), 53–61.

Rieckmann, K. H., and Lopez Antunano, F. J. (1971). Chloroquine resistance of *Plasmodium falciparum* in Brazil detected by a simple *in vitro* method. *Bull. W.H.O.* **45**, 157–167.

Rieckmann, K. H., Sax, L. J., Campbell, G. H., and Mrema, J. E. (1978). Drug sensitivity of *Plasmodium falciparum*: An *in vitro* microtechnique. *Lancet* **1**, 22–23.

Rowe, A. W., Eyster, E., and Kellner, A. (1968). Liquid nitrogen preservation of red blood cells for transfusion. *Cryobiology* **5**, 119–128.

Rudzinska, M. A., and Trager, W. (1959). Phagotrophy and two new structures in the malaria parasite *Plasmodium berghei*. *J. Biophys. Biochem. Cytol.* **6**, 103–112.

Ryley, J. F. (1953). The mode of action of proguanil and related antimalarial drugs. *Br. J. Pharmacol.* **8**, 424–443.

Scheibel, L. W., Ashton, S. H., and Trager, W. (1979). *Plasmodium falciparum*: Microaerophilic requirements in human red blood cells. *Exp. Parasitol.* **47**, 410–418.

Scheibel, L. W., and Pflaum, W. K. (1970). Carbohydrate metabolism in *Plasmodium knowlesi*. *Comp. Biochem. Physiol.* **37**, 543–553.

Sherman, I. W. (1977). Amino acid metabolism and protein synthesis in malarial parasites. *Bull. W.H.O.* **55**, 265–276.

Siddiqui, W. A. (1977). An effective immunization of experimental monkeys against a human malaria parasite, *Plasmodium falciparum*. *Science* **197**, 388–389.

Siddiqui, W. A., and Schnell, J. V. (1972). *In vitro* and *in vivo* studies with *Plasmodium falciparum* and *Plasmodium knowlesi*. *Proc. Helminthol. Soc. Wash.* **39**, Spec. Issue, 204–210.

Siddiqui, W. A., Schnell, J. V., and Geiman, Q. M. (1969). Nutritional requirements for *in vitro* cultivation of a simian malarial parasite, *Plasmodium knowlesi*. *Mil. Med.* **134**, Spec. Issue, 929–938.

Siddiqui, W. A., Schnell, J. V., and Geiman, Q. M. (1972). A model *in vitro* system to test the susceptibility of human malarial parasites to antimalarial drugs. *Am. J. Trop. Med. Hyg.* **21,** 392–399.

Strome, C. P. A., DeSantis, P., and Beaudoin, R. L. (1979). Cultivation of exoerythrocytic stages of *Plasmodium berghei* from sporozoite to merozoite. *In Vitro* **15,** 531–536.

Tonkin, I. M. (1946). The testing of drugs against exoerythrocytic forms of *Plasmodium gallinaceum* in tissue culture. *Br. J. Pharmacol. Chemother.* **1,** 163–173.

Trager, W. (1943). Further studies on the survival and development *in vitro* of a malarial parasite. *J. Exp. Med.* **77,** 411–420.

Trager, W. (1947a). The development of the malaria parasite *Plasmodium lophurae* in red blood cell suspensions *in vitro*. *J. Parasitol.* **33,** 345–350.

Trager, W. (1947b). The relation to the course of avian malaria of biotin and a fat soluble material having the biological activities of biotin. *J. Exp. Med.* **85,** 663–683.

Trager, W. (1950). Studies on the extracellular cultivation of an intracellular parasite (avian malaria). I. Development of the organism in erythrocyte extracts and the favoring effect of adenosine triphosphate. *J. Exp. Med.* **92,** 349–366.

Trager, W. (1957). The nutrition of an intracellular parasite (avian malaria). *Acta Trop.* **14,** 289–301.

Trager, W. (1958). Folinic acid and non-dialyzable materials in the nutrition of malaria parasites. *J. Exp. Med.* **108,** 753–772.

Trager, W. (1967). Adenosine triphosphate and the pyruvic and phosphoglyceric kinases of the malaria parasite *Plasmodium lophurae*. *J. Protozool.* **14,** 110–114.

Trager, W. (1971a). Further studies on the effects of antipantothenates on malaria parasites (*Plasmodium coatneyi* and *P. falciparum*) *in vitro*. *J. Protozool.* **18,** 232–239.

Trager, W. (1971b). A new method for intraerythrocytic cultivation of malaria parasites (*Plasmodium coatneyi* and *P. falciparum*). *J. Protozool.* **18,** 239–242.

Trager, W. (1971c). Malaria parasites (*Plasmodium lophurae*) developing extracellularly *in vitro:* Incorporation of labeled precursors. *J. Protozool.* **18,** 392–399.

Trager, W. (1973). Bongkrekic acid and the adenosinetriphosphate requirement of malaria parasites. *Exp. Parasitol.* **34,** 412–416.

Trager, W. (1974). Initial extracellular development *in vitro* of *Plasmodium falciparum*. *Proc. Int. Congr. Parasitol., 3rd, 1974* Vol. 1, p. 132.

Trager, W. (1976). Prolonged cultivation of malaria parasites (*Plasmodium coatneyi* and *P. falciparum*). *In* "Biochemistry of Parasites and Host-Parasite Relationships" (H. van den Bossche, ed.), pp. 427–434. North-Holland Publ., Amsterdam.

Trager, W. (1977). Cofactors and vitamins in the metabolism of malarial parasites. *Bull. W.H.O.* **55,** 285–290.

Trager, W. (1978). Cultivation of parasites *in vitro*. *Am. J. Trop. Med. Hyg.* **27,** 216–222.

Trager, W. (1979). *Plasmodium falciparum* in culture: An improved continuous flow method. *J. Protozool.* **26,** 125–129.

Trager, W., and Brohn, F. H. (1975). Coenzyme A requirement of malaria parasites: Effect of coenzyme A precursors on extracellular development *in vitro* of *Plasmodium lophurae*. *Proc. Natl. Acad. Sci. U.S.A.* **72,** 1834–1837.

Trager, W., and Jensen, J. B. (1976). Human malaria parasites in continuous culture. *Science* **193,** 673–675.

Trager, W., and Jensen, J. B. (1978). Cultivation of malarial parasites. *Nature (London)* **273,** 621–622.

Trager, W., and McGhee, R. B. (1950). Factors in plasma concerned in natural resistance to an avian malaria parasite (*Plasmodium lophurae*). *J. Exp. Med.* **91,** 365–379.

Trager, W., Langreth, S. G., and Platzer, E. G. (1972). Viability and fine structure of extracellular *Plasmodium lophurae* prepared by different methods. *Proc. Helminthol. Soc. Wash.* **39,** Spec. Issue, 220–230.

Trager, W., Robert-Gero, M., and Lederer, E. (1978). Antimalarial activity of S-isobutyl adenosine against *Plasmodium falciparum* in culture. *FEBS Let.* **85,** 264–266.

Trigg, P. I., and Shakespeare, P. G. (1976). Factors affecting the long-term cultivation of the erythrocytic stages of *Plasmodium knowlesi in vitro. In* "Biochemistry of Parasites and Host-Parasite Relationships" (H. van den Bossche ed.), pp. 435–440. North-Holland Publ., Amsterdam.

Walliker, D. (1976). Genetic factors in malaria parasites and their effect on host-parasite relationships. *Sym. Br. Soc. Parasitol.* **14,** 25–44.

World Health Organization (1975). Developments in malaria immunology. *W.H.O., Tech. Rep. Ser.* **579.**

Zuckerman, A. (1946). Infections with *Plasmodium gallinaceum* in chick embryos induced by exoerythrocytic and blood stage. *J. Infect. Dis.* **79,** 1–11.

Index